Dietitian's Pocket Guide to Nutrition

Nancie H. Herbold, EdD, RD, LDN
Simmons College
Boston, Massachusetts

Sari Edelstein, PhD, RD
Simmons College
Boston, Massachusetts

HERS
LONDON SINGAPORE

World Headquarters
Jones and Bartlett Publishers
40 Tall Pine Drive
Sudbury, MA 01776
978-443-5000
info@jbpub.com
www.jbpub.com

Jones and Bartlett Publishers
Canada
6339 Ormindale Way
Mississauga, Ontario L5V 1J2
Canada

Jones and Bartlett Publishers
International
Barb House, Barb Mews
London W6 7PA
United Kingdom

Jones and Bartlett's books and products are available through most bookstores and online booksellers. To contact Jones and Bartlett Publishers directly, call 800-832-0034, fax 978-443-8000, or visit our website www.jbpub.com.

Substantial discounts on bulk quantities of Jones and Bartlett's publications are available to corporations, professional associations, and other qualified organizations. For details and specific discount information, contact the special sales department at Jones and Bartlett via the above contact information or send an email to specialsales@jbpub.com.

The authors, editor, and publisher have made every effort to provide accurate information. However, they are not responsible for errors, omissions, or for any outcomes related to the use of the contents of this book and take no responsibility for the use of the products and procedures described. Treatments and side effects described in this book may not be applicable to all people; likewise, some people may require a dose or experience a side effect that is not described herein. Drugs and medical devices are discussed that may have limited availability controlled by the Food and Drug Administration (FDA) for use only in a research study or clinical trial. Research, clinical practice, and government regulations often change the accepted standard in this field. When consideration is being given to use of any drug in the clinical setting, the health care provider or reader is responsible for determining FDA status of the drug, reading the package insert, and reviewing prescribing information for the most up-to-date recommendations on dose, precautions, and contraindications, and determining the appropriate usage for the product. This is especially important in the case of drugs that are new or seldom used.

Production Credits
Publisher: Michael Brown
Production Director: Amy Rose
Associate Editor: Katey Birtcher
Editorial Assistant: Catie Heverling
Production Editor: Tracey Chapman
Associate Production Editor: Kate Stein
Marketing Manager: Jessica Faucher
Manufacturing and Inventory Control Supervisor: Amy Bacus
Composition: Graphic World
Cover Design: Scott Moden
Cover Image: © artida/ShutterStock, Inc.
Printing and Binding: Malloy, Inc.
Cover Printing: Malloy, Inc.

Library of Congress Cataloging-in-Publication Data
Dietitian's pocket guide to nutrition / [edited by] Nancie Herbold and Sari Edelstein.
p. ; cm.
Includes bibliographical references.
ISBN-13: 978-0-7637-6538-5 (pbk.)
ISBN-10: 0-7637-6538-4 (pbk.)
1. Nutrition--Handbooks, manuals, etc. 2. Dietetics--Handbooks, manuals, etc. I. Herbold, Nancie Harvey. II. Edelstein, Sari.
[DNLM: 1. Diet Therapy--Handbooks. 2. Dietetics--Handbooks. 3. Nutrition Physiology--Handbooks. WB 39 D5655 2009]
RM217.2.D543 2009
613.2--dc22

2008035232

6048

Printed in the United States of America
12 11 10 09 08 10 9 8 7 6 5 4 3 2 1

Table of Contents

Section 1 Maternal, Child, and Adult Normal Nutrition . . . 1

Basic Nutrition Through the Life Span . . . 1
- Infancy, the First Year of Life . . . 2
- Toddler Through Preschool Age (1–6 Years) . . . 7
- School Age (6–12 Years) Children . . . 11
- Adolescents . . . 14
- Adult Nutrition . . . 18
- Older Americans . . . 24
- Nutrition During Pregnancy . . . 33
- Nutrition During Lactation . . . 47
- Vegetarian Diet . . . 56
- Sports Nutrition . . . 62

Section 2 Adult Nutrition . . . 71

Chronic Nutrition Care Problems . . . 71
- Alzheimer's Disease . . . 72
- Cardiovascular Disease (CVD) . . . 77
- Cerebrovascular Accident (CVA) or Stroke . . . 80
- Chronic Obstructive Pulmonary Disease (COPD) . . . 83
- Congestive Heart Failure (CHF) . . . 86
- Decubitus Ulcers . . . 88
- Dehydration . . . 90
- Adults with Diabetes . . . 92
- Eating Disorders . . . 114
- Dysphagia . . . 119

Human Immunodeficiency Virus (HIV) and Acquired Immunodeficiency Syndrome (AIDS) 122
Malnutrition 127
Antianxiety Agents 130
ADHD Medications 132
Antidepressant Medications. 134
Common Issues with Mood Stabilizing Agents 138
Antipsychotic Drugs and Diet Interaction. 141
Chronic Renal Insufficiency 144
End Stage Renal Disease with Dialysis 150
Weight Management. 158

Section 3 Childhood Nutrition 161

Chronic Nutrition Care Problems. 161
Overweight/Obese in Children and Adolescents (Ages 2–20) 162
Type 1 Diabetes in Childhood 169
Type 2 Diabetes in Childhood 181

Section 4 Adult Nutrition 189

Acute Nutrition Care Problems. 189
Aspiration Pneumonia. 190
Gastric Bypass Surgery 193
Cancer (Nutrition During Chemotherapy and Radiation). 208
Adult Parenteral Nutrition (PN) Guide 215
Troubleshooting with Parenteral Nutrition (PN) 221
Adult Tube Feeding Guide 224
Troubleshooting with Adult Tube Feeding 232
Diverticulitis 238
Gastroesophageal Reflux Disease (GERD) 241
Lactose Intolerance. 243
Inflammatory Bowel Disease (IBD). 245

Celiac Disease or Celiac Sprue (Gluten Sensitive Enteropathy). 248
Cholecystitis (Inflammation of the Gallbladder) or Cholecystectomy (Gallbladder Removed). 250
Colostomy/Ileostomy 253
Short-Bowel Syndrome 257
Liver Disease. 260
Renal Calculi. 266

Section 5 Childhood Nutrition 271

Acute Nutrition Care Problems. 271
Acute Diarrhea Illness and Symptoms in Infants and Young Children 272

Section 6 Progressive Diets. 275

Progressive Diets. 275

Section 7 Appendices. 279

Appendix A: Total Fat 281
Appendix B: Caffeine Values 282
Appendix C: Calculations and Conversions. 284
Appendix D: Carbohydrates, Calories, and Glycemic Index of Commonly Consumed Foods 295
Appendix E: CPR 297
Appendix F: Dietary Guidelines for Americans 2005 298
Appendix G: Dietary Reference Intakes, 2000, and RDA, 1989. 301
Appendix H: Diet and Drug Interactions 309
Appendix I: Ethnic, Cultural, and Religious Food Considerations 320
Appendix J: Energy Equations. 326
Appendix K: Energy Expenditure of Activity 327
Appendix L: Exchange Lists for Meal Planning 328

Appendix M: Exchange List for Carbohydrate Counting. 345
Appendix N: Fast Food Nutrients. 346
Appendix O: Fat Sources. 356
Appendix P: Food Labels 358
Appendix Q: Foodborne Illness. 367
Appendix R: Glycemic Indexes for Foods 375
Appendix S: Growth Charts 376
Appendix T: Heimlich Maneuver 379
Appendix U: Herb Guide 381
Appendix V: Infant Formulas 385
Appendix W: Activity of Insulin Preparations 394
Appendix X: Micronutrients 396
Appendix Y: MyPyramid 398
Appendix Z: Normal Nutritional Lab Values 401
Appendix AA: Nutrition Assessment Sheet 415
Appendix BB: Physical Indicators of Nutritional Status . . 418
Appendix CC: Enteral Formula Selection 430
Appendix DD: Vitamin and Mineral Food Sources. 434
Appendix EE: Information Resources 435
Appendix FF: Food Sources of Selected Nutrients 446
Appendix GG: BMI Chart 458
Appendix HH: Super Recipes 459
Appendix II: Sodium Content of Foods 461

Index 463

Contributors

Sandra Allonen, MEd, RD, LDN
Beth Israel Deaconess Medical Center
Boston, Massachusetts

Donna Belcher, MS, RD, LDN
Northwestern Memorial Hospital
Chicago, Illinois

Joseph Carlin, MS, MA, RD, FADA
Federal Regions I, II, & III
U.S. Administration on Aging
Boston, Massachusetts

Linda S. Cashman, MS, RD, CNSD
South Shore Hospital
South Weymouth, Massachusetts

Sharon Collier, MEd, RD, LDN
Children's Hospital
Boston, Massachusetts

Kattia M. Corrales-Yauckoes, MS, RD, LDN
Joslin Clinic
Boston, Massachusetts

Kimberly Dong, MS, RD, LDN
School of Medicine
Tufts University
Boston, Massachusetts

Natalie Egan, MS, RD, CDE, LDN
Brigham and Women's Hospital
Boston, Massachusetts

Mary Emerson, MS, RD, LD
Spring Harbor Hospital
Gorham, Maine

Teresa Fung, ScD, RD, LDN
Simmons College
Boston, Massachusetts

Karlyn Grimes, MS, RD
Simmons College
Boston, Massachusetts

Amina Grunko, MS, RD, LDN
Children's Hospital
Boston, Massachusetts

Mary Rowan Harrity, MS, RD
Kindred Healthcare East
Hudson, Massachusetts

Patrick Healy, MS, RD, LD, CDE
Upham's Corner Health Center
Boston, Massachusetts

Michael Mansueto Leidig, RD, LDN
Children's Hospital
Boston, Massachusetts

Colleen McLean, CNSD, RD
Children's Hospital
Boston, Massachusetts

Yeemay Su Miller, MS, RD
Simmons College
Boston, Massachusetts

Nicola O'Brien, MS, RD, LDN
Long-Term Care Consultant
Milton, Massachusetts

Dianne Scheinberg, MS, RD, LD
DBS Consulting
Newton Upper Falls, Massachusetts

Elizabeth Scott, PhD
Simmons College
Boston, Massachusetts

Amy Sheeley, PhD, RD
Executive Office of Elders Affairs
Boston, Massachusetts

Deborah Shields, MS, RD, LDN
Metro West Wellness Center
Framingham, Massachusetts

Kendrin Sonneville, MS, RD, LDN
Children's Hospital
Boston, Massachusetts

Stephanie Vangsness, MS, RD, LDN, CNSD
Dana Farber Cancer Institute
Boston, Massachusetts

Janet Washington, MPH, RD, LDN
Simmons College
Boston, Massachusetts

Debra Wein, MS, RD, LDN, ACSM-HFI, NSCA-CPT
The Sensible Nutrition Connection, Inc.
Hingham, Massachusetts

Elizabeth Winthrop, MS, RD, CNSD
South Coast Medical Center
New Bedford, Massachusetts

SECTION 1

Maternal, Child, and Adult Normal Nutrition

Basic Nutrition Through the Life Span

Infancy, the First Year of Life 2
Toddler Through Preschool Age (1–6 Years) 7
School Age (6–12 Years) Children. 11
Adolescents 14
Adult Nutrition. 18
Older Americans 24
Nutrition During Pregnancy. 33
Nutrition During Lactation 47
Vegetarian Diet. 56
Sports Nutrition 62

Infancy, the First Year of Life

Authors: Sharon Collier, MEd, RD, LDN; Amina Grunko, MS, RD, LDN; Colleen Mclean, RD, CNSD, LDN

Infancy is a critical time of growth and development. Normal growth is expected to fall somewhere between the 10–90 percentile (%ile) on the Centers for Disease Control (CDC) growth charts. See growth charts in the appendix. However, more important is the trend of the individual and his or her own established "growth curve." Concern and further workup would be necessary for those who cross up or down 2 centiles from their own growth curve or if they were above the 90%ile or below the 10%ile weight for height. If there is a family history of allergy, consult with the primary medical doctor/registered dietitian (PMD). It is imperative that we take a proactive role in identifying and solving nutritional problems because the consequences may extend past the first year of life. There are many potential issues with this group, which follow:

Problem	*Do's and Don'ts*
Breast-feeding	**Do:** Encourage mother to drink plenty of fluids. Review the principles of supply and demand: the more an infant feeds, the more milk is produced. Instruct the mother to alternate initial breast for each feeding to facilitate equal emptying of breasts because infants have a more vigorous suck at the first breast. Discuss feeding frequency: an infant will nurse every 2–3 hours during first few weeks and typically takes 4–5 feedings per day after 3 months. Supplement infant with 200 IU vitamin D daily by 2 months of age with the physician's approval to prevent deficiency and rickets.* Use refrigerated expressed human milk within 48 hours or freeze for longer storage. Consult a lactation specialist, as needed. Ensure vegetarian mothers (especially vegan) receive adequate calcium, iron, and B_{12}. See the section on vegetarianism on page 56. See the section on nutrition during lactation on page 47. *The American Academy of Pediatrics (AAP) adjusted their recommendations for vitamin D from 200 IU/day beginning in the first two months of life to 400 IU/day beginning in the first few days of life. **Don't:** Don't supplement with unfortified milks (cow, goat, and soy milk) because they are nutritionally incomplete for infants less than 1 year of age.

Problem	Do's and Don'ts
	Don't overly diet.
	Don't allow alcohol or caffeine (coffee, most tea, and soft drinks).
	Don't allow medication or herbal supplements without first discussing with the PMD because they may pass into human milk.
Bottle Feeding	**Do:**
	Consult the PMD before making formula changes.
	Follow formula preparation instructions carefully; use only the scoop provided with the product (scoop sizes vary between products) unless otherwise instructed.
	Warm bottles using hot running water or in a bowl of warm water for no more than 15 minutes.
	Use a fresh bottle of formula at each feeding, discarding leftovers.
	Store mixed and opened ready-to-use formulas in a refrigerator; discard unused refrigerated concentrate and ready-to-use formula after 48 hours and formula prepared from powder after 24 hours.
	Supplement with fluoride when the infant is 6 months old after first consulting the PMD.
	Don't:
	Don't give a bottle to an infant without checking the temperature.
	Don't put an infant to bed with a bottle, which can lead to baby-bottle tooth decay.
	Don't leave the infant to feed him- or herself alone or with a propped up bottle.
	Don't provide low-iron formula unless prescribed by PMD, because this may lead to anemia.
	Don't heat bottles in a microwave, because they can heat unevenly and burn the baby.
	Don't supplement fluoride before age 6 months.
Introduction of Complementary Foods	**Do:**
	Initiate complementary feedings when the infant can sit with support, has good control of head and neck, leans forward, and can swallow food when fed by a spoon; provide 1–2 teaspoons of new foods, increasing quantity gradually.

Problem	*Do's and Don'ts*
	Provide rice cereal (single grain cereal) as the first complementary food, because it is least likely to cause an allergic reaction; introduce one new single-ingredient food item every 5–7 days to monitor for allergic reactions. Mix all warmed food thoroughly and check the temperature to avoid burning the infant's mouth. Limit fruit juice to 4 ounces per day after 6 months of age. **Don't:** Don't initiate complementary foods before age 4–6 months. Don't add salt, spices, or sugar to foods. Don't give honey or processed foods containing honey to infant until after 1 year of age because this places the infant at risk for botulism. (See the table on food safety on pages 367–374.) Don't add cereal to bottles or use "baby food nurser kits." Don't feed infants directly out of baby food jars because germs from the infant's mouth can contaminate the jar of food where the bacteria will continue to grow. Don't force infants to eat new foods they do not like. It can take up to 20 attempts before an infant accepts a new food. Don't give infants sweets (for example, candy, cake, or cookies); don't feed egg whites to infants until they are older than 1 year of age due to the possibility of food allergy.
Excessive Juice Intake	**Do:** Limit the intake of juice to 4–6 ounces per day because excessive quantities cause an osmotic diarrhea. Provide pasteurized 100% fruit juice. Serve juice only in a cup. **Don't:** Don't provide juice before 6 months of age or allow the infant to drink juice from a bottle.
Choking Risks	**Do:** Mash or puree foods to decrease the risk of aspiration. **Don't:** Don't provide the following foods: nuts, raisins or other small dried fruits, raw carrots, whole or round cut hot dogs, grapes, popcorn, potato chips, or rounded candies.

Problem	*Do's and Don'ts*
Poor Growth	**Do:** Assess the required intake as listed: the number of wet diapers (six to eight per day) and stool patterns are helpful in assessing the intake of the breast-fed infant; consult the PMD if patterns are severe or prolonged. Provide referrals to community and government programs to assist with food access if in financial hardship. Have as a base dietary reference intakes (DRI): Calories: 98–108 kilocalories per kilogram of body weight per day Protein: 1.5 gram per kilogram of body weight per day Vitamin D: 5 micrograms per day* Calcium: 210–270 milligrams per day Iron: 0.27–11 milligrams per day Zinc: 2–3 milligrams per day *In 2008 the AAP doubled the recommended amount of vitamin D for infants, children, and adolescents. Note: In infants less than 6 months old, base DRI for protein on the adequate intake (mean intake) of the breast-fed infant; therefore, it does not represent an upper limit or intend to meet the needs of 97–98% of estimated needs, as is the case with the recommended daily allowances (RDA). **Don't:** Don't forget to use corrected age when plotting infants who were born prematurely. Don't forget to use the correct age for weight through 24 months, height through 36 months, and head circumferences through 18 months of age. Don't provide more than 4 ounces of a juice per day or force feed.
Iron Deficiency Anemia	**Do:** Start on human milk or iron-fortified formula. Provide iron-fortified rice cereal as the first food followed by weaning foods high in iron; supplement with iron if prescribed by the PMD. **Don't:** Don't use formulas low in iron or unfortified milks (cow, soy, or goat milk).
Gas–Colic	**Do:** Ensure proper positioning of the bottle to decrease the amount of air present in the nipple during feeding. Verify that the mixture of formula is correct.

Problem	*Do's and Don'ts*
Gas–Colic	**Don't:** Don't overfeed the infant.
Spitting Up	**Do:** Discuss the normalcy of infants spitting up, and encourage burping. Verify that the mixture of formula is correct. **Don't:** Don't overfeed or force feed. Don't provide excessive movement after feeding or lay the infant flat on his or her back after feeding.
Constipation	**Do:** Determine adequacy of fluid intake. Verify that the mixture of formula is correct. Obtain diet history if taking complementary foods. **Don't:** Don't provide juice excessively, which may displace other nutrients.

Sources

American Academy of Pediatrics. "Policy Statement: Breastfeeding and the Use of Human Milk." *Pediatrics.* February 2005. 115(2), 496–506.

American Academy of Pediatrics. "Prevention of Rickets and Vitamin D Deficiency in Infants, Children, and Adolescents." *Pediatrics.* November 2008. 122, 1142–1152.

Butte, N., Cobb, K., Dwyer, J., Graney, L., Heird, W., & Rickard, K. "The Start Healthy Feeding Guidelines for Infants and Toddlers." *J Am Diet Assoc.* 2004. 104, 442–454.

Carruth, B., Ziegler, P., Gordon, A., & Hendricks, K. "Developmental Milestones and Self-Feeding Behaviors in Infants and Toddlers." *J Am Diet Assoc.* 2004. 104, S51–S56.

Hendricks, K. M., & Duggan, C. (Eds.). *Manual of Pediatric Nutrition* (4th ed.). Lewiston, NY: BC Decker. 2005.

Kleinman, R. E. (Ed.). *Pediatric Nutrition Handbook* (5th ed.). Elk Grove Village, IL: American Academy of Pediatrics. 2004.

Satter, E. *How to Get Your Kid to Eat…But Not Too Much.* Palo Alto, CA: Bull Publishing Company. 1987.

Story, M., Holt, K., & Sofka, D. *Bright Futures in Practice: Nutrition* (2nd ed.). Arlington, VA: National Center for Education in Maternal and Child Health. 2002.

Toddler Through Preschool Age (1–6 Years)

Authors: Sharon Collier, MEd, RD, LDN;
Amina Grunko, MS, RD, LDN;
Colleen Mclean, RD, CNSD, LDN

There are many challenges to assuring a young child's diet is healthy, adequate, and safe, which all could potentially impact appropriate growth and development. Normal growth is expected to fall somewhere between the 10–90 percentile (%ile) on the CDC growth charts. See growth charts in the appendix. However, more important is the trend of the individual and his or her own established "growth curve." Concern and further workup would be necessary for those who cross up or down 2 centiles from their own growth curve or if they were above the 90%ile or below the 10%ile weight for height. If there is a family history of allergy, consult with the PMD regarding guidelines/restrictions that may be necessary. Toddlerhood is the time for establishing independence, which may cause some of the following issues:

Problem	***Do's and Don'ts***
Bottle Dependency	**Do:**
	Offer a cup with every meal and put a very small amount of liquid in it; try giving the same liquid as in the bottle.
	Limit the bottle to specific times and places.
	Don't:
	Don't offer a bottle instead of cup when the child refuses the cup.
	Don't allow the child to run around with a bottle.
	Don't put juice in a bottle.
Picky Eating	**Do:**
	Offer small amounts of new food at least 10–14 times, which may be necessary to increase acceptance of new food.
	Offer choices selected by the parent/caregiver, but do let the child choose which one he or she wants from these.
	Offer new food along with one they already like.
	Remember portion sizes are much smaller for this group, one-fourth to one-third of an adult portion. Larger portions may be overwhelming.
	Offer new food at the beginning of a meal when the child may be hungrier.
	As the child gets older, allow him or her to participate in meal preparation, which can increase his or her acceptance of a new food.

Problem	*Do's and Don'ts*
Picky Eating	Provide a multi-vitamin with minerals if this will decrease parent anxiety and decrease battles at mealtimes. **Don't:** Don't interpret first food refusals as not liking the food. Don't be a short-order cook and provide substitutes because children usually make up calories on their own if they don't eat at a meal. Don't bribe or reward with treats or sweets. Don't force a child to eat or punish him or her for not eating. Don't make mealtime a battleground for controlling overeating.
Grazing	**Do:** Set times and places for eating, no matter if it is a snack or a meal. Give water only between a snack or meal if the child requests food or a drink. **Don't:** Don't allow the child to run around with food in his or her hand. Don't put large portions on the plate.
Poor Growth	**Do:** Choose whole milk and dairy products. Add monosaturated oil and/or butter to acceptable foods; feed nuts and seeds, which are higher in calories (for greater than 3 years old). Decrease distractions at mealtime to allow focus on eating/mealtime and have a set time and place for food consumption. Provide referrals to community and government programs to assist with food access if in financial hardship. Have evaluation by PMD if food avoidance is severe or prolonged. Dietary Reference Intake (DRI): Calories: 90–102 kilocalories per kilogram of body weight Protein: 1.1–1.2 grams per kilogram of body weight Vitamin D: 5 micrograms per day* Calcium: 500–800 milligrams per day Iron: 7–10 milligrams per day Zinc: 3–8 milligrams per day *In 2008 the AAP doubled the recommended amount of vitamin D for infants, children, and adolescents.

Problem	*Do's and Don'ts*
	Don't:
	Don't forget to use corrected age when plotting infants born prematurely; also use correct age for weight through 24 months, height through 36 months, and head circumferences through 18 months of age.
	Don't choose skim milk or low-fat dairy products.
	Don't allow unlimited juice or low-calorie foods/drinks because this can displace nutrient dense foods/drinks.
	Don't force feed.
Excess Weight Gain	**Do:**
	Offer healthy foods for meals and snacks.
	Offer low-fat or possibly skim milk and dairy products after 2 years of age.
	Let the child determine the amount they will eat at each meal or snack; however, the parent/caregiver makes the food choices from which they select.
	Decrease distractions at mealtime to focus on what is being eaten and how much.
	Increase activity.
	Have a set time and place for eating any food or calorie-containing liquid.
	Don't:
	Don't bribe to encourage weight loss.
	Don't allow greater than 2 hours of TV or computer time per day.
	Don't focus on calories or weight.
	Don't allow excessive soda and juice intake.
Choking Risks	**Do:**
	Cut up foods in very small pieces.
	Offer softer foods that are easy to chew.
	Mix gravy or broth with chewier/drier foods.
	Don't:
	Don't give peanuts, other nuts and seeds, hard candy, raisins or other small dried fruits, raw carrots, whole or round cut hot dogs, grapes, or apple skin.

Problem	*Do's and Don'ts*
Iron Deficiency Anemia	**Do:** Offer foods high in iron: red meats, dried beans, iron-fortified cereals. Evaluate further by the PMD if needed. **Don't:** Don't allow excess milk intake, which can displace other foods/nutrients.
Constipation	**Do:** Determine adequacy of fluid intake. Include more vegetables and fruits, whether cooked or raw, for the older child. Include also whole grain bread, pasta, rice, and cereals. See fiber in the Index. Incorporate regular physical activity. **Don't:** Don't serve refined starches (food containing sugar). Don't limit fluid intake unless medically necessary. Don't provide excess juice, which may displace other nutrients and/or provide excess calories.

Sources

American Academy of Pediatrics. "Prevention of Rickets and Vitamin D Deficiency in Infants, Children, and Adolescents." *Pediatrics.* November 2008. 122, 1142–1152.

Butte, N., Cobb, K., Dwyer, J., Graney, L., Heird, W., & Rickard, K. "The Start Healthy Feeding Guidelines for Infants and Toddlers." *J Am Diet Assoc.* 2004. 104, 442–454.

Food and Nutrition Board, Institute of Medicine. *Dietary Reference Intakes.* Washington, DC: National Academy Press. 1997–2001.

Hendricks, K. M., & Duggan, C. (Eds.). *Manual of Pediatric Nutrition* (4th ed.). Lewiston, NY: BC Decker. 2005.

Kleinman, R. E. (Ed.). *Pediatric Nutrition Handbook* (5th ed.). Elk Grove Village, IL: American Academy of Pediatrics. 2004.

Satter, E. *Child of Mine: Feeding with Love and Food Sense* (3rd ed.). Palo Alto, CA: Bull Publishing Company. 2000.

Satter, E. *How to Get Your Kid to Eat…But Not Too Much.* Palo Alto, CA: Bull Publishing Company. 1987.

School Age (6–12 Years) Children

Authors: Sharon Collier, MEd, RD, LDN;
Amina Grunko, MS, RD, LDN;
Colleen Mclean, RD, CNSD, LDN

There are many challenges to assuring a child's diet is healthy, adequate, and safe, which could potentially impact continued growth and development. Normal growth is expected to fall somewhere between the 10–90 percentile (%ile) on the CDC growth charts. See growth charts in the appendix. However, more important is the trend of the individual and his or her own established "growth curve." Concern and further workup would be necessary for those who cross up or down 2 centiles from their own growth curve or if they were above the 90%ile or below the 10%ile weight for height. Establishing good eating habits could be most effective in these earlier years to carry them into the future. There are many potential issues with this age group, which follow:

Problem	***Do's and Don'ts***
Poor Growth	**Do:**
	Emphasize high-calorie, dense foods including whole milk and dairy products.
	Provide referrals to community and government programs to assist with food access if in financial hardship.
	Explore further evaluation by PMD if experiencing severe or prolonged growth failure.
	Dietary Reference Intakes (DRI): Calories: 47–90 kilocalories per kilogram of body weight per day Protein: 1.0 gram per kilogram of body weight per day Vitamin D: 5 micrograms per day* Calcium: 800–1300 milligrams per day Iron: 8–10 milligrams per day Zinc: 5–8 milligrams per day
	*In 2008 the AAP doubled the recommended amount of vitamin D for infants, children, and adolescents.
Don't:	
	Don't force feed or bribe the child to eat.
	Don't allow unlimited juice/low-calorie drinks or foods.
	Don't choose skim or low-fat milk and dairy products, unless recommended by PMD.
Picky Eating	**Do:**
	Offer two to three varieties of foods each meal.
	Provide new food item with favorite/familiar foods.
	Decrease mealtime distractions.

Problem	*Do's and Don'ts*
Picky Eating	Provide a multivitamin with minerals to help decrease anxiety over adequacy of micronutrients. Offer praise when trying new foods. **Don't:** Don't force feed or punish for not eating. Don't bribe or reward with sweets or treats. Don't become a short-order cook to provide substitute foods.
Vegetable/ Fruit Refusal	**Do:** Offer new foods repeatedly in small amounts and ask the child to taste the food. Try a different form of the food, either raw or cooked, to help increase acceptance. Offer healthy dips (for example, low-fat dressings, hummus, or yogurt). Cut food in small pieces and incorporate in sauces and meats like meatloaf/meatballs, pizza, or casseroles. **Don't:** Don't force feed or punish for not eating. Don't bribe or reward with sweets or treats.
Skipping Breakfast	**Do:** Emphasize that breakfast is the most important meal of the day to provide the energy and nutrients for classroom work, which can translate into better test scores and overall healthier status. Provide quick, ready-to-eat items (for example, granola bar, fruit smoothie, yogurt, peanut butter sandwich, bagel with cheese, or cereal with fruit and milk). Prepare breakfast the night before if time is of the essence, or perhaps purchase school breakfast, if available, for the child. Allow the child leftovers if he/she prefers them versus "standard" breakfast items. **Don't:** Don't allow the excuse of not enough time to eat breakfast. Don't limit it to "standard" breakfast items.
School Lunch	**Do:** Involve the child in making choices about lunch items, whether buying at school or preparing at home. Discuss what he/she eats at school or snack and his/her lunch experiences.

Problem	*Do's and Don'ts*
	Don't:
	Don't assume the child is eating what is packed or brought for lunch.
Snacking	**Do:**
	Allow a healthy after-school snack, which can help in the interim until dinner time; provide fruit, cheese and crackers, vegetables with hummus, yogurt, popcorn, milk and cereal, baked tortilla chips with salsa, nuts, and seeds.
	Don't:
	Don't allow snacking in front of the TV or computer.
	Don't bribe the child with snacks to get him/her to do something else, like homework or housework.
Excess Weight Gain	**Do:**
	Encourage increased physical activity. Participate in favorite activities, involve the child in school sports, encourage family activities; focus on healthy eating.
	Limit time and place for meals and snacks.
	Decrease distractions around mealtimes to focus on amounts and foods consumed.
	Offer healthy foods for meals and snacks.
	Provide low-fat or skim milk and dairy products.
	Encourage the child to increase water intake.
	Don't:
	Don't allow greater than 2 hours of TV or computer time per day.
	Don't focus on calories and weight.
	Don't bribe or punish to encourage weight loss.
	Don't allow unlimited soda and juice consumption.

Sources

Food and Nutrition Board, Institute of Medicine. *Dietary Reference Intakes*. Washington, DC: National Academy Press. 1997–2001.

Hendricks, K. M., & Duggan, C. (Eds.). *Manual of Pediatric Nutrition* (4th ed.). Lewiston, NY: BC Decker. 2005.

Kleinman, R. E. (Ed.). *Pediatric Nutrition Handbook* (5th ed.). Elk Grove Village, IL: American Academy of Pediatrics. 2004.

Satter, E. *How to Get Your Kid to Eat…But Not Too Much*. Palo Alto, CA: Bull Publishing Company. 1987.

Adolescents

Authors: Sharon Collier, MEd, RD, LDN;
Amina Grunko, MS, RD, LDN;
Colleen Mclean, RD, CNSD, LDN

The following identified nutritional problems are common to adolescents due to their unique period in life. During adolescence, body changes affect their nutritional needs, and their physical and psychosocial development affects their food choices. Adolescents have increased independence, and their peers easily influence them, which makes it harder to plan healthy meals.

Normal growth is expected to fall somewhere between the 10–90 percentile (%ile) on the CDC growth charts. See growth charts in the appendix. However, more important is the trend of the individual and his or her own established "growth curve." Concern and further workup would be necessary for those who cross up or down 2 centiles from their own growth curve or if they were above the 90%ile or below the 10%ile weight for height.

Problem	***Do's and Don'ts***
Obesity	**Do:**
	Incorporate physical activity and healthy eating habits because daily and routine physical activities are strongly recommended to achieve adequate weight loss.
	Teach adequate portion sizes of foods, including grains, protein, vegetables, dairy, and fruits.
	Advocate three balanced meals a day, and keep healthy snacks available.
	Allow readily available healthy food choices.
	Encourage eating at home and less fast foods/processed foods.
	Encourage eating in one place without distractions.
	Provide referrals to community and government programs to assist with food access if in financial hardship.
	See the table on weight control on page 42.
	Dietary Reference Intakes (DRI): Calories: 2100–3100 kilocalories per day Protein: 0.85–0.95 gram per kilogram of body weight per day Vitamin D: 5 micrograms per day* Calcium: 1300 milligrams per day Iron: 8–15 milligrams per day Zinc: 8–11 milligrams per day
	*In 2008 the AAP doubled the recommended amount of vitamin D for infants, children, and adolescents.

Problem	*Do's and Don'ts*
	Don't: Don't allow adolescents to yo–yo diet or restrict certain food groups because it will deprive the body of important nutrients needed for growth and development.
Sports	**Do:** Suggest that adolescents eat a variety of foods from all food groups to provide the body with sufficient calorie and protein needs. Encourage nutritionally dense snacks between meals; drink plenty of fluids. See the section on sports nutrition on page 62. **Don't:** Don't allow overexercise and the use of protein powders or expensive supplements.
Vegetarianism	**Do:** Provide protein sources (for example, dairy, eggs, legumes, tofu, soy products, nuts, and grains). Provide adequate calcium, iron, and vitamin B_{12} sources found in some fortified foods and supplements. See the section on vegetarianism on page 56. **Don't:** Don't allow excessive restriction of protein and food choices or encourage the majority of foods from only one food group.
Eating Disorder	**Do:** Provide basic nutrition education on the need for the different food groups for adequate body function. Provide an interdisciplinary approach that includes nutrition, psychiatry, nursing, and PMD, as needed. Involve the patient in food selection and preparation; cover all food groups including dairy, fruits, vegetables, grains, and fat in food choices. See the section on eating disorders on page 114. **Don't:** Don't force feed or ignore behavior because feeding too much too fast may result in refeeding syndrome. Don't allow overexercise, unless approved by PMD.

Problem	*Do's and Don'ts*
Pregnancy	**Do:** Encourage adequate weight gain based on prepregnancy body mass index (BMI), wt/ht^2: BMI — Weight gain (pounds) Less than 19.8 — 28–40 19.8–26 — 25–35 26–29 — 15–25 Greater than 29 — at least 15 Explain importance of weight gain during pregnancy, and assess current diet and supplement intake. Start prenatal multivitamins if poor diet quality exists. Provide referrals to community and government programs to assist with food access if in financial hardship. Dietary Reference Intakes: Calories: 2400–2800 kilocalories per day Protein: 1.1 gram per kilogram of body weight per day Folic acid: 800 micrograms per day Vitamin D: 5 micrograms per day* Calcium: 1300 milligrams per day Iron: 10–27 milligrams per day Zinc: 12–13 milligrams per day *In 2008 the AAP doubled the recommended amount of vitamin D for infants, children, and adolescents. **Don't:** Don't forget to discuss diet concerns (for example, pica, *Listeria monocytogenes*, safe seafood consumption), limiting herbal tea and caffeine consumption, and the detrimental effects of alcohol during pregnancy.
Vitamin/ Herbal Supplements	**Do:** Communicate the use of any supplements to the PMD because the FDA does not regulate many over-the-counter vitamins and supplements, and when taken in excess they may be harmful. Single vitamin/mineral supplement is only necessary if the patient is on a restrictive diet. See the appendix on herbal supplements on pages 381–384. **Don't:** Don't recommend a particular herb or supplement without the approval of the PMD because some supplements may interact with common prescription medications.

Sources

American Academy of Pediatrics. "Prevention of Rickets and Vitamin D Deficiency in Infants, Children, and Adolescents." *Pediatrics*. November 2008. 122, 1142–1152.

Hendricks, K. M., & Duggan, C. (Eds.). *Manual of Pediatric Nutrition* (4th ed.). Lewiston, NY: BC Decker. 2005.

Kleinman, R. E. (Ed.). *Pediatric Nutrition Handbook* (5th ed.). Elk Grove Village, IL: American Academy of Pediatrics. 2004.

Satter, E. *How to Get Your Kid to Eat…But Not Too Much*. Palo Alto, CA: Bull Publishing Company. 1987.

Adult Nutrition

Author: Amy Sheeley, PhD, RD, LD

This list will assist the dietitian in answering general nutrition questions for adults. These guidelines outline nutrition recommendations for maintaining a healthy weight and preventing chronic diseases (for example, heart disease, osteoporosis, and diabetes).

Problem	*Do's and Don'ts*
Maintain a Healthy Weight and Prevent Chronic Diseases	**Do:**
	Encourage patients to choose a variety of different foods within each food group. Patients should consume a balanced diet of foods from all the different food groups including grains, fruits, vegetables, milk, and meat and beans.
	Control portion sizes to prevent excessive calorie intake and to allow for balance and variety in the diet.
	Consume at least 2 cups of fruit every day (fresh, frozen, canned, or dried fruit).
	Consume at least 2.5 cups of vegetables every day, varying intake by color, choosing dark green and orange vegetables, as well as legumes.
	Encourage patients to read the nutrition facts label on food products, especially noting the serving size and adjusting values based on the portion consumed. See page 358 for an example of a nutrition facts label.
	Consume 25–35 grams of fiber each day from a variety of foods, including whole grains (breads, rice, pasta, and crackers), legumes, and seeds.
	See MyPyramid on page 398.
	Don't:
	Don't assume that patients realize that restaurant and prepared foods are sold in recommended portion sizes.
	Don't allow fruit juices to be overconsumed due to their caloric content.
	Don't serve fried vegetables, such as french fries, or those in cream sauces.
	Don't select refined grains, such as white bread, in the place of whole grains.
Optimal Health to Prevent Dehydration	**Do:**
	Encourage patients to drink adequate fluids. Fluid needs vary depending upon an individual's size, activity level, and

Problem	*Do's and Don'ts*
	the climate. The average man needs an estimated 8–11 cups of fluids each day, while the average woman needs 6–9 cups. All sources can contribute to total fluid needs, including juices, soda, tea, coffee, and drinking water.
	Don't:
	Don't serve beverages high with added sugars, which add calories with few or no nutrients.
Gradual, Unhealthy Weight Gain, Inactivity	**Do:**
	Encourage patients to engage in approximately 60 minutes of moderate- to vigorous-intensity activity on most days of the week. To sustain weight loss, at least 60–90 minutes per day may be required. Patients should consult their PMD before beginning a new exercise regimen.
	Patients should choose activities that they enjoy with a backup plan for weather-dependent activities.
	To achieve physical fitness, patients should combine cardiovascular conditioning with stretching exercises for flexibility and resistance exercises for muscle strength and endurance. The patients' PMD may recommend specific activities that are best for them.
For Heart Health (especially those with risk factors of high serum lipids and hypertension)	**Do:**
	Recommended patients keep total fat intake between 20% to 35% of calories. See the appendix on page 281 to figure this amount, with most fats coming from polyunsaturated and monounsaturated fat sources (for example, fish, nuts, and vegetable oils). Encourage patients to follow these guidelines:
	Consume less than 10% of calories from saturated fat, less than 300 mg per day of cholesterol, and keep trans-fatty acid consumption as low as possible.
	Consume less than 2300 mg of sodium per day (approximately 1 tsp. of salt).
	Consume 4700 mg of potassium each day by choosing potassium-rich foods, including fresh fruits and vegetables, meats, grains, and legumes.
	Consume at least two servings of omega-3-rich fish per week (for example, mackerel, salmon, bluefish, sablefish, herring, lake trout, sardines, and tuna). See section regarding mercury contamination in fish on page 22. Other good sources of omega-3 fatty acids include flaxseed and flaxseed oil, canola oil, soybean oil, and nuts.

Problem	Do's and Don'ts
For Heart Health	**Don't:** Don't provide foods high in saturated fat, such as whole dairy products, butter, and fatty meats as well as processed foods high in saturated and trans fats, including chips, cakes, and cookies. Don't provide high-sodium canned or frozen foods as well as processed meats and salty snacks (for example, pretzels, nuts, and chips).
Microbial Foodborne Illness	**Do:** Encourage patients to use the following safe food handling techniques: Clean hands, food contact surfaces, and fruits and vegetables. Separate raw, cooked, and ready-to-eat foods while shopping, preparing, or storing foods. Cook foods to a safe temperature to prevent the growth of micro-organisms. Keep cold food cold (below 41°F) and hot food hot (above 135°F). Set the refrigerator at no higher than 41°F and the freezer at 0°F. Check these temperatures with an appliance thermometer. See the appendix on foodborne illness on pages 367–374. **Don't:** Don't rinse or wash meat and poultry. Don't allow raw (unpasteurized) milk or any products made from unpasteurized milk, raw or partially cooked eggs or foods containing raw eggs, raw or undercooked meat and poultry, unpasteurized juices, and raw sprouts. Don't forget to refrigerate leftovers right away because they can become unsafe. Don't forget to dispose of food if there is a question about whether or not a food is safe to eat. "If in doubt—throw it out."
Alcohol Intake	**Do:** Advise patients who choose to drink alcoholic beverages to do so sensibly and in moderation, up to one drink per day for women and up to two drinks per day for men. Evaluate patients with alcoholism. They may require folic acid, thiamin, vitamins B_6, and B_{12} supplementation, with the agreement of the PMD.

Problem	*Do's and Don'ts*
	Don't: Don't forget that alcoholic beverages should not be consumed by pregnant and lactating patients, or those who could become pregnant, children and adolescents, or those taking medications that can interact with alcohol. Don't allow alcoholic beverages for patients engaging in activities involving attention or skill (for example, driving or operating heavy machinery).
Bone Health (Osteoporosis Prevention)	**Do:** Advise patients to consume 1000 mg of calcium per day (1200 mg for those greater than 51 years old) to achieve and maintain dense bones. Encourage sources of vitamin D to maximize calcium absorption. Good sources of calcium include dairy products (for example, milk, yogurt, and cheese). Other sources of calcium are calcium-fortified cereals, orange juice, and calcium precipitated tofu. In addition, oysters, sardines (with bones), and green vegetables (broccoli, bok choy, kale, parsley, watercress, and turnip greens) are rich sources of calcium. Dairy products are typically fortified with vitamin D, but other good sources are egg yolks, saltwater fish, and liver. Advise the patient that a diet rich in other nutrients, including vitamin K, magnesium, and potassium may also help to maintain bone mineral density. Good sources of vitamin K are leafy green vegetables (for example, Swiss chard, kale, broccoli, spinach, and dark green lettuce). Other rich sources are liver, egg yolks, cabbage, and brussels sprouts. Foods high in magnesium include halibut, artichokes, legumes, seeds, nuts, yogurt, milk, and leafy green vegetables. Foods high in potassium include fruits (fresh and dried) and vegetables (for example, bananas, cantaloupe, raisins, potatoes, tomato products, winter squash, and lima beans). Encourage weight training and weight-bearing activities to help maintain bone density. **Don't:** Don't advocate that a patient displace milk in the diet with cola products. Don't forget to remind the patient that smoking and excessive alcohol consumption increase the risk of osteoporosis.

Problem	*Do's and Don'ts*
Anemia	**Do:** Explain to the patient that anemia is any condition that occurs when there are too few, small, or immature red blood cells. Nutrient deficiencies of vitamin B_6, B_{12}, folate, or iron may result in anemia. Encourage good sources of vitamin B_6, including protein-rich foods (for example, meat, fish, and poultry as well as non-citrus fruits, fortified cereals, liver, and soy products). Encourage foods high in vitamin B_{12}, including animal products (for example, meat, fish, poultry, shellfish, cheese, and eggs) as well as fortified cereals. Vegetarians may require supplements. Encourage good sources of folate, including fortified cereals, leafy green vegetables (for example, spinach and broccoli) and legumes (for example, black beans, kidney beans, and black-eyed peas). Other good sources are liver, seeds, and citrus fruits. Encourage foods high in iron, such as meats, fish, poultry, shellfish, and eggs. Other good sources are legumes, fortified cereals, dark greens, such as broccoli, and dried fruits, such as raisins.
Vegetarian Diets	**Do:** Ensure that patients who are on strict vegetarian diets receive adequate intake of protein, iron, zinc, calcium, vitamin D, and B_{12}.
Additional Recommendations for Older Adults	**Do:** Evaluate older patients for a lack of calcium, vitamin D, iron, and vitamin B_{12}. Achieve adequate intakes by including foods from all food groups in the diet. Suggest fortified foods or supplements in some cases. Evaluate older patients for increased risk of dehydration and high blood sodium levels. Encourage adequate fluid intake of at least eight 8-ounce glasses per day. All persons older than 60 years of age are eligible for meals served at congregate meal sites or home-delivered meals provided by the Elderly Nutrition Program (US government funded).
Mercury Contamination	**Do:** Teach pregnant and lactating patients about the high risk of mercury toxicity causing damage to the developing brain.

Problem	*Do's and Don'ts*
	• Fish that are relatively high in mercury include tilefish, swordfish, king mackerel, and shark. • Fish relatively low in mercury include cod, haddock, pollock, salmon, sole, and most shellfish. **Don't:** Don't forget to avoid fish highest in mercury and limit ocean, coastal, and commercial fish to 12 oz. (cooked) per week; limit freshwater fish caught by friends and family to 6 oz. cooked.

Sources

American Heart Association. *Healthy Lifestyle.* 2005. http://www.americanheart.org.

Clark, N. *Nancy Clark's Sports Nutrition Guidebook*. Champaign, IL: Leisure Press. 1990.

Department of Health and Human Services & United States Department of Agriculture. *Dietary Guidelines for Americans.* 2005. http://www.health.gov/dietaryguidelines.

United States Department of Agriculture. 2005. http://www.mypyramid.gov.

Whitney, E., & Rolfes, S. R. *Understanding Nutrition* (10th ed.). Belmont, CA: Wadsworth. 2005.

Older Americans

Author: Joseph M. Carlin, MS, MA, RD, LDN, FADA

This list will assist the dietitian to be more alert to the physical and nutritional concerns of America's fastest growing population: people over the age of 60 years. These do's and don'ts for adults overlap the recommendations for good health. See specific disease conditions in other tables for more detailed recommendations.

Problem	*Do's and Don'ts*
Optimum Nutrition for Older Americans	**Do:**
	Ask what older patients had to eat during the past 24 hours.
	Seek out valid and science-based advice on how to choose a diet compatible with good health.
	Brainstorm with older people to identify current eating practices.
	Try to identify any barriers to proper nutrition.
	Try to identify caregivers, family members, and others who can assist the older person in solving food- and nutrition-related problems.
	Don't:
	Don't hesitate to refer older patients to an area agency on aging for a thorough assessment.
	Don't ignore the "Determine Your Nutritional Health Checklist" (www.aafp.org/afp/980301ap/edits.html) as a tool for determining nutritional risks.
Adequate Nutrients	The USDA Dietary Guidelines for Americans and the MyPyramid Plan are useful nutrition education tools. See the appendix or go to www.mypyramid.gov.
	Do:
	Limit portion sizes to prevent excessive calorie intake and to allow for balance and variety in the diet.
	Advocate consumption of a variety of nutrient-dense foods and beverages. Recommend a daily multivitamin and mineral supplement, particularly one that contains vitamin B_{12} and vitamin D. Consult with the PMD about the supplement usage.
	Consider extra vitamin D and vitamin D-fortified foods (for example, milk, salmon, canned tuna, raisin bran cereal, and/or supplements), particularly if the patient has dark skin or is exposed to insufficient sunlight. (The upper level of vitamin D is 50 mcg per day.)

Problem	*Do's and Don'ts*
	Recommend less than 10% of calories from saturated fats and eat less than 300 mg of cholesterol per day and a reduction of trans fatty acids. Limit total fat intake to between 20% to 35% of calories. Suggest polyunsaturated and monounsaturated fats from sources such as fish, nuts, and vegetable oils (canola and olive oils are excellent).
	Check for the use of "health foods," vitamin and mineral supplements, herbals, and botanicals.
	Assess the patient's belief of curative powers and use of foods, ingredients, or supplements and educate accordingly. Talk about the accuracy of health claims made on TV infomercials and advertisements in popular magazines.
	Seek advice from the PMD if there is a suspicion in the accuracy of diet recommendations the patient is following.
	Don't:
	Don't forget to discuss overeating in restaurants and the consumption of foods and beverages that are high in fats and added sugars.
	Don't forget to check for an overconsumption of nutrient supplements because older patients may fall victim to false claims for the curative effects of unproven foods, ingredients, or supplements.
	Don't forget that nutritional supplements are not a substitute for a balanced nutritious diet.
Weight Management	Being overweight puts older people at risk for diabetes, cardiovascular diseases, and other diseases.
	Do:
	Assess what the patient's ideal weight should be.
	Balance caloric intake from foods and beverages with calories expended through physical activity.
	Make preventing weight gain a high priority as patients age.
	Make small decreases in food and beverages consumed.
	Advocate safe exercise.
	Consult with PMD for the presence of chronic disease and/or any medications before recommending changes in diet or an exercise program.
	Notify the PMD if there is an unexpected weight loss.

Problem	Do's and Don'ts
	Don't:
	Don't ignore the importance of a regular program of physical activity, even if it is only walking.
	Don't ignore the importance of seniors staying active.
Physical Activity	Regular physical activities help older people to reduce or maintain their proper weight.
	Do:
	Make physical activity a part of a daily strategy to improve the older person's cardiovascular and bone health.
	Ask the PMD about appropriate levels of regular physical activity, including resistance training. A successful intervention can be a step meter (with the PMD's approval), which tracks steps taken per day. The senior can try to reach 10,000 steps a day (depending on age and health).
	Don't:
	Don't ignore the importance of increasing fluid intake during and after exercising.
Healthful Foods	Consume fruits, vegetables, and whole grain cereals for optimum nutritional health.
	Do:
	Add more variety to the foods seniors consume daily.
	Encourage purchasing foods in smaller quantities to help add variety and recommend new foods frequently.
	Recommend increasing consumption of enriched and whole-grain products (for example, wheat bread, brown rice, and whole-grain breakfast cereals).
	Advocate consumption of fat-free or low-fat milk or dairy products daily.
	Recommend foods rich in dietary fiber. Fiber has excellent laxative properties thereby reducing the incidence of constipation. Nuts and whole grains are an excellent source of fiber.
	Serve vegetables and other foods rich in calcium (for example, broccoli, sardines).
	Encourage the consumption of an adequate amount of liquids daily to prevent dehydration. Recommend about eight 8-ounce glasses each day. Physical activity levels and medication usage will influence fluid needs.

Problem	*Do's and Don'ts*
	Don't: Don't serve foods that are not nutrient dense (for example, white bread, sugars, and alcohol). Don't neglect to read the labels on packaged foods and beverages to ensure the older person is getting the highest level of fiber in the diet. Don't forget that water contained in soups and other foods count toward fluid needs.
Sodium and Potassium	Decreased consumption of sodium and increased consumption of potassium rich foods are linked to good nutritional health. **Do:** Reduce the use of salt at the table and in cooking. Cut back on foods high in sodium (for example, pickles, canned soups, luncheon meats, snack foods). Compare sodium contents of packaged foods. "Low-sodium," "reduced-sodium," and "no-sodium added" food products may be helpful for some older adults. Recommend daily sodium intake of less than 2300 mg, and have blood pressure checked frequently. Encourage potassium-rich foods, such as fruits and vegetables (bananas, cantaloupe, grapefruit, oranges, tomato or prune juice, honeydew melons, prunes, molasses, and potatoes). See the appendix on page 446 for more sources of nutrients in food. **Don't:** Don't forget to ensure prescribed medication is taken for high blood pressure.
Alcohol	Consuming alcoholic beverages sensibly and in moderation contributes to health benefits. **Do:** Talk to the PMD about medications that might interact with alcohol. Advocate drinking alcohol in moderation. A daily intake of one to two drinks daily has been associated with decreased mortality. **Don't:** Don't allow alcohol when clients are engaged in activities requiring attention or coordination.

Problem	*Do's and Don'ts*
Alcohol	Don't ignore the caloric content of alcoholic beverages.
Social Environment	Social isolation has demonstrated to be a risk factor for poor nutrition. **Do:** Encourage older people to take every opportunity to eat with friends, family, or others. **Don't:** Don't forget to encourage caregivers to eat with older people.
Psychological Health	Optimum mental health is essential for maintaining nutritional health. **Do:** Look for the signs of depression because it may result in a lack of motivation to cook or to seek nutritional help. **Don't:** Don't ignore cognitive problems that might interfere with a person's ability to cook, shop for food, or go to a senior meal site for help.
Food Safety	Older adults have reduced immune function and are at increased risk of foodborne illness. **Do:** Review food safety practices. See the appendix on pages 367–374. Clean hands and food-contact surfaces and rinse fruits and vegetables under running water. Wash hands frequently. Cook food to a safe temperature to kill harmful micro-organisms. Use a food thermometer. Keep perishable food properly refrigerated. Avoid unpasteurized milk or apple cider. Keep a supply of shelf-stable foods on hand in case of emergencies (a week's supply of bottled water, tuna fish, canned soups, crackers, canned fruits, etc.). **Don't:** Don't serve raw or partially cooked eggs. Don't prepare raw foods on cutting boards or work surfaces without cleaning them.

Problem	*Do's and Don'ts*
	Don't serve undercooked meats or raw shellfish. Don't defrost foods outside the refrigerator. Don't serve any food you suspect could be spoiled.
Food Insecurity/ Hunger	In every community, there are state and/or federal programs to help older Americans meet their nutritional needs. **Do:** Call the local Area Agency on Aging, senior center, or neighborhood (congregate) meal program in the community for recommendations. Inquire about meals delivered to the home (Meals on Wheels) when the client is homebound or immobile. Inquire about other help (for example, food stamps, in-home services, shopping assistance, and chore services). **Don't:** Don't hesitate to call the local Area Agency on Aging for patient services.
Diabetes	**Do:** Assess the senior's meal plan. Educate the person on optimal diabetes care, blood sugar levels, and sick-day plans. Develop a strategy to reach the older person's ideal weight. Encourage foods that are low in fat, salt, and sugar. Eating right will help maintain weight or reduce weight if the senior is overweight. Reduced weight will keep blood glucose in a desirable range and prevent heart and blood vessel disease. Reinforce the need for three meals per day and snacks as needed depending on medications. **Don't:** Don't skip meals. Don't think that people with diabetes need to eat special foods.
Eye Health	Proper nutrition is essential to prevent oxidative damage to eye tissue. **Do:** Encourage increased consumption of fresh fruits and vegetables, vitamin C, vitamin E, carotenoids (yellow and orange fruits and vegetables, dark green leafy vegetables such

Problem	*Do's and Don'ts*
Eye Health	as spinach, kale, romaine lettuce), and flavonoids (found in citrus fruits, apples, grapes, wine, tea, and chocolate). They have been associated with decreased risk of cataracts and macular degeneration. Zinc intake is also important. Sources of zinc include beef, eggs, poultry, shellfish, nuts, and beans. **Don't:** Don't think that carrots are the only eye-healthy food.
Dental Health	Optimum oral hygiene practices are fundamental to the pleasure of eating and the avoidance of chewing problems. **Do:** Consider chopped or pureed foods for problems chewing or swallowing. Reduce exposure of fermentable carbohydrates (sucrose, starch, etc.), a major contributor to dental caries. **Don't:** Don't ignore the importance of providing fluoridated water and/or fluoride-containing dental products. Both reduce the risk of dental caries.
Osteoporosis	Keeping bones healthy decreases the risk of developing osteoporosis, a disease that causes weak, brittle bones that are prone to breakage. **Do:** Consult with the PMD about the risk for osteoporosis (fragile bones). Recommend consumption of foods rich in calcium, such as dairy products and vegetable greens (for example, spinach, kale, and broccoli) and vitamin D-rich foods (for example, salmon and fortified dairy products). Evaluate the physical environment to help prevent falls. Suggest purchasing nonslip shoes, installing grab bars in the home where necessary, and removing any hazard in the home that might cause falls. Advise eating lactose-reduced and lactose-free dairy products if there is lactose intolerance. **Don't:** Don't forget that some plant foods, such as legumes and soybean products, are good sources of calcium. Don't hesitate to refer the patient to physical therapy if there are any problems with mobility. Don't forget dark green leafy vegetables and calcium-precipitated or fortified soy products as a source of calcium.

Problem	*Do's and Don'ts*
Osteoarthritis	**Do:** Encourage optimal weight maintenance. Assess diet adequacy, paying particular attention to calcium- and vitamin-D rich foods (low-fat milk, cheese, and yogurt). Suggest increasing foods containing omega-3 fatty acids, canola oil, flaxseed oil, salmon, mackerel, tuna, walnuts, and soy. If advised by the PMD, try glucosamine (500 mg) and chondroitin sulfate (400 mg) three times a day. Some patients may find it helpful. (Check with the PMD before using glucosamine if the patient is allergic to shellfish, which produces glucosamine.) Check blood sugars frequently if diabetes is present. Glucosamine is an amino sugar. Check clotting time more often when using chondroitin sulfate with blood thinners or aspirin. **Don't:** Don't continue glucosamine and chondroitin sulfate after 6–8 weeks if no help is evident from their use. Pregnant women, women of childbearing age, and children should not use it.
Rheumatoid Arthritis	**Do:** Suggest adaptive equipment if small and large joint involvement impairs ability to prepare and eat food. Suggest prechopped or sliced foods. Suggest foods with soft consistency if temporomandibular joint problems cause difficulty in chewing. Suggest taking with milk or food to avoid stomach irritation for patients on aspirin therapy. Assess food intolerances due to esophageal and GI disturbances. Encourage use of omega-3 fatty acids: canola and flaxseed oil, salmon, mackerel, tuna, walnuts, and soy. Suggest a folic acid supplement if the patient is on immunosuppressives (methotrexate). Evaluate patients on steroids (prednisone) for calcium and vitamin D supplements. Steroids can cause reduced absorption and increased excretion of calcium. Check with the PMD before making any supplement recommendations. Check patients for elevated blood sugars and edema also caused by steroid use. Suggest a diabetic diet if necessary and encourage low-sodium foods to alleviate edema.

Problem	*Do's and Don'ts*
Rheumatoid Arthritis	Discuss flare-ups and the foods eaten preceding the episode for possible food allergies. Fasting (under medical supervision) for a short period may alleviate symptoms for some. Encourage a balanced diet (www.MyPyramid.gov) with adequate calories, protein, and the use of omega-3 fatty acids. For additional information on supplement use in arthritis, see the Arthritis Foundation's Web site (www.arthritis.org). **Don't:** Don't overlook the possibility of xerostomia and secondary dysphasia. Don't ignore the possibility of anorexia due to medications. Don't serve high-salt foods (for example, processed and canned foods, luncheon meats, and cheese). Don't use alfalfa, copper salts, or zinc because these can cause harmful side effects.

Sources

American Academy of Family Physicians. *Determine Your Nutritional Health Checklist.* http://www.aafp.org/x16138.xml.

American Society on Aging. *Live Well, Live Long: Health Promotion & Disease Prevention for Older Adults.* http://www.asaging.org/cdc/index.cfm.

Arthritis Foundation. *Diet and Your Arthritis.* http://www.arthritis.org/resources/nutrition/diet.asp.

Arthritis Foundation. *Glucosamine and Chondroitin Sulfate.* http://www.arthritis.org/conditions/alttherapies/Glucosamine.asp.

Augustin, A. J. (Ed.). *Nutrition and the Eye: Basic and Clinical Research.* Basel, Switzerland: Karger. 2005.

Department of Health and Human Services & U.S. Department of Agriculture. *Nutrition and Your Health: Dietary Guidelines for Americans.* http://www.health.gov/dietaryguidelines/.

Mahan, K. L., & Escott, S. *Krause's Food, Nutrition and Diet Therapy* (11th ed.). Philadelphia, PA: Saunders. 1122–1133. 2004.

NIH Senior Health. National Institute of Diabetes and Digestive and Kidney Diseases. http://nihseniorhealth.gov.

U.S. Department of Agriculture. http://www.mypyramid.gov.

U.S. Food and Drug Administration & U.S. Department of Agriculture. *To Your Health! Food Safety for Seniors.* http://www.fightbac.org.

Nutrition During Pregnancy

Author: Yeemay Su Miller, MS, RD

Healthcare providers need to be both supportive and knowledgeable about nutrition during pregnancy. The following table will guide the provider through many nutritional and physiological issues.

Problem	*Do's and Don'ts*
Nausea and Vomiting	**Do:**
	Recommend that the patient eat small, frequent meals and snacks (every 1.5–2 hours).
	Suggest the patient have crackers or dry toast at the bedside if nauseous upon waking. Have the patient carry food and keep snacks in the car.
	Recommend plenty of fluids between meals and nutritious shakes, if this is easier than eating solids. In general, try any foods that are appealing to the patient.
	Suggest the patient try smelling fresh lemon, squeezing lemons into sparkling water, lemon sour candies, lemonade, ginger ale, or ginger tea.
	Increase food sources of vitamin B_6 (for example, meat, poultry, fish, potatoes, bananas, watermelon, acorn squash, and fortified cereal).
	Suggest foods that are easier to digest.
	Encourage the patient to take the prenatal vitamin at night as a feasible option.
	See Table 1-1 on page 42.
	Don't:
	Don't allow the patient to stop eating and drinking altogether even if they have no appetite because this can worsen nausea.
	Don't let more than 2–3 hours pass before eating.
	Don't give any medication, over-the-counter products, or supplements (including vitamin B_6) without the PMD's approval.
	Don't provide high-fat or oily foods, which take longer to digest.
	Don't serve caffeinated beverages (coffee, some teas, and some soft drinks).
	Don't stop taking a multivitamin; instead, see if taking it at another time of day helps the patient feel better.

Problem	*Do's and Don'ts*
Nausea and Vomiting	Don't allow the patient to stay in poorly ventilated rooms or places with bothersome smells (for example, cigarette smoke or strong perfume/cologne).
Vomiting/ Hyperemesis Gravidarum	**Do:** Have the patient stay well hydrated by drinking plenty of fluids, including a rehydrating drink containing electrolytes (for example, Gatorade) and juices in small amounts throughout the day. Try adding ginger root to foods and drink ginger root tea or red raspberry tea. Suggest low-fat foods that are easy to digest. Recommend snacks with high water content (for example, watermelon, canned fruit, gelatin, fruit juice bars, Popsicles, sorbet, and Italian ices). The PMD may initiate intravenous rehydration if the patient is unable to keep any fluids down. Hospitalization may be necessary. Get psychosocial support in addition to physical support for the patient. **Don't:** Don't provide caffeinated beverages (coffee, some teas, and soft drinks).
Hypo- and Hyperglycemia	**Do:** Encourage the patient to eat a diet consisting proportionally of complex, high-fiber carbohydrates (for example, whole-grain breads and cereals, brown rice, legumes, and fresh fruits and vegetables). Provide smaller meals with appropriate snacks between meals. Include some source of protein (for example, milk, yogurt, cheese, meat, poultry, eggs, or nut butters) in all meals and snacks. **Don't:** Don't eat or drink fruit juice or highly sweetened beverages and concentrated sweet foods.
Low Maternal Weight (BMI less than 19.8), Low Weight Gain/ Weight Loss	**Do:** Identify cause (for example, lack of food, body image concerns, an eating disorder, poor appetite, prolonged nausea and vomiting, and stress). Offer frequent meals and snacks consisting of nutrient-dense, high-kilocalorie foods (for example, cheese, yogurt, milk shakes, granola, dried fruits, starchy vegetables, and

Problem	*Do's and Don'ts*
	muffins) or what appeals to the patient if appetite is poor. Try Carnation Instant Breakfast, Ensure, or homemade shakes (blend yogurt, milk powder, and fresh fruit).
	Ask the PMD to prescribe approved medication if nausea or vomiting is preventing adequate intake. See section on nausea/vomiting on page 33.
	Problem solve ways to minimize stress or to slow down if patient is "too busy" to eat.
	Provide referrals to community and government programs to assist with food access if in financial hardship.
	Consult with PMD if weight gain remains poor.
	See Table 1-2 on page 43.
	Don't:
	Don't allow the patient to skip meals.
	Don't allow the patient to do excessive exercise or physical activity.
High Maternal Weight (BMI greater than 29) or Weight Gain	**Do:**
	Establish a healthy eating pattern of regular meals and snacks with nutrient-dense foods lower in calories.
	Encourage high-fiber choices (for example, vegetables, fruits, beans, legumes, whole-grain cereals/breads).
	Brainstorm easy ways to get more fruits and vegetables on a regular basis.
	Provide low-fat or nonfat dairy foods, seafood, chicken, or lean meat for the patient.
	Suggest more water and caffeine-free, noncaloric beverages. If the patient likes soft drinks, try club soda mixed with some fruit juice.
	Suggest frozen yogurt, light ice cream, and sugar-free puddings for dessert.
	Recommend moderate exercise on a regular basis (for example, walking, swimming, dancing, and prenatal yoga).
	Encourage breast-feeding as a helpful means of "burning" maternal fat stores.
	Examine ways to decrease stress, fatigue, and anxiety in the patient's life. Increased food intake positively correlates with these psychosocial factors.
	See Table 1-1 on page 42.

Problem	*Do's and Don'ts*
High Maternal Weight	**Don't:** Don't impose skipping meals or severe calorie restrictions to lose weight.
Poor Appetite	**Do:** Recommend small amounts of food frequently. Snacking may be easier if meals seem too difficult. Patients can try sipping fruit juices/nectars and nutritious shakes (for example, Carnation Instant Breakfast or homemade shakes using yogurt and fruit). Take advantage of times when appetite is better and provide more food. Remind patient of the importance of eating for nutrition and not only for hunger or appetite. Try increasing physical activity to stimulate appetite and metabolism.
Heartburn	**Do:** Suggest eating small, frequent meals and low-fat snacks in a relaxed setting. Recommend eating slowly and staying upright after eating. Suggest taking a walk after meals. The patient should wait at least 2 hours before lying down and elevate the upper body when sleeping. **Don't:** Don't allow high-fat, spicy food and foods that tend to "revisit." Don't allow spearmint, peppermint, and caffeine. Don't allow antacids without consulting the PMD first.
Edema or Fluid Retention	**Do:** Monitor weight gain and blood pressure. Rule out hypertension and the appearance of proteinuria. Assess amount of sodium in diet. Suggest the patient elevate feet whenever possible and wear support pantyhose, especially for work or when standing for long periods. **Don't:** Don't limit fluid intake, which will only worsen the problem, when approved by the PMD. Don't salt foods.

Problem	*Do's and Don'ts*
	Don't allow processed foods and high-sodium items (for example, soups, salty snacks, pickles, cured meats, cold cuts, and some fast foods). Don't use diuretics unless prescribed by the PMD.
Iron Deficiency Anemia	**Do:** Provide high-iron foods (for example, beef, liver, fish, clams, cooked oysters, poultry, dried peas, beans, lentils, and fortified cereals); accompany with vitamin C-rich food to aid iron absorption from meats. The PMD may order a daily ferrous iron supplement of 60–120 mg. Decrease the dose if side effects (for example, nausea, cramps, constipation, and diarrhea) persist, or try a slow-release preparation at mealtime if approved by the PMD. Continue with prenatal vitamin. **Don't:** Don't consume any raw oysters, clams, or any uncooked seafood. Don't allow coffee or teas, which can inhibit iron absorption. Don't give an iron supplement with milk products.
Meeting Nutrient Needs	**Do:** Increase food sources and/or supplements of the following nutrients: • Iron (See iron deficiency anemia in the previous section.) • Folate (for example, leafy, dark green vegetables, legumes, dried beans and peas, citrus fruits and juices, most berries, and fortified breakfast cereals). The recommended intake of folate is 600 mg per day. A supplement of 400 mg per day of folic acid is advisable with the PMD's approval. • Vitamin B_{12} (for example, cooked clams, oysters, liver, herring, crab, liver, salmon, lobster, beef, and all bran cereal). If vegan, the patient must consume a reliable vitamin B_{12} source (for example, fortified soymilk or a supplement). • Zinc (for example, cooked oysters, crab, ground beef, beef liver, porterhouse steak, dark meat of turkey, wheat bran flakes cereal, and Cheerios). See Table 1-3 on page 44 for recommended servings of foods from each group.

Problem	*Do's and Don'ts*
Meeting Nutrient Needs	**Don't:** Don't supply supplements without approval from the PMD. Don't allow fish over 12 oz. per week to avoid overconsumption of mercury. See the following section and foodborne illness in the appendix on pages 367–374.
Constipation	**Do:** Advocate plenty of vegetables and fruits in all meals and snacks, 100% whole wheat bread, bran, and whole-grain cereals or muffins. Suggest plenty of fluids (at least eight 8-oz. glasses per day). Try dried apricots, prunes, and prune juice. Consider how to increase iron-rich foods to substitute for the supplement (with the PMD's approval), which may be binding, if the patient is taking an iron supplement. Recommend regular, appropriate physical activity. **Don't:** Don't use mineral oil or other "natural" remedies. Don't allow laxatives.
Use of Artificial Sweeteners	**Do:** Use natural sugar in moderate amounts, unless contraindicated by the PMD. For those with gestational diabetes or needing to control calories, discuss the various choices of artificial sweeteners. **Don't:** Don't use artificial sweeteners without an approval from the PMD. Women with phenylketonuria should not use aspartame (Equal).
Food Safety	**Do:** **Meats and Seafood** Separate raw meat, poultry, and seafood from ready-to-eat foods in the grocery shopping cart, refrigerator, and while preparing and handling foods. Consider placing raw meats inside plastic bags in the shopping cart to keep the juices contained while shopping. Cook meats and seafood thoroughly before eating. Check with the PMD for the portion and a variety of cooked fish each week that is safe to serve.

Problem	*Do's and Don'ts*
	Dairy and Eggs Check labels on all the dairy and egg products to be certain they are pasteurized. Cook eggs thoroughly until the yolks and whites are firm. **Fruits and Vegetables** Wash thoroughly all raw produce with running water, especially fruit rinds that are removed (for example, melons, oranges). Serve only pasteurized juice (found in the refrigerated section of the store) or shelf-stable juices (for example, juice boxes). Follow the 2-hour rule. Discard perishable foods left at room temperature for over 2 hours. On hot days, 90°F or higher, discard food after one hour. **Eating Out** Encourage eating out only at clean, reputable places that practice food safety rules. Refrigerate leftovers/doggie bags within 2 hours. Call the US Food and Drug Administration Food Information Line at 1-888-SAFE FOOD for more information regarding food safety. See the appendix on pages 367–374. **Don't:** Don't allow raw or undercooked (rare) meats, poultry, or seafood (for example, oysters, sushi, or sashimi). Don't allow swordfish, tilefish, king mackerel, and shark due to the high methyl-mercury content. Don't serve unpasteurized milk or milk products such as imported feta, brie, or goat milk cheese, which could contain *Listeria*. Don't allow the patient to taste raw batter, filling, or raw cookie dough that contains eggs. Don't use Caesar dressing, sauces (for example, béarnaise, hollandaise, aioli), and desserts made with raw eggs (for example, mousse, meringue, tiramisu) if at all possible. Don't serve raw sprouts of any kind (for example, alfalfa, clover, radish, and mung bean) if at all possible. Don't provide hot dogs or luncheon meats unless reheated to steaming hot.

Problem	*Do's and Don'ts*
Food Safety	Don't serve pâtés or meat spreads due to the risk of *Listeria*. Don't eat at parties where food may be sitting at room temperature for over 2 hours and is risky to eat.
Alcohol Use	**Do:** Recommend abstaining from the use of any alcoholic beverages. No safe level has been determined for pregnant women; therefore, most health professional organizations recommend abstaining. **Don't:** Don't allow any type of alcoholic beverages.
Caffeinated Beverages	**Do:** Encourage moderate intake of teas, coffee, and cola. **Don't:** Don't serve more than a maximum of 2–3 cups per day of coffee and tea. Do not allow herbal tea.
Medications and Other Supplements	**Do:** Discuss use of any medication, over-the-counter or prescription, and supplements with the PMD.
Geophagia and Pica	**Do:** Complete a thorough nutritional assessment. Increasing iron-rich foods may be important. Problem solve and explore possible substitutions for pica substances and behaviors (chew gum or suck fruit juice ice cubes).
Preventing Pediatric Food Hypersensitivities and Allergies	**Do:** Warn the patient to reduce the number of times exposed to possible allergens that exist in the family history. **Don't:** Don't eat nuts if there is a family history of environmental and/or food allergies.

Sources

Carey, J. C., & Rayburn, W. F. *Obstetrics & Gynecology* (4th ed.). Philadelphia, PA: Lippincott Williams & Wilkins. 6–7. 2002.

Carlsson, C. P., et al. "Manual Acupuncture Reduces Hyperemesis Gravidarum: Placebo-controlled, Randomized, Single-blind, Crossover Study." *J Pain Symptom Management*. 2002. 20, 273–279.

Erick, M. *Managing Morning Sickness: A Survival Guide for Pregnant Women.* Boulder, CO: Bull Publishing. 2004.

Holistic Healing. http://www.holisticmed.com.

Hurley, K. M., Caulfield, L. E., Sacco, L. M., Costigan, K. A., & Depietro, J. A. "Psychosocial Influences in Dietary Patterns during Pregnancy." *J Am Diet Assoc.* 2005. 105, 963–966.

International Food and Nutrition Council Foundation. http://ific.org/publications/brochures/pregnancybroch.cfm.

Knight, B., et al. "Effect of Acupuncture on Nausea of Pregnancy: A Randomized, Controlled Trial." *Obstetrics & Gynecology.* 2001. 97, 184–188.

Koren, G. & Bishai, R. (Ed.). *Nausea and Vomiting of Pregnancy: State of the Art 2000.* Vol. 1, p. 219. Toronto: Motherisk. 2000.

National Academy of Sciences, Institute of Medicine, Food and Nutrition Board, Committee on Nutritional Status During Pregnancy and Lactation. *Nutrition During Pregnancy and Lactation, An Implementation Guide.* Washington, DC: National Academy Press. 1992.

Sahakian, V., et al. "Vitamin B_6 Is Effective Therapy for Nausea and Vomiting of Pregnancy: A Randomized, Double-Blind Placebo-Controlled Study." *Obstetrics & Gynecology.* 1991. 78, 33–36.

Sampson, H. A. "Update on Food Allergy." *J Allergy Clin Immunol.* May 2004. 113(5), 805–819.

U.S. Food and Drug Administration, Center for Food Safety and Applied Nutrition/Office of Food Safety, Defense, and Outreach. http://www.cfsan.fda.gov/list.html.

U.S. Food and Drug Administration, Center for Food Safety and Applied Nutrition/Office of Food Safety, Defense, and Outreach. http://www.mchlibrary.info/pubs/PDFs/ nutritionupdate.pdf.

Vutyavanich, T., Kraisarin, T., & Ruangsri, R. "Ginger for Nausea and Vomiting in Pregnancy: Randomized, Double-Masked, Placebo-Controlled Trial." *Obstet Gynecol.* 2001. 97, 577–582.

Table 1-1 Recommended Weight Gain Chart

Recommended Weight Gain for Pregnant Women by Pre-Pregnancy Body Mass Index (BMI)[a]

Weight-for-Height Category	Recommended Total Weight Gain Kilograms	Pounds
Underweight (BMI < 19.8) or 90% wt/ht	12.5–18	28–40
Normal weight (BMI 19.8 to 25) or 90–120% wt/ht	11.5–16	25–35
Overweight (BMI 26 to 29) or 120–135% wt/ht	7–11.5	15–25
Obese (BMI > 29) or 135% wt/ht	7	No more than 15
Twin gestation (any BMI)	16–20	35–45
Triplet gestation (any BMI)	23	50

Monitor women at greater risk for delivering low birth weight babies, including adolescents, African-American women, and others for optimal weight gain and dietary quality throughout pregnancy.

[a]BMI is an indicator of nutritional status based on two common measurements; height and weight. Because it reflects body composition, such as body fat and lean body mass, consider BMI a more accurate indicator than height/weight tables.

BMI in this table is based on metric calculations, using the following formula:

$$\text{BMI} = \text{wt/ht}^2 \text{ (metric)} = \text{body weight in kilograms/height in meters}^2$$

Reprinted with permission from *Recommended Dietary Allowances*, 10th ed., ©1989, by the National Academy of Sciences, courtesy of the National Academies Press, Washington, DC.

Reprinted with permission from Dietary Reference, ©2000, by the National Academy of Sciences, courtesy of the National Academies Press, Washington, DC.

Table 1-2 Sample Shopping List to Help Stop Nausea

Fill in blanks with appealing foods and drinks of patient's personal favorites
soft (mashed potatoes, custard, applesauce, ______________________)
smooth (milk, yogurt, pudding, ______________________)
crunchy (celery, crackers, nuts, ______________________)
salty (potato chips, pretzels, nuts, ______________________)
sweet (grapes, raisins, dates, jam, ______________________)
sour (pickles, lemons, sauerkraut, sour candies, ______________________)
citrus (oranges, grapefruit, lemons, ______________________)
bitter (radishes, seltzer, tonic water, ______________________)
pungent (blue cheese, ginger, vinegar, Italian dressing, ______________________)
spicy (cinnamon tea, hot salsa, Tabasco sauce, ______________________)
bland (rice, pasta, bread, ______________________)
cold (salads, ice cream, Popsicles, sorbet, ______________________)
hot (soup, tea, prepared hot entrées, ______________________)
wet (juices, seltzer, water with a slice of lime, ______________________)
dry (crackers, dry cereal, bread, ______________________)
thick (stew, frappe, oatmeal, chowder, ______________________)
thin (juices, broth, broth-based soups, ______________________)
favorites: ______________________

Table 1-3 Recommended Foods and Portions for Pregnant Women

MyPyramid: A Guide to Daily Choices for Pregnant Women

Food Group	Recommended Servings	What Counts as a Serving?
Breads, cereal, rice, and pasta group— especially whole grain and refined (enriched)	6–11 servings	• 1 slice bread • 1/2 hamburger bun or English muffin • 3–4 small or 2 large crackers • 1/2 cup cooked cereal, pasta, or rice • About 2 cups ready-to-eat cereal
Fruit	2–4 servings	• 3/4 cup juice • 1 medium apple, banana, orange, pear • 1/2 cup chopped, cooked, or canned fruit
Vegetables (Eat dark green, leafy, yellow, or orange vegetables and cooked dry beans and peas often.)	3–5 servings	• 1 cup raw leafy vegetables • 1/2 cup other vegetables—cooked or raw • 3/4 cup vegetable juice
Meat, poultry, fish, dry beans, eggs, and nuts— preferably lean or low-fat	3–4 servings	• 2–3 ounces cooked lean meat, poultry, fish • 1/2 cup cooked, dry beans[b] or 1/2 cup tofu counts as 1 ounce lean meat • 2 tablespoons peanut butter or 1/3 cup nuts counts as 1 ounce meat
Milk, yogurt, and cheese—preferably fat free or low fat	3–4 servings[a]	• 1 cup milk • 1 cup buttermilk • 8 ounces yogurt • 1 1/2 ounces natural cheese • 2 ounces processed cheese • 1 cup calcium-fortified soy milk
Fats and sweets	Use sparingly	• Limit fats and sweets
Water	10 cups per day	• 1 cup = 8 ounces
Alcohol	None	• Avoid alcoholic beverages

[a] During pregnancy and lactation, the recommended number of milk group servings is the same for nonpregnant women. A soy-based beverage with added calcium is an option for those who prefer a nondairy source of calcium.

[b]Count dry beans, peas, and lentils as servings in either the meat and beans group or the vegetable group. As a vegetable, 1/2 cup cooked, dry beans counts as one serving. As a meat substitute, one cup cooked, dry beans counts as one serving (2 ounces meat).

Adapted from *Dietary Guidelines for Americans*, 5th ed., ©2000, U.S. Department of Agriculture and the U.S. Department of Health and Human Services and MyPyramid, U.S. Department of Agriculture, 2005.

Table 1-4 Dietary Reference Intakes: Recommended Intakes for Pregnant Women

2000 DRIs	< 18 years	19–30 years	31–50 years
Calcium (mg/d)	1,300*	1,000*	1,000*
Potassium (mg/d)	1,250	700	700
Vitamin D[1] (mg/d)	5*	5*	5*
Fl (mg/d)	3*	3*	3*
Thiamin (mg/d)	1.4	1.4	1.4
Riboflavin (mg/d)	1.4	1.4	1.4
Niacin (mg/d)	18	18	18
Vitamin B_6 (mg/d)	1.9	1.9	1.9
Folate (mg/d)	600	600	600
Vitamin B_{12} (mg/d)	2.6	2.6	2.6
Pantothenic Acid (mg/d)	6*	6*	6*
Biotin (mg/d)	30*	30*	30*
Choline (mg/d)	450*	450*	450*
Vitamin C (mg/d)	80	85	85
Vitamin E (mg/d)	15	15	15
Se (mg/d)	60	60	60
Mg (mg/d)	400	350	360
Vitamin A (mg RE)	750	770	770
Vitamin K (mg)	75*	90*	90*
Iron (mg)	27	27	27
Zinc (mg)	12	11	11
Iodine (mg)	220	220	220

* The asterisk (*) indicates adequate intakes; all other nutrient amounts are Recommended Dietary Allowances (RDA).

[1]As cholecalciferol. 1 mg cholecalciferol = 40 IU vitamin D and in the absence of exposure to sunlight.

Table 1-5 DRIs for Pregnant Women

	Kcal per day[1]	Carbohydrate (g/d)	Total Fiber (g/d)	Total Fat	Protein
14–18 years old		175	28*	ND[2]	71[3] (1.1 g/kg/d)
1st trimester	2368				
2nd trimester	2708				
3rd trimester	2820				
19–50 years old		175	28*	ND[2]	71[3] (1.1 g/kg/d)
1st trimester	2403				
2nd trimester	2743				
3rd trimester	2855				

* The asterisk (*) indicates adequate intakes; all other nutrient amounts are Recommended Dietary Allowances (RDAs).

[1] These energy requirements assume an active lifestyle.

[2] ND = Not determined.

[3] Protein requirements are based on a reference female: 5′4″ tall, 119 lbs. (14–18 years old), or 126 lbs. (19–30 years old).

Reprinted with permission from *Recommended Dietary Allowances*, 10th ed., ©1989 by the National Academy of Sciences, courtesy of the National Academies Press, Washington, DC.

Reprinted with permission from *Dietary Reference*, ©2000, by the National Academy of Sciences, courtesy of the National Academies Press, Washington, DC.

Nutrition During Lactation

Author: Yeemay Su Miller, MS, RD

Healthcare providers need to be both supportive and knowledgeable about breast-feeding. The following table will guide the provider through many nutritional and physiological issues.

Problem	*Do's and Don'ts*
Caloric Requirements–Weight Concerns	**Do:**
	Approximately 500 kcal more are needed per day than a nonpregnant, non–breast-feeding woman.
	Recommend a minimum of 1800 kcal per day. If exclusively breast-feeding, recommend 2500–3300 kcal per day depending on physical activity.
	Advise healthful foods and eating according to appetite, especially for the first 2 months.
	Initial weight loss will usually occur without conscious caloric restriction during lactation. Gradual weight loss of 0.5–2.0 lb per week is best. Remember, returning to prepregnancy weight normally takes many months and could take up to a year.
	Don't:
	Don't severely limit calories in the effort to lose weight, which could affect milk supply. Weight loss should not exceed over 2 pounds per week.
	Don't follow diets or use medications that promise rapid weight loss.
	Don't recommend consuming less than 1800 kcal per day because nutrient needs will most likely not be met.
Nutrient Needs	**Do:**
	Increase foods rich in vitamins A, E, C, and D, as well as the B vitamins and folate, zinc, calcium, and magnesium. See the table in the Appendix on pages 446–457.
	Recommend a prenatal vitamin or other comparable multivitamin, with the PMD's input. In general, recommend a generous intake of nutrients from fruits and vegetables, whole-grain breads and cereals, calcium-rich dairy products, and protein-rich foods (for example, meats, fish, and legumes).
	Recommend an exclusively breast-fed infant be supplemented with 200 IU of vitamin D (available as liquid drops

Problem	*Do's and Don'ts*
Nutrient Needs	per the PMD's direction) or be exposed to sunlight on the face and hands for approximately 15 minutes a few times per week. Assure the patient that even if her diet is lacking in nutrients, her breast milk will still be of ideal composition to foster proper growth for her baby.
Lactose Intolerance/ Low Intake of Milk Products	**Do:** Suggest calcium-containing foods, such as leafy greens (for example, collard and mustard greens, broccoli, watercress, bok choy, and kale), cauliflower, some brands of tofu, beverages (for example, calcium-fortified orange juice, soymilk), corn tortillas, sardines with bones, almonds, and blackstrap molasses.
Baby Reacting to Mother's Diet	**Do:** Evaluate diet if the baby gets symptoms (fussy, gassy, cries more, appears uncomfortable or colicky) every time a certain type of food is eaten. Eliminate that particular item from the diet. Try reintroducing the food to see if baby appears symptomatic again at a later date. Milk and other dairy foods tend to be the most likely culprit for some babies, so eliminate dairy first. Other problem foods could include gassy vegetables (for example, broccoli, cauliflower) or spicy foods.
Caffeinated Beverages	**Do:** Suggest moderate intake of teas, coffee, and cola. Be aware that decaffeinated coffee still contains some caffeine. **Don't:** Don't allow the patient to exceed two cups per day of coffee, tea, or colas. Excessive caffeine could cause baby to be restless and irritable.
Alcohol Intake	**Do:** Recommend no alcohol because it does reach the baby via breast milk if the mother drinks. It can also affect the milk letdown and ejection reflex, thereby decreasing the amount of milk baby gets. **Don't:** Don't allow the intake of alcohol for all breast-feeding mothers; alcohol via breast milk can affect baby's motor skill development and can impair baby's growth.

Problem	*Do's and Don'ts*
Adequate Milk Supply	**Do:** Recommend breast-feeding often—at least 8 to 10 times per day in the early postpartum period. The more frequently the baby feeds, the more milk the body will produce. Suggest feeding on one side as long as the baby wants or until he/she falls asleep, and then offer the other breast. Arouse the baby if necessary to receive enough breast milk. Suggest enough rest and the keeping of stress levels down to promote the letdown reflex. Promote eating well and drinking plenty of fluids. Mothers should relax and find a comfortable place to breast-feed. Advocate pumping or expressing milk if separated from baby for more than 3 hours. Ensure that any birth control prescription is compatible with successful lactation. Delay the introduction of any solids to the baby until at least 4–6 months. Ensure that baby is wetting six to eight diapers per day and gaining 4–8 ounces of weight per week as a sign of adequate supply and intake of breast milk. Supplementing with infant formula may be necessary if all other strategies to increase milk supply are not successful. **Don't:** Don't allow any supplements or natural herbal remedies (for example, fenugreek, fennel seed, and blessed thistle) that claim to increase milk production, unless approved by the PMD. Don't let more than 3 hours pass before feeding the baby. Supplementing with infant formula may further diminish mother's milk supply. Don't forget that some oral contraceptive agents may negatively affect milk supply. Don't introduce solid foods to baby prior to 4 months of age.
Engorgement/ Overabundance of Milk	**Do:** Recommend that the mother express/pump just enough milk to relieve any breast pain. Use ice packs or frozen peas or corn as ice packs for pain relief because they mold well to the breast. Suggest a warm shower and a gentle massage or warm compresses to allow the outflow of some milk to relieve the pressure. Nursing the baby is the best remedy.

Problem	*Do's and Don'ts*
Engorgement/ Overabundance of Milk	Assure the patient that with a newborn, initial engorgement is normal and improves on its own for most people when the mother's body adjusts to the infant's actual needs. Engorgement can also happen when baby sleeps through the night (that is, no middle of the night feeding). For incessant engorgement, refer patient to a lactation consultant. **Don't:** Don't suggest overpumping, which later increases milk supply and worsens engorgement.
Sore/Cracked Nipples	**Do:** Assure the patient that pain and soreness in the initial 2–3 weeks of breast-feeding is normal until the nipples are able to toughen up from the frequent feedings. Therefore, be certain that baby is positioned correctly at the mother's breast and taking the areola into his/her mouth and not just the nipple. Pain during the initial weeks of breast-feeding can be quite severe even when done in a completely correct manner. Remind the mother that breast milk makes the best salve; expression of a little milk on the nipple after each feeding and air drying is ideal. Recommend continued use of breast milk as a salve for cracked nipples. Encourage the use of Lansinoh cream for cracked nipples. Recommend pumping milk into a bottle and feeding the baby this milk until the cracks improve. **Don't:** Don't let the baby suck on the nipple, which may lead to cracked nipples.
Fluid Intake	**Do:** Suggest drinking plenty of fluids to prevent dehydration. Recommend additional fluids above what patient normally drinks while not pregnant or lactating. As a good guideline, drink a glass of water, milk, or juice each time the baby is breast-fed. **Don't:** Don't assume excessive fluids will necessarily increase milk supply. Don't advise herbal teas.
Safe Foods	**Do:** Recommend an upper limit of 12 ounces of certain fish or seafood per week, such as shrimp, catfish, pollack, and

Problem	*Do's and Don'ts*
	salmon. Check with the government sources often because list can vary from time to time.
	Don't:
	Don't serve fish high in methyl mercury (for example, swordfish, shark, tilefish, mackerel, and tuna).
Complete Vegetarianism/ Vegan Diet	**Do:**
	Suggest a source of vitamin B_{12}—either food with added B_{12} or a separate vitamin supplement.
Postpartum Anemia	**Do:**
	Advocate high-iron foods (for example, beef, liver, fish, clams, oysters, poultry, dried peas, beans, lentils, fortified cereals); accompany with vitamin C-rich food to aid heme iron absorption. A daily ferrous iron supplement of 60–120 mg may be needed and should be approved by the PMD. Notify the PMD if side effects occur (for example, nausea, cramps, constipation, and diarrhea). PMD will recheck blood levels to assess continuation of ferrous iron.
	Don't:
	Don't provide coffee or teas, which can inhibit iron absorption by mother and baby.
Baby Having Inadequate Weight Gain	**Do:**
	Refer mother to a lactation consultant. The mother may need to feed baby longer on each breast to ensure baby receives hind milk, which is higher in fat content.
	Evaluate baby's sucking strength and determine whether letdown reflex is occurring while baby is on breast.
	Assess mother's stress and anxiety levels, her ability to relax while feeding baby, any substance use (for example, alcohol, other drugs), and her confidence level to breast-feed successfully.
	Recommend plenty of rest, sleeping when baby sleeps, eating well, and drinking plenty of fluids.
	Consider supplementing with formula if the mother has tried all solutions to help promote successful breast-feeding and the baby is still not gaining adequate weight. If the mother has a low BMI and the maternal diet is severely restricted calorically, then milk volume could diminish. However, an inadequate maternal diet alone is not likely the cause. Consult with the pediatrician and lactation consultant regarding the need to supplement the infant's diet.

Problem	*Do's and Don'ts*
Diabetes	**Do:** Referred patients should have careful monitoring and counseling to ensure successful lactation. Adjustment of caloric intake and insulin or oral hypoglycemic agent doses by the PMD is also necessary to meet heightened needs of milk production.
Preventing Pediatric Food Hypersensitivities and Allergies	**Do:** Suggest purposeful reduction of exposure to possible allergens. **Don't:** Don't forget the most common allergenic foods, such as peanuts and tree nuts (for example, almonds, walnuts, hazelnuts, Brazil nuts, cashews, pistachios). Remind the patient not to consume these foods, especially if there is a family history of food or environmental allergies.
Medications and Supplements	**Do:** Review the safety and compatibility of any medication/supplement with breast-feeding. If the mother is taking any PMD-recommended medicines, the baby should be breast-fed first, and then the mother should take the medicine.
Food Taboos	**Do:** Inquire about food restrictions that have been self-imposed due to family/cultural beliefs, notions, or superstitions. On the converse, inquire about excessive consumption of particular foods for the same reasons. **Don't:** Don't have the mother eat excessive amounts of any one particular food due to the increased risk of predisposing the baby's hypersensitivity to the food item.
Smoking/Illicit Drugs/HIV/AIDS Infection	**Do:** Advise mothers who smoke or take illicit drugs to quit. Babies exposed to cigarette smoke or illicit drugs are at much greater risk of Sudden Infant Death Syndrome (SIDS). **Don't:** Don't allow mothers who are HIV positive or have AIDS to breast-feed their babies.

Sources

Auckland Allergy Clinic. *Allergy Prevention*. http://www.allergyclinic.co.nz/guides/27.html.

Collier, S., Fulhan, J., & Duggan, C. "Nutrition for the Pediatric Office: Update on Vitamins, Infant Feeding, and Food Allergies." *Pediatrics*. June 2004. 16(3), 314–320.

Dewey, K. G. "Energy and Protein Requirements During Lactation." *Annual Review of Nutrition*. 1997. 17, 19–36.

Institute of Medicine. *Nutrition During Lactation*. Washington, DC: National Academy Press. 1991.

Medline Plus. U.S. Library of Medicine–National Institutes of Health. http://www.nlm.nih.gov/medlineplus/ency/article/002454.htm.

Mofidi, S. "Nutritional Management of Pediatric Food Hypersensitivity." *Pediatrics*. June 2003. 111(6), 1645–1653.

Sampson, H. A. "Managing Peanut Allergy." *BMJ*. Apr 27, 1996. 312(7038), 1050–1051.

Sicherer, S. H. "The Impact of Maternal Diets During Breastfeeding on the Prevention of Food Allergy." *Current Opinion in Allergy & Clinical Immunology*. 2002. 2(3), 207–210.

Whitney, E. N., & Rolfes, S. R. *Understanding Nutrition* (9th ed.). Wadsworth Group, Thomson Learning. United States. 2002.

http://www.lalecheleague.org/NB/NBMarApr04p44.html.

http://www.eatright.org.

http://www.womenshealth.gov/Breastfeeding/print-bf.cfm.

Table 1-6 Food Sources of Nutrients Needed in Increased Amounts During Lactation

Calcium: Milk; cheese; yogurt; fish with edible bones; tofu processed with calcium sulfate; bok choy; broccoli; kale; collard, mustard, and turnip greens; breads made with milk

Zinc: Meat, poultry, seafood, eggs, seeds, legumes, yogurt, whole grains (Bioavailability from this source is variable.)

Magnesium: Nuts, seeds, legumes, whole grains, green vegetables, scallops, and oysters (In general, this mineral is widely distributed in food rather than concentrated in a small number of foods.)

Vitamin B_6: Bananas, poultry, meat, fish, potatoes, sweet potatoes, spinach, prunes, watermelon, some legumes, fortified cereals, and nuts

Thiamin: Pork, fish, whole grains, organ meats, legumes, corn, peas, seeds, nuts, fortified cereal grains (widely distributed in foods)

Folate: Leafy vegetables, fruit, liver, green beans, fortified cereals, legumes, and whole-grain cereals

Table 1-7 Food Guide for Lactating Women

Nutrient-Rich Food Group	Servings Needed	What Equals a Serving
Milk and high-calcium foods	Adult pregnancy: 3–4 servings (low fat is best) Teen pregnancy: 4–5 servings (low fat is best) Lactation: 4–5 servings (low fat is best)	• 1 cup milk or yogurt • 2 cups cottage cheese • 1½ oz cheese • 1 cup fortified soy beverage • 1½ cups ice cream • 1 cup calcium-fortified fruit juice
Protein foods	2–3 servings (lean is best)	• 3 oz cooked meat, fish, or poultry • 2 eggs • 1 cup cooked beans • 4 Tbsp peanut butter
Breads and grains	6 or more servings (whole grains are best)	• One slice bread (1 oz) • One small tortilla • ½ cup cooked cereal • ¾–1 cup cold cereal • ½ cup cooked pasta • ⅓ cup cooked rice • ½ English muffin • ½ small bagel
Fruits and vegetables	5 or more servings (fresh is best)	• 1 cup raw fruit or vegetables • ½ cup cooked vegetables • 1 medium piece fresh fruit • 1 cup green salad • ¼ cup dried fruit • ½ cup fruit juice • ⅛ avocado
Fats and oils	2–3 servings (unsaturated is best)	• 1 tsp vegetable oil (olive or canola oils are best) • 1 tsp mayonnaise • 6 almonds (¼ oz nuts) • 1 Tbsp sunflower seeds

Vegetarian Diet

Author: Janet L. Washington, MPH, RD, LDN

The following list will assist the dietitian in understanding the different types of vegetarian diets that patients may wish to maintain.

Problem	*Do's and Don'ts*
Vegetarian	**Do:** Ask what foods are consumed and what foods are avoided. Clarify the interpretation or application of the vegetarian definition. Typically, vegetarians avoid meat, poultry, and fish. Self-described "almost" vegetarians occasionally include meat, fish, or poultry. Patients can follow restrictions at home and allow food intake variations in the work site or in a social setting. Inform patient of successfully developed meal plans for modified diets (that is, renal, diabetes, weight management, etc.) and athletic programs. Encourage variety. Vegetarian meal plans tend to be high in fiber, potassium, folate, vitamin C, vitamin E, and phytochemicals. Encourage meal planning ahead of time and stock the pantry with quick-fix foods that will aid in varied and nutritious vegetarian meals.
Vegan	**Do:** Clarify the interpretation or application of the vegan definition. Typically, vegans avoid animal products (for example, dairy, eggs, casein, whey, and honey), and some vegans can avoid refined sugar because of the bone-char-filter processing. Include a variety of grains, legumes, vegetables, nuts, and seeds. Snack suggestions: • Scrambled tofu • Rye bread toast with fruit spread • Fresh fruit • Leftover pasta and vegetables • Bean chili with vegetables Encourage women's calcium intakes to meet the recommendations of at least 1000 mg of calcium per day. See the calcium section in the appendix on pages 450–451.

Problem	*Do's and Don'ts*
	Assess calories and calcium intake to promote birth outcomes similar to the nonvegetarian population. Check the daily supplements of B_{12} (or reliable source) and vitamin D.
Lacto-ovo	**Do:** Clarify the interpretation or application of the vegetarian definition. Typically, lacto-ovo vegetarians avoid animal products (for example, meat, poultry, and fish). Include a variety of grains, legumes, vegetables, nuts, seeds, dairy, and eggs. Snack suggestions: • Cereal with low-fat milk • Whole-wheat toast with fruit spread • Fruit • Vegetable sticks • Veggie burger • Small bean burrito • Macaroni and cheese Assess pregnant women for sufficient calories to promote birth outcomes similar to nonvegetarian population. **Don't:** Don't overdo whole-fat dairy and eggs because they may contribute to a higher fat intake.
Macrobiotic	**Do:** Clarify the interpretation or application of the vegetarian definition. Typically, the macrobiotic vegetarian avoids animal products, dairy products, eggs, nightshade vegetables (for example, potatoes, tomatoes, peppers, and eggplant), tropical fruits (for example, mango, papaya, banana, and coconut), processed sweeteners, and sometimes fish. Include a variety of grains, legumes, vegetables, sea vegetables, soy products (nuts, seeds, fruits to a lesser extent); consume some seafood. Snack suggestions: • Miso soup with vegetables • Oatmeal • Steamed vegetables Check the supplement of B_{12} and vitamin D. See calcium and vitamin D section in the appendix on pages 450–451.

Problem	*Do's and Don'ts*
Fruitarian	**Do:** Clarify the interpretation or application of the vegetarian definition. Typically, the fruitarian avoids animal products, grains, legumes, and many vegetables. Diet includes fruits, vegetables that are botanical fruits (for example, tomatoes, eggplant, peppers, avocado, and squash), nuts, and seeds. Check on supplement of B_{12} and vitamin D. See calcium and vitamin D section in the appendix on pages 450–451. Check diet adequacy because the diet may be low in protein, iron, zinc, and other nutrients. Snack suggestions: • Dried fruit and nuts • Nut mix • Sliced fruit • Steamed vegetables • Almond milk **Don't:** Don't allow fruitarian diets for infants and children, because it may be associated with growth delays.
Raw Foods	**Do:** Clarify the interpretation or application of the vegetarian definition. Typically, the raw foods diet does not contain animal products and cooked plant foods. This diet includes raw vegetables, fruits, nuts, seeds, sprouted grains, and sprouted beans. Some adherents can use raw dairy products. Snack suggestions: • Fresh fruit salad • Fruit and nut bars • Vegetable salads **Don't:** Don't allow a raw foods diet for infants and children.

	Nutritional Concepts
Benefits of vegetarian diets	Note that diet and lifestyle choices affect chronic diseases. Understand plant protein replacing animal protein results in lower cholesterol levels. Limit food choices that are high in saturated fat and trans-fatty acids. Vegetarians tend to have lower blood pressure and lower rates of hypertension.
Vitamin B_{12}	Select three servings per day. Vitamin B_{12}-fortified foods include some brands of cereal (Cheerios, Total, and Wheaties), meat analogues, soy milk, and nutritional yeast. Eggs and dairy products also have vitamin B_{12}. Patients following a vegan diet need B_{12}-fortified foods or vegan supplements. Lacto-ovo vegetarians eating dairy products and eggs occasionally may need B_{12}-fortified foods or supplements. Vegetables are not a reliable source of B_{12}. Popular literature can offer sources of B_{12}—including tempeh, sea vegetables, etc. These may interfere with absorption and do not meet vitamin B_{12} needs. B_{12} deficiency is sometimes irreversible. Chewing vitamin B_{12} supplements increases absorption. The pharmacist is a resource to recommend a vegan supplement. Companies clearly label vegan supplements.
Vegetarian sources of protein	Eat a variety of plant foods daily, including soy foods, grains, legumes, and nuts. Relax about protein needs. Special combinations of protein foods are not required at each meal. Conscious combining of foods at meals is not necessary. Adding protein powder is not a requirement of a healthy vegetarian diet.
Calcium and vitamin D	Vegetarians who use dairy products have calcium intake similar to the general population. Nondairy calcium sources include greens like kale and collards, broccoli, calcium-set tofu, and calcium-fortified foods, including orange juice, soy/rice milks, and breakfast cereals.

	Nutritional Concepts
Calcium and vitamin D	Patients may need calcium supplements. The pharmacist will recommend which calcium salt is best absorbed. Age, medications, and health conditions may change the supplement recommended. Spread calcium supplements over the day. Vitamin D sources include fortified soy/rice milks, fortified cow's milk, and fortified breakfast cereal. Sunlight exposure promotes vitamin D production (10 minutes a day).
Fats	Linoleic acid (LA) and alpha-linoleic acid (ALA) are essential fatty acids. Soybeans, whole grains, nuts, and vegetable oils have LA. Flaxseed, walnuts, soybeans, and soybean/canola oils have ALA. Seeds and nuts are a healthy alternative to foods that contain trans-fatty acids. Vegetarian diets are not necessarily low in fat. Avoid restricting fat in infant meal plans.
Iron	Good sources of iron include whole grains, fortified cereals, dried beans, and soy products. Continue use of iron-fortified infant cereals through the infant's first year. Vitamin C is abundant in vegetarian diets. Include vitamin C sources (for example, orange juice, tomato, or peppers) at every meal to increase iron absorption of nonheme iron by reducing dietary ferric iron to ferrous iron. The incidence of iron deficiency anemia is similar among vegetarians and nonvegetarians.
Decreased appetite	Offer small portions of nutrient-rich foods: • Soy smoothie with fruit • Hot cereal with dried fruit • Peanut butter noodles • Whole-grain bread with nut butters • Soy milkshakes
Teenagers and eating disorders	All children (except infants) can follow a vegetarian diet and remain healthy as long as parents/caregivers are aware of good sources of calcium, iron, zinc, omega-3 fatty acids, and vitamins D and B_{12}. Consider referring to an RD who specializes in eating disorders.

Nutritional Concepts

Vegetarian meal choices do not predict eating disorders. Eaters with a disorder may disguise their change in eating behavior by this initial restriction.

Sources

Mangels, A. R., Messina, V., & Melina, V. "Position of the American Dietetic Association and Dietitians of Canada: Vegetarian Diets." *J Am Diet Assoc*. 2003. 103, 748–765.

Messina, V., Mangels, R., & Messina, M. *The Dietitian's Guide to Vegetarian Diets*. (2nd ed.). Jones and Bartlett Publishers. 2004.

Vegetarian Nutrition. A Dietetic Practice Group of the American Dietetic Association (ADA). http://www.vegetariannutrition.net.

Realities concerning vegetarian diets. Seventh-Day Adventist Dietetic Association. http://www.sdada.org.

Vegetarian Resource Group. http://www.vrg.org.

Sports Nutrition

Author: Debra Wein, MS, RD, LDN, ACSM-HFI, NSCA-CPT

This section provides the dietitian with guidelines for energy, protein, carbohydrate, fat, and fluid needs of those participating in sports.

Problem	*Do's and Don'ts*
Energy/Calories	**Do:** Supply the appropriate amount of calories: • Active women: 2500–4000 calories per day • Active men: 3000–6000 calories per day • Less active women (ages 18–35): 1800–2100 calories per day • Less active men (ages 18–35): 2200–2500 calories per day **Don't:** Don't undersupply energy that also provides vital nutrients for athletes. The energy requirements may be even higher during growth, and there is a slight decrease with advancing age. Certain activities require a larger energy intake during competition or intense training.
Protein	**Do:** Recommend adults consume 10–35% of their calories from protein per the Institute of Medicine. Functions of proteins: • Structural component of cells • Contractile apparatus in muscles • Catalyst (enzymes) for reactions • Precursors for hormone synthesis Protein needs of various athletes/lifestyles: • Sedentary adults: 0.8 g per kg of body weight (0.4 g per lb) • Recreational exerciser, adult: 1.0–1.5 g per kg of body weight (0.5–0.75 g per lb) • Competitive athlete: 1.2–1.8 g per kg of body weight (0.6–0.9 g per lb) • Growing teenage athlete: 1.8–2.0 g per kg of body weight (0.9–1.0 g per lb) • Adult building muscle mass: 1.4–1.8 g per kg of body weight (0.7–0.9 g per lb) • Athlete restricting calories: 1.4–2.0 g per kg of body weight (0.7–1.0 g per lb) • Maximum usable amount for adults: 2.0 g per kg of body weight (1.0 g per lb) **Don't:** Don't use protein as an energy source.

Problem	Do's and Don'ts
	Don't forget that all foods carry some micronutrients (see appendix on pages 396–397) that are especially needed by athletes.
Carbohydrates/ Glycemic Index (GI)	**Do:** Recommend adults consume 45–65% of their calories from carbohydrates per the Institute of Medicine. The role of carbohydrates before exercise is to: • Prevent low blood sugar before exercise. • Provide fuel by topping off muscle glycogen stores. • Settle the stomach, absorb gastric juices, and prevent hunger. • Instill confidence in the athlete's ability. Carbohydrate (CHO) recommendations surrounding exercise: • Choose low GI foods before activity and high GI foods afterward (see appendix on page 375 for list). • Choose 1 g of CHO per kg of body weight, 1 hour prior to exercise. • Choose 2 g of CHO per kg of body weight, 2 hours prior to exercise. • Choose 3 g of CHO per kg of body weight, 3 hours prior to exercise. • Choose 4 g of CHO per kg of body weight, 4 hours prior to exercise. • For fast recovery after a hard workout or competition, eat 1.0–1.2 grams of carbohydrates per kg body weight (0.45–0.55 g per lb) each hour for the first 4 hours of recovery. **Don't:** Don't ignore the need of carbohydrates in sport performance and recovery. Don't forget that all foods carry some micronutrients (see appendix on page 396) that are especially needed by athletes.
Fat	**Do:** Recommend that adults should consume 20% to 35% of their calories from fat per the Institute of Medicine. Type of fat and recommendation: • Monounsaturated: Up to 20% (olive, sesame, and canola oils) • Polyunsaturated: Up to 10% (safflower, sunflower, corn, and cottonseed oils)

Problem	*Do's and Don'ts*
Fat	• Saturated: Less than 7% (animal fat sources) • Trans fat: Less than 1% (read labels to see trans fat content) • Cholesterol: Less than 300 mg **Don't:** Don't conclude that athletic performance means a free pass to the consumption of dietary fat. Don't forget that all foods carry some micronutrients (see appendix on pages 396–397) that are especially needed by athletes.
Hydration	**Do:** Provide adequate fluid support needed in the sport. Requirements: • Men: 3.7 liters (125 oz) • Women: 2.7 liters (90 oz) Drinking fluids should account for about 80% of hydration needs, while foods account for about 20% of these requirements. However, some individuals, and athletes in particular, may have higher than average fluid and electrolyte needs. Guidelines: • 2 hours before exercise: 500 ml (about 17 oz) • During exercise: Start drinking early and at regular intervals Consume fluids at a rate sufficient to replace all the water lost through sweating (that is, body-weight loss), or consume the maximal amount that can be tolerated. Exercise lasting longer than 1 hour: • Ingest carbohydrates at a rate of 30–60 g per hour. • Drink 600–1200 ml per hour of solutions containing 4–8% carbohydrates. The carbohydrates can be sugars (glucose or sucrose) or starch (for example, maltodextrin). See Table 1-8 on page 68. • Beverage should contain sodium (0.5–0.7 grams per liter of water) to enhance palatability, promote fluid retention, and possibly prevent hyponatremia. See Table 1-9 on page 69. After exercise: Include carbohydrates and/or electrolytes in the fluid replacement solution. Exercise lasting less than 1 hour: There is little evidence of performance enhancement between consuming a carbohydrate-electrolyte drink and plain water. Temperature: Ingest fluids cooler than ambient temperature between 15°–22°C (59°–72°F).

Problem	*Do's and Don'ts*
	After exercise: For each pound of body weight lost, drink 20 oz. of water. To ensure optimal hydration: • Hydrate daily with adequate fluids. • Monitor morning weight to check on overall hydration status. • Monitor the color of your urine to check on hydration status. Light color urine is a gross indicator of adequate hydration. Dark urine indicates dehydration. • Weigh before and after exercise to determine fluid losses during training. **Don't:** Don't ignore the critical nature of providing the appropriate fluids, electrolytes, and carbohydrates in intense sports.
Preventing the Female Athlete Triad	**Do:** Suggest these guidelines by the American Dietetic Association for preventing the female triad in the Team Prevention Strategies of 1994. • Separate food- and weight-related behaviors from feelings and psychological issues. Appreciating the difference can help the athlete to learn to separate facts and move toward a better understanding of how to get better. • Teach the connection between food intake and health and the requirement of nutrients in food for the optimal functioning of women's bodies. • Incorporate education with behavior changes. For example, teach the need for nutrients and energy before suggesting an increase in caloric intake. • Work on small changes rather than making gross alterations in the athlete's lifestyle. Discourage the athlete from wanting to change everything at once. Small changes are more likely to be adapted and maintained. • Explain that setbacks are normal and can be used as learning tools to sculpt responses to cures. • Teach self-monitoring techniques, such as a food diary and behavior record, so the individual can feel a sense of control over her treatment and choices. Include in the diary food, exercise, and behaviors, such as frequent binging and/or purging as well as weight gain/fluctuation. • Use weight and eating contracts, but avoid using these techniques if the individual becomes too overly involved because it may be counterproductive.

Problem	*Do's and Don'ts*
Preventing the Female Athlete Triad	• Slowly increase weight to prevent feelings of a loss of control and potentially cause her to withdraw from therapy. • Encourage regular meal times, variety/moderation of intake, and gradual reintroduction of foods. The best received foods are typically those most recently excluded from the diet. **Don't:** Don't forget to maintain a weight that is healthy. Teaching the athlete this is very important.

Sources

American College of Sports Medicine. "Position stand on exercise and fluid replacement." *Med Sci Sports Exerc.* 1996. 28, i–vii.

American College of Sports Medicine, American Dietetic Association, Dieticians of Canada. "Nutrition and Athletic Performance." *Med Sci Sports Exerc.* 2000. 32, 2130–2145.

Bjorck, I., & Elmstahl, H. L. "The Glycemic Index: Importance of Dietary Fiber and Other Food Properties." *Proc Nutr Soc.* 2003 Feb. 62(1), 201–206.

Burke, L. M., Slater, G., Broad, E. M., Haukka, J., Modulon, S., & Hopkins, W. G. "Eating Patterns and Meal Frequency of Elite Australian Athletes." *Int J Sport Nutr Exerc Metab.* 2003 Dec. 13(4), 521–538.

Coyle, E. "Fluid and Fuel Intake During Exercise." *J Sports Sci.* 2004 Jan. 22(1), 39–55.

Deutz, R. C., Benardot, D., Martin, D. E., & Cody, M. M. "Relationship Between Energy Deficits and Body Composition in Elite Female Gymnasts and Runners." *Med Sci Sports Exerc.* 2000 Mar. 32(3), 659–668.

Food and Nutrition Board, Institute of Medicine. *Dietary Reference Intakes for Water, Potassium, Sodium, Chloride, and Sulfate.* Washington, DC: National Academies Press. 2004. http://www.nap.edu.

Hargreaves, M., Hawley, J., & Jeukendrup, A. "Pre-Exercise Carbohydrate and Fat Ingestion: Effects on Metabolism and Performance." *J Sports Sci.* 2004 Jan. 22(1), 31–38.

Hargreaves, M. "Pre-Exercise Nutritional Strategies: Effects on Metabolism and Performance." *Can J Appl Physiol.* 2001. 26 Suppl, S64–S70.

Hawley, J. A., & Burke, L. M. "Effect of Meal Frequency and Timing on Physical Performance." *Br J Nutr.* 1997 Apr. 77 Suppl 1, S91–S103.

Jebb, S. A., Prentice, A. M., Goldberg, G. R., Murgatroyd, P. R., Black, A. E., & Coward W. A. "Changes in Macronutrient Balance During Over- and

Underfeeding Assessed by 12-d Continuous Whole-Body Calorimetry." *Am J Clin Nutr.* 1996 Sep. 64(3), 259–266.

Jentjens, R. L., Cale, C., Gutch, C., & Jeukendrup, A. E. "Effects of Pre-Exercise Ingestion of Differing Amounts of Carbohydrate on Subsequent Metabolism and Cycling Performance." *Eur J Appl Physiol.* 2003 Jan. 88(4–5), 444–452.

Jeukendrup, A. E., Jentjens, R. L., & Moseley, L. "Nutritional Considerations in Triathlon." *Sports Med.* 2005. 35(2), 163–181.

Koopman, R., et al. "The Combined Ingestion of Protein and Free Leucine With Carbohydrate Increases Post Exercise Muscle Protein Synthesis in Vivo in Male Subjects." *Am J Physiol Endocrinol Metab.* Nov 23 2004.

Lambert, C. P., Frank, L. L., & Evans, W. J. "Macronutrient Considerations for the Sport of Bodybuilding." *Sports Med.* 2004. 34(5), 317–327.

Lemon, P. W. R. "Effects of exercise on dietary protein requirements." *International Journal of Sport Nutrition.* 1998. 8, 426–447.

Myszkewyez, L., & Koutedakis, Y. "Injuries, Amenorrhea, and Osteoporosis in Active Athletes: An Overview." *J Dance Med Sci.* 1998. 2, 88–94.

Rosenbloom, C. *Sports Nutrition, A Guide for the Professional Working with Active People* (3rd ed.). Chicago, IL: The American Dietetic Association. 2000.

Rosenbloom, C. "Why Don't Athletes Drink Enough During Exercise, and What Can Be Done About It?" *J Sports Sci Exchange.* 2001. 12.

Sahyoun, N. R., et al. "Dietary Glycemic Index and Load, Measures of Glucose Metabolism, and Body Fat Distribution in Older Adults." *Am J Clin Nutr.* 2005 Sep. 82(3), 547–552.

Sands, R., Tricker, J., Sherman, C., Armatas, C., & Maschette, W. "Disordered Eating Patterns, Body Image, Self-Esteem, and Physical Activity in Preadolescent School Children." *Int J Eat Disord.* 1997. 21, 159–166.

Shisslak, C. M., et al. "Potential Risk Factors Associated with Weight Control Behaviors in Elementary and Middle School Girls." *J Psychosom Res.* 1998. 44, 301–313.

Stevenson, E., Williams, C., & Biscoe, H. "The Metabolic Responses to High Carbohydrate Meals with Different Glycemic Indices Consumed During Recovery From Prolonged Strenuous Exercise." *Int J Sport Nutr Exerc Metab.* 2005 Jun. 15(3), 291–307.

Volek, J. S. "Influence of Nutrition on Responses to Resistance Training." *Med Sci Sports Exerc.* 2004 Apr. 36(4), 689–696.

Volek, J. S., Vanheest, J. L., & Forsythe, C. E. "Diet and Exercise for Weight Loss: A Review of Current Issues." *Sports Med.* 2005. 35(1), 1–9.

Table 1-8 How to Determine Carbohydrate Content in a Beverage

	Fluids Conversion: 12 oz = 355 ml
Sports drinks	14–16 g CHO/8 oz serving $\frac{14 \text{ grams}}{236 \text{ ml}} \times 100 = {\sim}6\%$ CHO
Fruit juices	$\frac{35\text{–}42 \text{ grams}}{355 \text{ ml}}$/ 12 oz serving = 10–12 % CHO

Table 1-9 Nutrient Breakdown of Selected Sport Drinks

Product (8 oz)	Calories	Carbohydrates (g)	Carbohydrate Concentration	Sodium (mg)	Potassium (mg)
Gatorade	50	14	6%	110	30
Powerade	70	19	8%	55	30
All Sport	70	20	8–9%	80	50
Accelerade	105	19.5	8%	142.5	43
Cytomax	50	10	4%	50	55
GU2O	50	13	6%	120	35
Shaklee Performance	100	25	10%	115	50
Amino	35	8	7%	10	35
Ultima Replenisher	20	5	2%	25	150
Extran Thirstquencher	45	11	5%	61	50

SECTION 2

Adult Nutrition

Chronic Nutrition Care Problems

Alzheimer's Disease 72
Cardiovascular Disease (CVD) 77
Cerebrovascular Accident (CVA) or Stroke 80
Chronic Obstructive Pulmonary Disease (COPD) 83
Congestive Heart Failure (CHF) 86
Decubitus Ulcers 88
Dehydration 90
Adults with Diabetes 92
Eating Disorders 114
Dysphagia 119
Human Immunodeficiency Virus (HIV) and Acquired Immunodeficiency Syndrome (AIDS) 122
Malnutrition 127
Antianxiety Agents 130
ADHD Medications 132
Antidepressant Medications 134
Common Issues with Mood Stabilizing Agents 138
Antipsychotic Drugs and Diet Interaction 141
Chronic Renal Insufficiency 144
End Stage Renal Disease with Dialysis 150
Weight Management 158

Alzheimer's Disease

Author: Mary Rowan Harrity, MS, RD

This list will assist the dietitian in addressing nutritional issues for patients with Alzheimer's disease or related dementias. Common concerns include distraction at mealtimes, chewing and swallowing problems, failure to recognize food or utensils, and weight loss.

Problem	*Do's and Don'ts*
Distractions	**Do:** Evaluate dining situations. If dining with others, seat the person in a quiet part of the dining area. Consider whether tablemates would be helpful or not, and if so, choose carefully. A smaller group may be helpful. Maintain supervision, and redirect to the table if the person gets up and wanders away. Offer smaller, frequent feedings to offset the short attention span. Include high–nutrient-density foods. When serving dinner in courses, offer only one food item at a time. Change any environmental factors that cause distractions. Consider the following: • Reduce noise level if possible. • Try playing soft music. • Turn off the TV. • Limit overhead pages, if any. • Ensure the temperature is properly controlled. • Offer meals at regular times. • Use solid colored plates and tablecloths to minimize visual clutter. Color contrast may be helpful for the visually impaired. • Use color to distinguish between the plate and tablecloth or placemat. • Try warm reds and oranges to increase appetite. **Don't:** Don't isolate the individual more than necessary. Don't let background noise interfere with a calm dining experience. Don't use patterned plates, tablecloths, and placemats that may confuse and distract the person.

Problem	Do's and Don'ts
Failure to Effectively Use Eating Utensils	**Do:**
	Consider whether occupational therapy may be helpful.
	Provide lip or high-wall plates to prevent excess spillage, and built-up or weighted utensils may compensate for tremors.
	Substitute bowls for plates. Set bowls or plates on a nonskid surface (a cloth, towel, or nonskid mat).
	Use straws or cups with lids for drinking.
	Consider a finger-food regimen (for example, sandwiches, bite-sized pieces of vegetables and fruit, bread and rolls, cookies for dessert, or ice cream cones to hold softer desserts) for minimal or little use of utensils.
	Serve soup and cereal in mugs with handles.
	Puree vegetables, and thin with warm milk to make a cream soup with a full serving of vegetables.
	Offer simple, clear instructions. Cue the patient to put food on the fork, and raise it to the mouth. Assist if needed. Putting your hand over the person's hand on the utensils, then lifting it to his or her mouth may "model" the process and get the patient started eating on his or her own. Be patient, noncritical, and repeat if necessary. Allow plenty of time.
	Encourage good posture, sitting straight with the head slightly forward.
	Know the Heimlich maneuver. See appendix on page 379.
	Check the mouth after meals and snacks to be sure the patient swallowed all food. Food left in the mouth can cause choking later on.
	Don't:
	Don't resort to feeding patients if they are able to feed themselves adequately with appropriate modifications.
	Don't forget that the head should not be tilted backward.
Swallowing Difficulty	**Do:**
	Involve speech therapy.
	Modified textures of some foods and beverages may help to prevent choking or aspiration. Foods may need to be ground or pureed; thicken liquids if needed.
	Ask a pharmacist to review medications that might affect the swallow process; possibly reduce or omit some medications.
	Patients may need a meal supervision regimen. Discuss with the PMD.

Problem	*Do's and Don'ts*
Swallowing Difficulty	**Don't:** Don't reduce the amount of food or fluids offered. Malnutrition and dehydration would become bigger risks. Don't make any medication changes without consulting the PMD.
Reduced Appetite	**Do:** Monitor which foods are best accepted, and try to provide these more often. If sweets are preferred, consider serving extra sugar, jam, jelly, honey, or syrup with all meals, even those not usually associated with these sweeteners. Many taste buds may be less effective, but the preference for sweets often outlasts other tastes. Note which meal of the day is best accepted, which foods the patient selects, and which he/she refused. This may help to identify patterns for planning future meals. Involve a pharmacist in reviewing medications. Many medications may have an impact on appetite, both favorable and unfavorable. Some medications used in Alzheimer's care may cause nausea unless given with food. Offer smaller, more frequent feedings to avoid overwhelming the individual with large quantities at any one time and to maximize the opportunity for nutrient intake. Keep healthy snacks on hand and in sight to entice the appetite. Consider using concentrated nutritional supplements or meal replacements. Use fortified foods with meals to maximize nutrient density, and take advantage of preferences for sweet tastes. These may include cereals, soups, puddings, or casseroles with added milk powder, cream, sugar, and other calorie sources. Keep dietary restrictions to a minimum to allow more variety in the diet. Offer breakfast foods throughout the day if the person frequently asks about breakfast. These might include toast with peanut butter, cereal with milk, banana, juice, and eggs. **Don't:** Don't assume that long-term favorites will be well accepted. Often, the patient loses interest in old favorites, and different foods are better accepted. Don't recommend excess medication, which may cause adverse side effects.

Problem	*Do's and Don'ts*
Variety of Foods	**Do:** Try to ensure a variety of foods to provide all essential nutrients. Folic acid, vitamins B_6 and B_{12}, calcium, and protein are important in preventing cognitive decline, maintaining heart health, preventing fractures, and maintaining skin integrity and immune competence. If the diet does not include a good variety of foods, including milk, fruits, and vegetables, check with the PMD about a balanced multivitamin, calcium supplements, or calorie and protein supplements. **Don't:** Don't start a supplement without checking for food/drug interactions.
Depression	**Do:** Advise the patient that depression is common in elderly individuals, including those with memory loss. This is especially true in those who are aware of their condition. Treatment of depression may improve appetite, and some antidepressants may have appetite-stimulating effects. **Don't:** Don't encourage use of antidepressants that can reduce appetite.
Constipation	**Do:** Advise the patient that constipation can result from reduced activity, medications, or a low-fiber diet. It may cause a sense of fullness, further reducing appetite. Encourage high-fiber foods, like whole grain breads and cereals, fruit and vegetables (fresh, if possible), and plenty of fluids. Prune juice may be helpful. Recommend laxatives if dietary adjustments are not enough or are not feasible. Encourage activity when possible. Increases in activity may help with bowel function. **Don't:** Don't forget that complaints of being "full" may signal constipation. Don't underestimate the risk of falls.
Dehydration	**Do:** Remind the person to drink all fluids at meals, and give extra fluids with medications. The sense of thirst may not

Problem	*Do's and Don'ts*
Dehydration	be as acute as it once was in the elderly, and someone with dementia may not recognize the need to drink fluids. Encourage between-meal fluids. Ensure that those fluids the individual likes best are available. **Don't:** Don't allow alcoholic beverages and excess caffeine (but it need not be withdrawn if caffeinated beverages are favorites). The sense of thirst will not be a reliable indicator of need to drink.
Preventing New Problems	**Do:** Avoid temperature extremes. The person may not be able to tell if the food or beverage is too hot or too cold. Avoid highly salted foods or sweets if the person has hypertension or diabetes. Monitor food intake. In the event that the person is often hungry, weight gain could be a problem. Serve smaller portions, with healthy snacks. Maintain good oral hygiene. Use oral swabs if a toothbrush is too difficult. Continue regular dental visits. **Don't:** Don't overly restrict the person who has little interest in food.

Sources

Alzheimer's Association. (2004). *About Eating*. Fact Sheet. ED247ZH.

American Dietetic Association. "Liberalized Diets for Older Adults in Long-term Care." *Journal of the American Dietetic Association*. 2002. 102, 1316–1323.

———. "Nutrition, Aging, and the Continuum of Care." *Journal of the American Dietetic Association*. 2000. 100, 580–595.

Changes and Challenges: Providing Alzheimer's Disease Care. Novartis. http://AlzheimersDisease.com.

Dunne, T., Cronin-Golomb, A., Neargarder, S., & Cipolloni, P. *Colored Cups, Plates Spur Food, Beverage Consumption in Advanced Alzheimer's Disease*. Boston University. http://EurekAlert.org.

Fisher Center for Alzheimer's Disease Research Foundation. *Treatment of Alzheimer's Disease*. http://www.alzinfo.org/treatment/maintaining/default.aspx.

Cardiovascular Disease (CVD)

Author: Donna Belcher, MS, RD, LDN

This list will assist the dietitian in answering nutrition questions and serve as a guide to assist patients who have CVD, also known as Coronary Artery Disease (CAD). The recommendations that follow are for patients who have had a myocardial infarction (MI) or have had coronary artery bypass grafting (CABG). Associated risk factors include hypertension (HTN), diabetes mellitus (DM), high cholesterol, excessive weight gain or obesity, smoking, and inactivity.

Nutrition therapy for CVD encourages use of healthful fats, replacing saturated and trans fat with monounsaturated fat wherever possible, as well as encouraging use of omega-3 fatty acids. It encourages use of whole grains, fruits, and vegetables to increase soluble and insoluble fiber intake. In addition, calories should be at a level intended to maintain or achieve appropriate weight.

To maintain artery health and prevent further progression of the disease, lifestyle changes are essential, and medication is often necessary. The goal is to keep the blood flowing freely through the arteries. The National Cholesterol Education Program's (NCEP) third Adult Treatment Panel (ATP III) and the Therapeutic Lifestyle Changes (TLC) address all the known factors affecting the process.

The indicated TLCs are as follows (ATP III, 2001):

- Consume less than 7% of calories from saturated fat per day and avoid trans-fatty acids.
- Consume less than 200 mg of cholesterol per day.
- Consume 25% to 35% of energy from fat, using up to 20% monounsaturated and 10% polyunsaturated fats, including omega-3 fatty acids.
- Consume 50% to 60% of other energy from carbohydrates and approximately 15% from protein.
- Consider increasing soluble fiber to 10–25 g per day and adding plant stanols/sterols (2 g per day).
- Energy intake should maintain desirable body weight or prevent weight gain.
- Include enough moderate exercise to expend at least 200 kcal per day.
- Sodium may be limited to 2400 mg for hypertension or to control edema.

SECTION 2

Problem	***Do's and Don'ts***
Decreased Appetite, Following CABG or MI	**Do:** Encourage intake and try to determine source/cause of diminished appetite (that is, nausea, constipation, weakness/fatigue, taste changes, depression).
Food Lists for TLC Guidelines (CAD, MI, s–p CABG)	**Do:** Choose 5–6 oz of lean meat, poultry, fish, and meat alternatives daily. Bake, broil, or grill meats.

Problem	*Do's and Don'ts*
Food Lists for TLC Guidelines (CAD, MI, s–p CABG)	Try to have fish twice a week. Remove the skin from chicken. Look for less than 3 g fat per ounce in lunch meat. Limit eggs to three yolks per week; use egg whites or low-fat egg substitutes more often if desired. Choose two to three servings of low-fat dairy products daily (for example, skim or 1% milk, low-fat or fat-free sour cream, yogurt, or frozen yogurt). Choose cottage cheese, ricotta, mozzarella, or low-fat cheeses. Choose three to five servings of fresh, frozen, or canned vegetables without added salt, fat, or sauce daily. Choose two to four servings of fresh or frozen fruit/fruit juice daily, dried fruit, or fruit canned in water or juice. Choose 6–11 servings of breads, cereals, rice, or pasta daily. Choose whole-grain and high-fiber products (low-fat crackers such as graham or animal crackers or products with no trans fat). Use 6–8 teaspoons of fat per day, choosing monounsaturated or polyunsaturated fats from the following: • Monounsaturated: Olive or peanut oils; avocados, almonds, cashews, peanuts, pecans, sesame seeds, and tahini • Polyunsaturated: Tub or squeeze margarine from oils, select brands with zero trans fats listed on the label (for example, canola, corn, safflower, sesame, sunflower), walnuts, and pumpkin and sunflower seeds **Don't:** Don't recommend fried or breaded versions of fish, shellfish, chicken, or veal patties/cutlets. Don't serve heavily marbled prime grades of beef/prime rib or fatty meat. Avoid bacon, sausage, hot dogs, and processed meats (that is, bologna, salami). Don't provide whole or 2% milk, regular yogurt, regular cheeses, ice cream, half and half, whipping cream, nondairy creamer, or sour cream. Don't fry vegetables or serve with added fat, sauce, cheese, or butter.

Problem	*Do's and Don'ts*
	Don't purchase fruit canned in heavy syrup. Don't serve fruit with cream.
	Don't serve fried fruit.
	Don't provide high-fat breads, such as croissants and biscuits, high-fat crackers, and commercially prepared pastries and desserts.
	Don't forget to avoid saturated fats and trans fats (for example, butter, lard, shortening, stick margarine, regular salad dressings).

Sources

American Dietetic Association. *American Dietetics Association Nutrition Care Manual*. Chicago, IL. http://www.eatright.org.

American Heart Association. http://www.americanheart.org.

TLC Diet. http://www.nhlbi.nih.gov/chd/lifestyles.htm.

National Institutes of Health. "Third Report of the National Cholesterol Education Program Expert Panel on Detection, Evaluation, and Treatment of High Blood Cholesterol in Adults" (Adult Treatment Panel III). *National Institutes of Health*. 2001. NIH Publication 01-3670.

NCEP. http://www.nhlbi.nih.gov/about/ncep/index.htm.

NHLBI (DASH Diet)."Facts About the DASH Eating Plan." *NIH Publication* No. 03-4082. May 2003. http://www.nhlbi.nih.gov/health/public/heart/hbp/dash/.

Cerebrovascular Accident (CVA) or Stroke

Author: Donna Belcher, MS, RD, LDN

This table will assist the dietitian in answering food tolerance questions and serve as a guide to assist patients who have had a stroke. Following a stroke, patients may have difficulty chewing or swallowing and may need assistance with their meals. Address high blood pressure, heart disease, and diabetes as risk factors for stroke.

Problem	*Do's and Don'ts*
Chewing or Swallowing Problems	**Do:** Obtain a speech therapy/occupational therapy evaluation. Monitor patient's tolerance and apply aspiration precautions. Thicken liquids to a nectar, honey, or pudding consistency as needed. Food thickeners (Thick It) or prethickened beverages are available—check with food services for availability. Recommend appropriate texture modification, as found in the National Dysphagia Diet. There are four defined diet levels: Level 1: Dysphagia pureed (pureed, homogenous, cohesive, puddinglike) Level 2: Dysphagia mechanically altered (cohesive, moist, semisolid; requires some chewing ability; ground or minced meats with fork-mashable fruits and vegetables; exclude most bread products, crackers, and other dry foods) Level 3: Dysphagia advanced (soft solids; requires more chewing ability; easy-to-cut meats, fruits, and vegetables; excludes hard crunchy fruits and vegetables, sticky foods, and very dry foods) Level 4: Regular (any solid textures) **Don't:** Don't feed before assessing ability to chew and swallow. Don't leave food with patient or family members if patient's tolerance has not been established.
Vision or Mobility Impairment	**Do:** Move the tray for the patient; there can be a field of vision issue where the patient cannot see part of his or her food tray. Use adaptive equipment (for example, weighted utensils, two-handled cups) as needed for the patient to feed him- or herself. Assist patient with meals and supervise feedings.

Problem	*Do's and Don'ts*
	Don't: Don't expect that patients will be able to open all containers and feed themselves. Assess their abilities first.
Decreased Appetite	**Do:** Encourage intake and try to determine source/cause of diminished appetite (that is, nausea, constipation, swallowing difficulty, taste changes, depression). Consider supplements (liquid or pudding), especially when giving medications. **Don't:** Don't assume that the patient requires a tube feeding.
Alternate Nutrition	**Do:** Assess feeding needs that are in the patient's best interest. If the patient is unable to swallow safely, tube feedings may be required. Adequate nutrition includes adequate feeding volume, as well as adequate hydration. Free-water flushes are necessary and may help to prevent clogged tubes when provided before and after medication administration. Check residuals and keep bed elevated according to your hospital standards for enteral feeding. See table on enteral feedings on pages 430–433. **Don't:** Don't forget ethics. Tube feedings are for the patient's nutrition, although we sometimes feed for the family's comfort. Don't crush a medication if there is a liquid form available for administration via tubes.
Food/Drug Interactions	**Do:** Be aware of the warfarin (Coumadin) and vitamin K interaction. Encourage consistent amounts of vitamin K foods (dark green leafy vegetables). Check prothrombin time (PTT) and international normalized ratio for clotting time (INR) regularly to keep in therapeutic range. **Don't:** Don't eliminate vitamin K-containing foods from the patient's diet (for example, broccoli, brussels sprouts, spinach, asparagus, lettuce, scallions, plums, turnips, and collard and beet greens).

Problem	*Do's and Don'ts*
Prevent Recurrence; Control Blood Pressure, Treat Heart Disease and Diabetes, if Present	**Do:**
	Consider recommending the DASH diet, which limits intake of sodium, saturated and trans fats, and cholesterol, increases intake of monounsaturated fats (olive/canola oils, avocados, nuts, and nut butters) and omega-3 fatty acids (salmon, tuna, walnuts, and flaxseeds), and fiber from grains, fruits, and vegetables.
	Choose whole grains, dried beans and peas, and lean protein foods, such as fish and poultry.
	Bake, broil, roast, steam, or boil foods to avoid frying.
	Monitor portion sizes of meats, 3–4 oz per serving.
	Limit alcohol intake to one drink per day because it may raise blood pressure.
	Don't:
	Don't allow salty foods, monosodium glutamate (MSG), or salted snack foods, pickles, or foods high in salt, such as sauerkraut. Don't add salt or salt seasonings.
	Don't serve canned foods (soups, vegetables, or meats).
	Don't serve other processed or packaged foods with more than 300 mg of sodium per serving.
	Don't provide high saturated fats (for example, bacon, sausage, salami, hot dogs, egg yolks, regular hamburger, butter, margarine, shortening, gravy, sauces, salad dressings, whole-fat milk and ice cream, and desserts high in fat and sugar).

Sources

American Dietetic Association Nutrition Care Manual. *National Dysphagia Diet: Standardization for Optimal Care.* Chicago, IL: American Dietetic Association. 2005.

American Stroke Association and American Heart Association. *Facts About the DASH Eating Plan*. NIH Publication No. 03-4082. May 2003. http://www.nhlbi.nih.gov/ health/public/heart/hbp/dash/.

National Cholesterol Education Program (NCEP). *USDA National Nutrient Database for Standard Reference*. 2005. http://www.nal.usda.gov/fnic/foodcomp/ Data/.

Chronic Obstructive Pulmonary Disease (COPD)

Author: Donna Belcher, MS, RD, LDN

This list will assist the dietitian in answering food tolerance questions and serve as a guide to assist patients who have COPD, emphysema, or chronic bronchitis. Smoking is the primary risk factor for COPD, and smoking cessation is crucial for prevention and halting its progression. Current treatment for COPD is limited to relieving symptoms. Weight loss usually occurs in those with severe COPD, mostly related to poor oral intake rather than changes in metabolism. Other associated comorbidities include cardiovascular disease (CVD), lung cancer, and sleep-disordered breathing.

Problem	*Do's and Don'ts*
Adequate Intake	**Do:**
	Eat first high-calorie, high-protein foods (for example, eggs, whole milk, custard, pudding, yogurt, ice cream, cheese, cream cheese, butter, mayonnaise, vegetable oils, peanut and other nut butters, granola and other energy bars). See cancer section on page 208.
	Offer foods that are easy to chew (that is, pudding, ice cream, meatloaf, eggs).
	Encourage slow eating and chewing, taking small bites while breathing, and resting between bites.
	Offer meal replacement supplements and more calorie-dense options for the smaller volume in addition to meals.
	Don't:
	Don't choose low-fat or low-calorie foods, unless otherwise indicated.
	Don't suggest consumption of nonnutritious beverages and foods (that is, soda, black coffee or tea, potato chips, candy, or other snack foods).
	Don't allow alcohol, which is of minimal nutritional value, can interact with medications, and can impair breathing and the ability to cough productively.
Maintain a Healthy Weight	**Do:**
	Monitor weight weekly, or even daily, if the patient has been prescribed diuretics or steroids. Patients with COPD expend up to 10 times more energy (calories) to breathe than someone with normal pulmonary musculature.
	Evaluate for depression, which can impair appetite.

Problem	*Do's and Don'ts*
Maintain a Healthy Weight	**Don't:** Don't forget that being overweight makes breathing more difficult because the heart and lungs work harder, and being underweight causes weakness and fatigue, which also hinders breathing.
Controlling Fluid Balance	**Do:** Restrict sodium/salt intake to prevent fluid retention. Use seasonings that do not contain salt or MSG. Choose foods with less than 300 mg of sodium per serving. See table in the appendix on page 461. Monitor potassium levels if the patient is on medications that are potassium losing, and encourage intake of potassium foods (that is, bananas, citrus, potatoes, and tomatoes). **Don't:** Don't add salt to foods or eat high sodium/salty foods. Don't avoid fluids where the patient becomes dehydrated because fluid overload also impairs breathing ability.
Abdominal Discomfort	**Do:** Be aware of how foods affect the patient. Distending/bloating can make breathing uncomfortable. Have the patient sit up to eat. Offer frequent small meals and snacks. Offer liquids at the end of meals. **Don't:** Don't offer gas-forming foods (for example, beans, peas, cabbage, cauliflower, broccoli, brussels sprouts, peppers, onions, apples, avocados, and melons; also, deep-fried, high-fat, and highly seasoned foods). Don't overeat, which can make breathing uncomfortable.
Oxygen Saturation	**Do:** Have air cannula on during meals if continuous oxygen is ordered. Digestion requires oxygen and energy. Clear airway within an hour of eating. **Don't:** Don't remove oxygen source because it is inconvenient.

Sources

Chronic Obstructive Pulmonary Disease (COPD) Data Fact Sheet. NIH Publication No. 03-5229.

Croxton, T. L., Weinmann, G. G., Senior, R. M., Wise, R. A., Crapo, J. D., & Buist A. S. "Clinical Research in Chronic Obstructive Pulmonary Disease: Needs and Opportunities, NHLBI Workshop Summary." *Am J Respir Crit Care Med.* 2003. 167, 1142–1149.

Ferreira, I. M., Brooks, D., Lacasse, Y., & Goldstein, R. S. "Nutritional Support for Individuals with COPD: A Meta-Analysis." *Chest.* 2000. 117, 672–678.

National Heart, Lung, and Blood Institute. US Department of Health and Human Services. National Institutes of Health. http://www.nhlbi.nih.gov/health/public/lung/.

Nutritional Guidelines for People with COPD. http://www.clevelandclinic.org/health/health-info/docs/2400/2411.asp?index=9451.

Congestive Heart Failure (CHF)

Author: Donna Belcher, MS, RD, LDN

This list will assist the dietitian in answering food tolerance questions and serve as a guide to assist patients who have CHF. Manage fluid retention needs to decrease workload on the heart and to maintain blood pressure. A 2–3 g sodium restriction usually accomplishes this and possibly a fluid restriction in a progressed disease.

Problem	***Do's and Don'ts***
Adequate Intake	**Do:** Monitor weights weekly, or even daily, if fluid balance has been an issue. Evaluate for depression, which can impair appetite. Have the patient sit up to eat. Offer frequent small meals and snacks. Drink allowable liquids at the end of meals. Offer foods that are easy to chew (that is, yogurt, meat loaf, and eggs). Encourage slow eating and chewing, taking small bites while breathing, and resting between bites. **Don't:** Don't forget that being overweight makes breathing more difficult because the heart and lungs work harder. Being underweight causes weakness and fatigue, which also hinders breathing.
Hyponatremia	**Do:** Restrict fluids to 1500 ml daily and restrict sodium to 2 g daily, as per the PMD's orders.
Control Fluid Balance	**Do:** Restrict sodium/salt intake to prevent fluid retention. Use seasonings that do not contain salt or MSG. Choose foods with less than 300 mg of sodium per serving. Monitor potassium levels if the patient is on potassium-losing medications, and encourage intake of potassium foods (that is, bananas, citrus, potatoes, tomatoes). **Don't:** Don't add salt to foods or eat high-sodium or salty foods. Don't avoid fluids where the patient becomes dehydrated because fluid overload also impairs breathing ability.

Problem	Do's and Don'ts
DASH Eating Plan for Maintenance at Home	**Do:** Reduce sodium in diet including fruits, vegetables, and whole grains. Limit fats consistent with TLC diet on the Cardiovascular Disease Table to lower blood cholesterol. This diet provides an eating pattern that is high in potassium, calcium, magnesium, and fiber, while limiting sodium to levels between 1500 mg–2400 mg per day. Types of foods included daily are as follows: • Seven to eight servings of whole grains • Four to five servings of fruits • Four to five servings of vegetables • Two to three servings of low-fat or fat-free dairy • Two or less servings of meat **Don't:** Don't allow alcohol, especially if this contributed to CHF. Otherwise, limit to one drink per day.

Sources

American Dietetics Association Nutrition Care Manual. 2005.

American Heart Association. http://www.americanheart.org.

National Institutes of Health. "Third Report of the National Cholesterol Education Program Expert Panel on Detection, Evaluation, and Treatment of High Blood Cholesterol in Adults (Adult Treatment Panel III)." NIH Publication 01-3670. 2001.

TLC Diet. http://www.nhlbi.nih.gov/chd/lifestyles.htm.

NCEP. http://www.nhlbi.nih.gov/about/ncep/index.htm.

National Institutes of Health. "Facts About the DASH Eating Plan." NIH Publication No. 03-4082. May 2003. http://www.nhlbi.nih.gov/health/public/heart/hbp/dash/.

Decubitus Ulcers

Author: Nicki O'Brien, MS, RD, LDN

A major concern of skin integrity is avoiding the development of pressure-related ulcers. The following information will assist in the healing of decubitus via nutritional interventions.

Problem	*Do's and Don'ts*
Decubitus	**Do:**
	Determine the stage of the decubitus. Request a serum albumin level should a recent level not be available.
	Review the patient's meal completion record. The degree or lack of meal completion will determine use of some interventions.
	Review the patient's weight status and history.
	Recalculate the patient's basal energy expenditure (BEE). Ascertain level of activity factor (bedfast/bedrest = 1.2, wheelchair/ambulatory = 1.3, active = 1.5).
	Calculate the protein needs based on the stage of the decubitus and the serum albumin level.* Depleted serum albumin may have higher protein needs.
	Ascertain daily fluid needs, using the following formula:
	Actual weight/kg multiplied by *(×)* fluid factor = ml fluids.
	(Fluid factors are: normal = 30 ml/kg, CHF = 25 ml/kg, UTI = 40 ml/kg.)
	Review medications the patient receives. If not already on a daily multivitamin, recommend it.
	Interview the patient for food preferences, especially for foods that are good sources of protein. If the patient enjoys eggs at breakfast, have them served at every breakfast. Should the patient drink milk at meals, increase the amount served. Suggest yogurt at meals or as a between-meal snack.
	Increase the protein portion at the patient's meals, such as cottage cheese with meals. Provide nutrient-dense foods that the patient already enjoys, or fortified Super Cereal, Super Pudding, Super Spuds, Super Muffins, and Super Soup. See recipes in the appendix on pages 459–460.
	Consider protein powder supplements if the patient does not agree to food adjustments.

Problem	*Do's and Don'ts*
	If the decubitus is staged a III or IV, include vitamin C (500 mg) and zinc (220 mg) every day with a PMD's order.
	Consider supplemental arginine, with PMD input.
	Assess the use of nutrient-dense supplements between meals.
	Don't:
	Don't overlook the stage of the skin.
	Don't ignore the expertise you can share.
	Don't forget there are medical conditions that will alter protein needs—renal disease, for example.
	Don't forget to interview the patient and/or family for food ideas.
	Don't use zinc for longer than 30 days because extended use may deplete copper and iron stores.

*To establish protein needs, determine the patient's ideal body weight (IBW) range, using the patient's height. Employ the following formula:
- For males, use 106 lbs for the first 60 inches of height, plus 6 lbs for each additional inch of height. If the patient's height is less than 60 inches, subtract 3 lbs for each inch less than 60 inches.
- For females, use 100 lbs for the first 60 inches of height plus 5 lbs for each additional inch of height. If the patient's height is less than 60 inches, subtract 2.5 lbs for each inch less than 60 inches.
- Convert pounds to kg (weight divided by 2.2). This will be the base protein needs in grams.

Take into account protein factors:
Normal = 0.8–1.0 per kg of body weight
Decubitus = 1.2–1.5 per kg of body weight
Fracture/surgery = 1.0–2.0 per kg of body weight
Burns/multiple fractures = 2.0–2.5 per kg of body weight

Sources

Thomas, D. R. *Nutrition and Chronic Wounds*. (2004). Prevention and treatment of pressure ulcers. *J Am Med Dir. Assoc*. 2006. 7(1), 46–59.

Fleishman, A. "Adult Wound Care." *Today's Dietitian*. 2005. 1, 39–41.

Initial Nutritional History–Assessment Form. (1992). Briggs Corporation.

New England Diet Manual for Extended Care. (2003). Boston, MA.

Dehydration

Author: Nicki O'Brien, MS, RD, LDN

Patients and the elderly population are more likely to have insufficient intake of fluids; the reasons for this include diminished sense of thirst, decreased ability to perform daily functions, and diminished cognition. The elderly sometimes self-limit fluid intake because of incontinence or to decrease trips to the bathroom. The following list will help the dietitian examine ways to increase the availability of fluids to patients at risk for dehydration and identify some symptoms of dehydration.

Problem	***Do's and Don'ts***
Dehydration	**Do:**
	Observe the patient for skin turgor, dry mouth, cracked lips, and if possible, color of urine.
	Determine the daily fluid needs of the patient, based on actual body weight. Convert weight in pounds to kg (weight divided by 2.2). Weight in kg × 30 ml = daily fluid needs under normal metabolic conditions.
	Place the patient on intake and output (I and O) for a prescribed length of time to ascertain an average daily intake.
	Compile a fact sheet for the staff that lists the volume of commonly used receptacles—juice glasses, mugs, coffee cups, and soup bowls—to aid in the calculation of the patient's daily fluid intake.
	Interview the patient and/or family members to identify favored fluids.
	Encourage family members and visitors to bring in favored fluids.
	Provide bedside water containers; encourage and/or assist the patient to drink.
	Refill the containers twice daily. Include a glass of water at all meals—be it in a dining room or on meal trays.
	Offer the patient a drink or encourage them to drink from the bedside water container each time a nursing assistant or nurse enters a patient's room. Assist the patient as necessary with drinks.
	Offer Popsicles or sherbet as snacks between meals. Offer season-appropriate fluids between meals—lemonade in warm weather or hot cocoa or hot cider in cool weather.

Problem	*Do's and Don'ts*
	Place a water fountain or water dispenser with cups provided in a patient gathering place or public place.
	Increase the amount of fluids offered during a medication pass; encourage the patient to complete the fluids given to them.
	Don't:
	Don't forget to remind family members to inform the nursing assistant or nurse of fluids consumed.
	Don't ignore possible use of straw or adaptive cup.
	Don't place cups where difficult to reach. Leave the drinks sitting next to the bed or on the tray table.
	Don't forget to check with the PMD for agreed upon fluid needs of the patient to confirm no underlying medical conditions, such as renal disease.

Sources

Initial Nutritional History–Assessment Form. Briggs Corporation. 1992.

Aucoin, J. W. *Nutrition and Hydration; Advance for Providers of Post-Acute Care*. 57–59. 2005.

New England Diet Manual for Extended Care. Boston, MA. 2003.

Adults with Diabetes

Authors: Natalie Egan, MS, RD, CDE, LDN;
Patrick Healy, MPH, CDE, RD, LDN

Persons with diabetes require a broad spectrum of care with regard to diet, exercise, and self blood-glucose monitoring. This chapter will assist the dietitian in guiding the patient toward healthy diet, exercise, and blood sugar goals in adults with Type 1 Diabetes and Type 2 Diabetes.

Note: Because of the complexity of managing diabetes and diet, please note that an RD and PMD should be involved in all areas of patient care.

Problems	***Do's and Don'ts***
Self Management Blood Sugar Testing	**Do:** Encourage the patient to check blood sugars as a means of evaluating glycemic control. Evaluate patient's ability and technique of using a glucose-monitoring machine. Recommend a testing schedule of three times per day for non–insulin-dependent patient: • Fasting • Before a meal • Two hours after that same meal (vary meal tested from day to day) Review blood sugar goals with patients. See table on page 113. Encourage Type 1 or insulin-dependent Type 2 patients to check blood sugars before and after each meal to determine meal effects on glycemic control. Evaluate glucometer prescribed and patient's needs, such as limited sight or neuropathy. Be sure glucometer prescribed is compatible with insurance coverage for strips. **Don't:** Don't provide a meter that does not meet patient needs. Don't provide a meter without reviewing its use with the patient. Don't forget to provide a concrete testing schedule.
Diet Therapy General	**Do:** Prescribe caloric restriction to achieve ideal body weight. Reinforce how different foods, amounts/types of foods, and timing of foods affect blood sugar.

Problem	*Do's and Don'ts*
	Prescribe macronutrient goals to help normalize blood glucose and lipid levels. • Consider degree of obesity and/or BMI. See the appendix on page 458. • Current lipid levels including HDL, LDL, and triglyceride • Presence of kidney disease • Presence of elevated blood pressure Reinforce the need for dietary follow-up visits to help individualize meal plans for lifestyle changes. Individualize diet therapy with stated and achievable goals. Educate patients on the benefits of a multidisciplinary program. Educate all patients in the following areas: • Diabetes disease process • Meal planning • Record keeping of blood sugars and dietary intake • Use of insulin and oral diabetes medications • Management for sick days • Management and prevention of hypoglycemia • Safe physical activity • Complications that may occur and preventions • Total health monitoring for patients with diabetes, including checking blood pressure, visiting professionals for eye and foot care, monitoring heart and kidney health Refer patient for multiple one-on-one follow-up visits. **Don't:** Don't prescribe generic meal plan without individualized calorie level. Don't neglect to take into account fat intake and sources of fat. Don't assume that one visit with the nutritionist will provide all the necessary information for diet and lifestyle changes. Don't end education attempts if patient refuses to attend classes.
Diet Therapy Treatment Goals for Type 1 Diabetes	**Do:** Strive for glycemic control near normal and avoid episodes of severe hypo- or hyperglycemia. Strive to delay onset of long-term complications related to poor blood sugar control.

SECTION 2

Problem	*Do's and Don'ts*
Diet Therapy Treatment Goals for Type 1 Diabetes	Teach carbohydrate counting. Determine carbohydrate to insulin ratio (CIR): • CIR = 2.8 × weight in lbs divided by total daily dose. • On the average, 1 u of insulin covers 7–25 gm of carbohydrate, but individualize as much as possible. Do aim for normal blood pressure control: • 130/80 mm/Hg BP goal. • Keep sodium intake to less than 3 gm per day. • Limit sodium intake to 2 gm per day or less if patient has neuropathy or hypertension. Aim for blood lipid control: • LDL should be below 100 mg/dl. • HDL should be above 40 mg/dl for men and 50 mg/dl for women. • Triglycerides should be less than 150 mg/dl. Maintain appropriate weight goal. Keep in mind that insulin given to manage blood sugars without taking into account calories and carbohydrate can encourage weight gain. **Don't:** Don't administer insulin without taking into account diet and eating habits. Don't provide a blanket meal plan without taking into consideration carbohydrate content and distribution. Don't provide patient with a fixed meal plan. Don't underestimate the importance of blood pressure monitoring and diet related to blood pressure control. Don't continually administer correction insulin without looking at the root cause of hyperglycemia. Don't forget to point out sources of sodium in the diet. See appendix on page 461.
Diet Therapy Treatment Goals for Type 2 Diabetes	**Do:** Encourage moderate weight loss to help reduce hyperglycemia, dyslipidemia, and hypertension. Inform the patient that weight control will likely improve blood sugar control and delay onset of complications. Aim for normal blood pressure control: • 130/80 mm/Hg BP goal. • Keep sodium intake to less than 3 gm per day.

Problem	*Do's and Don'ts*
	• Limit sodium intake to 2 gm per day or less if patient has neuropathy or hypertension. Aim for blood lipid control: • LDL should be below 100 mg/dl. • HDL should be above 40 mg/dl for men and 50 mg/dl for women. • Triglycerides should be less than 150 mg/dl. Maintain appropriate weight goal. Keep in mind that without appropriate caloric restriction, sulfonylureas and thiazolidinediones (TZDs) can minimize weight loss. Encourage moderate caloric restriction of 250–500 fewer calories per day. Reinforce not skipping meals and eating about the same amount at about the same time each day. Encourage patients to eat healthy foods. Reinforce the need to measure portions of foods. Encourage an increase in physical activity. Encourage client to enroll in a weight-loss program that encompasses behavior modification, exercise, and monitoring. **Don't** Don't inform patient that weight loss will cause diabetes to go away without looking at the cause, duration of diabetes, or glycemic control. Don't inadvertently discourage patient from taking medicine to avoid weight gain. Don't encourage patient to skip meals to lose weight. Rather, encourage consistent intake with smaller portions. Don't encourage patient to enroll in or subscribe to fad diets or diets that have unbalanced macronutrient distribution to facilitate weight loss.
Dietary Carbohydrate	**Do:** Instruct patient on sources of dietary carbohydrate in foods. See table on page 345. Differentiate between refined and higher-fiber carbohydrates. Include information on the glycemic index and carbohydrates or information about how rapidly carbohydrates affect your blood sugar. See appendix on page 375.

Problem	*Do's and Don'ts*
Dietary Carbohydrate	Base total carbohydrate intake on specified calorie level. Individually assess total calories from carbohydrates, though typically 40–50% is normal. Fiber intake should be 25–35 gm per day. Instruct on carbohydrate counting if patient is on insulin. **Don't:** Don't forget to point out healthier carbohydrate choices and the difference in refined and fiber-containing carbohydrates. Don't increase fiber intakes quickly. Consider increasing fiber slowly at 5 gm per week to prevent constipation. Don't forget to increase fluid intake along with fiber intake. Don't prescribe a blanket increase in fiber intake without reviewing past medical history for issues with gastrointestinal tract, such as diverticulitis, Crohn disease, or inflammatory bowel disease. See other tables.
Dietary Protein	**Do:** Protein should be 16–20% of total calories. Aim for 0.8 gm–1.0 gm per kilogram; use adjusted weight if patient is over 120% of ideal body weight. If patient has nephropathy, protein should be 0.8 gm per kg or less as assessed. **Don't:** Don't underestimate protein intake because it may have delayed effect on blood glucose.
Dietary Fat	**Do:** Encourage patients to use healthy fat in appropriate amounts for their meal plans. Choose monounsaturated (olive oil) and polyunsaturated fats (corn, safflower, canola oil). Avoid foods that have significant amounts of saturated fats (animal fats) and trans fats (read labels). Adhere to general fat intake guidelines at about 25–50 g per day, though individual assessment is key. Maintain normal blood lipid levels: • Percentage of fat is variable based on calorie needs. • Review lipid levels (HDL, LDL).

Problem	*Do's and Don'ts*
	• Study triglyceride levels and dietary intake. Prescribe individualized diet therapy based on results. • Keep less than 10% of fat calories from saturated fats. See appendix on page 281. • Try to avoid minimizing or eliminating trans-fat intake. • Keep cholesterol intake to less than 200 mg/dl per day if LDL is greater than 100 mg/dl.
	Don't: Don't assume that blanket reduction of fat intake will correct hyperlipidemia. Correlate the laboratory values with diet therapy. Don't forget to differentiate between different types of fat in the diet. Don't assume reduction in total fat intake will solve hypertriglyceridemia. Consider carbohydrate intake and blood sugar control as well.
High Blood Sugar Before Meal—Type 1 Diabetes	**Do:** Aim for good control of premeal blood sugars. • Premeal goal is between 70–130 mg/dl if the patient does not have a history of severe hypoglycemia. • If the patient has history of hypoglycemia and significant microvascular disease, premeal blood sugar goals are 80–160 mg/dl. Make sure patient is taking insulin. Evaluate if patient is properly mixing insulin doses or if bottles are being cross contaminated. Evaluate that patient's technique for administering insulin is appropriate. This will determine if underdosing of insulin is occurring or if site given is appropriate. Evaluate patient for changes in medical history, including sight or dexterity since last visit when prescribed insulin. Make adjustments as needed. Increase time between giving fast-acting insulin and starting the meal by 15–20 minutes with the PMD's approval. Determine correct dose of short- or rapid-acting insulin with PMD's approval. Add or subtract the correction dose to the planned dose of bolus insulin based on blood sugar before a meal. The correction dose is the number of points or mg/dl per one unit of fast-acting insulin will decrease the blood sugar.

Problem	*Do's and Don'ts*
High Blood Sugar Before Meal— Type 1 Diabetes	The correction is equal to: Actual blood sugar minus desired blood sugar (100 mg/dl), divided by correction factor (1700 = total daily dose of insulin). Take note of correction factors and TDD differences. Check with the PMD or CDE if 1700 is the correct number to use for this patient. Evaluate carbohydrate intake at prior meal and plan accordingly for next meal. Consider that protein intake may contribute to elevated blood sugar by causing a delayed effect. Therefore, evaluate portions of protein. Encourage 15–30 minutes of activity before or after the meal to potentiate insulin action if blood glucose levels are within safe ranges for exercise. **Don't:** Don't have the patient eat large meals; substitute smaller, more frequent meals and snacks. Don't randomly increase short-acting bolus insulin to lower blood sugar. Don't allow the patient to skip a meal and give full short-acting insulin dose to correct blood sugar. Don't assume patient is taking insulin appropriately. Don't assume patient technique is reliable; ask the patient to demonstrate insulin administration. Don't have the patient exercise if blood sugar levels are greater than 300 mg/dl or greater than 250 mg/dl and urine ketones are present. Don't change more than one variable at one time until effects of the change are better known.
High Blood Sugar Before Meal— Type 2 Diabetes	**Do:** Aim for good blood glucose control before a meal, 70–130 mg/dl. Evaluate meal or snack prior to blood glucose check for carbohydrate content and portion of protein. Consider that protein intake may contribute to elevated blood sugar by causing a delayed effect and evaluate portions of protein.

Problem	*Do's and Don'ts*
	Encourage 15–30 minutes of activity before or after the meal to potentiate insulin action if blood glucose levels are within safe ranges for exercise.
	Don't:
	Don't have the patient take an additional oral medication to control blood sugar.
	Don't have the patient skip a meal to control blood sugar.
Low Blood Sugar Before Meal—Type 1 Diabetes	**Do:**
	Aim for good blood sugar control. At premeal, consider less than 70 mg/dl a low blood sugar.
	Start the meal with a food high in carbohydrate because it is more quickly absorbed (that is, potato, rice, bread, pasta, 4 ounces of fruit juice, fruit).
	Take fast-acting insulin just before eating or just after starting the meal.
	Have food prepared before taking insulin.
	Allow a small increase in portion sizes.
	Correct low blood sugar first, based on the correction factor. (Example: The patient needs 15 gm carbohydrate to increase blood glucose by 50 mg/dl. Eat 15 gm of carbohydrate to correct blood sugar, and then proceed with the meal.)
	Encourage weight loss with a reduction of fast-acting insulin dose along with carbohydrate intake.
	Evaluate activity or meal prior to the low blood sugar for necessary changes.
	Evaluate the condition of the insulin, including storage area for appropriateness.
	Evaluate if patient is properly mixing insulin doses or if bottles are being cross contaminated.
	Evaluate whether patient's technique for administering insulin is appropriate. This will determine if underdosing of insulin is occurring or if site given is appropriate.
	Evaluate patient for changes in medical history, including sight or dexterity since prescribing insulin at last visit. Make adjustments as needed with the PMD's approval.
	Don't:
	Don't take insulin before the meal if blood glucose is too low.

Problem	*Do's and Don'ts*
Low Blood Sugar Before Meal—Type 1 Diabetes	Don't delay the meal without eating a snack if the blood glucose is too low. Don't overeat carbohydrates in an attempt to correct blood sugar. Don't correct low blood sugar with a fatty food or only protein because it may delay absorption and correction. Don't give insulin and then prepare a meal because cooking or preparation time may further decrease blood sugar. Don't assume the patient's technique is reliable. Ask the patient to demonstrate insulin administration. Don't assume the patient is storing the insulin appropriately.
Low Blood Sugar Before a Meal—Type 2 Diabetes	**Do:** Evaluate meal and activity intake prior to blood sugar check to determine if additional carbohydrate at the prior meal or snack between meals is necessary. Aim for proper blood sugar control. At premeal, consider less than 70 mg/dl a low blood sugar. Start the meal with a food high in more quickly absorbed carbohydrate (that is, potato, rice, bread, pasta, 4 ounces of fruit juice, fruit). Keep a food record to determine actual amounts of food eaten. Consider any changes in timing of medications that may have occurred. **Don't:** Don't have the patient overeat carbohydrates in an attempt to correct blood sugar. Don't avoid correcting low blood sugar with a fatty food or only protein because it may delay absorption and correction.
Elevated Postprandial Glucose (blood sugars over 180 mg/dl)	**Do:** Aim for proper blood sugar control following a meal. Postprandial blood sugar goals are between 140–180 mg/dl. Elevated blood sugars following a meal could indicate unbalanced carbohydrate intake with the medication taken. Evaluate blood sugar before the meal. Premeal hyperglycemia may be the cause of postprandial hyperglycemia and should have been corrected prior to the meal.

Problem	*Do's and Don'ts*
	Evaluate the meal plan for carbohydrate content. Consider that carbohydrate content of the meal may have been too high.
	Encourage the patient to keep a food record that includes: • Food and amount eaten • Time of meal • Grams of carbohydrates
	If carbohydrate content of meal was on target, including portions, consider reevaluation of meal plan.
	Suggest a 15–30 minute activity (walking) for the hypoglycemic effect.
	Remind the patient to increase the preprandial fast-acting insulin depending on the carbohydrate consumption.
	Consider using the CIR for meal-related bolus in patients using an insulin pump or those who have the ability to do so. Tailoring insulin requirements better meets the patient's needs.
	CIR = (2.8 × weight in pounds) divided by total daily dose of insulin (TDD).
	Example: A patient with a 1:15 CIR needs 1 unit of insulin to cover 15 gm of carbohydrate. Therefore, 45 gm of carbohydrate will require 3 units of insulin to cover.
	Introduce this equation only if the patient has the level of understanding of the disease process and medication interactions and with the PMD's approval.
	See table in the appendix on pages 394–395 for fast-acting insulin duration times.
	Don't:
	Don't forget to check postprandial blood sugars. These often contribute most to elevated hemoglobin A1c.
	Don't provide "coverage" with extra-fast-acting insulin for 3 hours or until before next meal because this could lead to hypoglycemia.
	Don't use correction factor without considering that fast-acting insulin has not finished working.
	Don't estimate portion sizes if postprandial blood sugar control is repeatedly elevated.
	Don't suggest exercise if blood sugar is too high or if patient has not been properly evaluated for safety during exercise.

Problem	*Do's and Don'ts*
Elevated Post-prandial Glucose (blood sugars over 180 mg/dl)	Delay exercise if blood glucose is greater than 300 mg/dl or if greater than 250 mg/dl and urine ketones are present. If the insulin level is too low, hyperglycemia and potential ketosis may occur. Don't utilize carbohydrate to insulin ratio if not clear or unsure of how to calculate ratios or if patient will do more harm than good to blood glucose control.
Blood Sugar Less than 100 mg/dl Before Bed	**Do:** Consider before bed snack of protein- or fat-containing foods (for example, peanut butter, nuts, cheese, and whole milk) in addition to a carbohydrate to prevent nocturnal hypoglycemia. Evaluate carbohydrate content of meal eaten prior to bedtime to determine if adequate. Evaluate activity level following last meal and prior to bedtime to determine cause of low blood sugar. Reduce rapid-acting insulin taken before bed or have it coincide with foods eaten. **Don't:** Don't allow the patient to overeat to correct for a low blood sugar. Foods eaten within 2 hours of bed can continue to cause the blood sugar to rise. Overeating to correct low blood sugar may increase morning blood sugars. Don't allow the patient to skip the evening snack.
Dehydration, High Specific Gravity Urine, or Dark, Strong Odor Urine	**Do:** Increase consumption of no- or low-calorie beverages (for example, water, sugar-free soft drinks, sugar-free flavored waters, diet gelatin, broth, or diet juices). Consuming light (50%) juices will require consideration of carbohydrate content. Inform the patient that on sick days, the beverages will need to contain carbohydrates. Check blood sugar and ketones for elevated levels. **Don't:** Don't use thirst as the only indicator of dehydration.
Medication-Associated Weight Gain	**Do:** Combine increase in activity with reduction in calories to restore calorie balance. Ask patient to keep a food record for 3 days.

Problem	*Do's and Don'ts*
	Evaluate emotional eating component of weight gain and the presence of stressors contributing to increased intake. Increase low-calorie beverages (less than 20 calories per serving). Evaluate calorie consumption, specifically hidden fat calories, or calorie-dense foods. Replace refined carbohydrates with high-fiber foods, like fresh fruits, vegetables, whole grains, beans, and legumes within carbohydrate allotments. Reduce portion sizes, fatty foods, animal fats, and meat. Exercise 2–3 hours per week at a brisk pace, if approved by the PMD. Measure portion sizes. Evaluate if you are overcompensating for low blood sugars with additional portions. Use glucose testing with exercise to increase safety. Medications may have caused a reduced urinary glucose excretion resulting in weight gain. Remember that insulin stimulates appetite and may have had an effect. Discourage diet pills and fad diets. **Don't:** Don't allow the patient to skip meals. Instead, use lower-calorie foods and beverages with exercise.
Dyslipidemia	**Do:** Keep blood lipids in good control. DCCT Research group recommends: • LDL cholesterol should be less than 100 mg/dl • HDL cholesterol should be greater than 45 mg/dl in men and greater than 55 mg/dl in women • Triglycerides should be less than 150 mg/dl Evaluate each component of the total cholesterol and make interventions where needed. Record a 24-hour food history and/or food frequency to help identify possible changes. Recommend moderate physical activity (30–60 minutes, 3–6 days per week) for high-density lipoproteins increase. This will also help lower triglycerides.

SECTION 2

Problem	*Do's and Don'ts*
	If LDL is elevated: • Focus on lowering saturated and trans fats in diet. • Reduced fried and fast foods. • Focus on healthy fat choices, including monounsaturated and polyunsaturated fats. Explore need for statin with the PMD's approval. Present diabetes standards call for statin use in treatment. If HDL level is low: • Determine if lack of exercise may be contributory or if there is a genetic component to low HDL. • Consider that males and postmenopausal females may have lower HDL levels. • Encourage exercise if safe. If triglyceride is elevated: • Identify foods that may increase triglyceride level, such as simple carbohydrates. • Encourage exercise if safe. • Keeping glucoses near normal will reduce lipids in blood. Consider referral to an exercise and diet group. Consider adding omega-3 fats (tuna, salmon, and sardines) if safe to do so. **Don't:** Don't rely solely on statin use to lower lipids. Don't wait beyond 3–6 months for diet to lower blood lipids. Don't assume lowering cholesterol intake will automatically lower total cholesterol or lipid components. Don't take fat completely out of the diet. Rather, focus on the individual's needs.
Chronic Renal Failure	**Do:** Keep blood glucose control near normal (80–140 mg/dl). See table on page 113 for hemoglobin A1c values. Aggressively achieve blood pressure control with medications and low-sodium diet control. Consume low-fat protein of high biologic value, such as eggs, animal protein, fish, seafood, tofu, within protein recommendations. Consider changing multivitamin to renal vitamin.

Problem	*Do's and Don'ts*
	Don't: Don't use kidney-damaging medications or diagnostic dyes (insulin is excreted by the kidneys, thus working longer). Don't provide the patient with high-potassium foods (see appendix on pages 446–447) to correct blood sugar if potassium levels are elevated. Don't use high-potassium foods solely to compensate for diuretics. Don't provide high-sodium foods (see appendix on page 461) and fluids if patient has significant fluid retention.
Gastroparesis	**Do:** Treat nausea and vomiting as follows: • Eat five to six small meals a day or eat every few hours. • Eat slowly. • Avoid greasy, fried, or spicy foods. • Eat simply prepared foods or have food prepared for you; the smell of food cooking can cause nausea. • Drink fluids between meals. Consult with the PMD for patients with severe vomiting. Check the PMD about the use of medications (antiemetics). Encourage patients with diarrhea to decrease fiber in diet. Encourage patients with constipation to increase fiber and water. Physical activity, such as walking, also improves constipation. Consult the PMD regarding medications that may assist with gastric emptying. If severe and persistent, the PMD may consider a study to evaluate gastric emptying and motility or refer to a gastroenterologist. **Don't:** Don't give insulin before meals. Instead, wait for gastric motility to clear food from stomach before using fast-acting insulin.
Hypoglycemia	**Do:** Test blood glucose to verify low blood sugar. Utilize the following formula: $100 - \text{blood glucose (BG)} \times 0.2 = \text{grams of glucose needed.}$ If patient is conscious, treat with 10–15 gm of oral glucose: • Feed 15 grams of readily available carbohydrates. See Table 2-1 on page 112 for suggested carbohydrate sources. Retest blood sugars and check symptoms in 10–15 minutes.

Problem	*Do's and Don'ts*
Hypoglycemia	• If glucose is not up or still below 70, feed another 15 gm of carbohydrates. • If a meal is more than 1 hour away, eat a snack that contains protein and carbohydrates (for example, a half sandwich and glass of milk or yogurt and fruit). • If meal is less than 1 hour away, eat early. Ask patient to carry readily absorbable carbohydrate source such as: • Two to three glucose tablets (5 gm glucose each) • Five Lifesavers • A small juice box (4 ounces) or 4 ounces of regular soda • 1 tablespoon of honey or sugar If patient is not conscious or cannot swallow, administer 0.5–1.0 mg of IM glucagons. Administer glucagons if: • Unable to eat • Unconscious • Does not improve following eating a sugar-sweetened product In a hospital setting, if the patient cannot safely swallow, parenteral treatment is required. Ideally, use 50% dextrose solution. $100 - BG \times 0.4 =$ cc of 50% dextrose given. If IV access is not available, monitor the following possible causes of hypoglycemia: • Weight loss reduces need for insulin and some medications. • Alcohol can cause low blood sugar. • Exercise lowers blood sugar for 24 hrs afterward by restoring glycogen stores in muscles. • Eating at the wrong time for the medications taken. • Skipping or not finishing meals or snacks. Review methods to prevent hypoglycemia with patient, including: • Eating meals on time • Not skipping meals or snacks • Testing on schedule • Performing extra tests if feeling different from normal • Conferring with PMD and diabetes educators on how to adjust medications and food with exercise, weight loss, changes in schedule, or other lifestyle changes

Problem	*Do's and Don'ts*
	Don't:
	Don't try to increase blood sugar with chocolate or nuts—the fat slows digestion and results in slower glucose rise.
	Don't allow the patient to drink alcohol on an empty stomach because it may lower blood sugar and cause hypoglycemia.
	Don't continue giving the same dosage of insulin with major changes in the diet or body habits.
	Don't allow the patient to exercise without properly checking blood sugar and providing an appropriate snack.
Improper Dentition	**Do:**
	Take a 24-hour recall to determine a typical meal plan and types of foods eaten.
	Change consistency of diet to soft or ground if appropriate.
	Evaluate foods using a food frequency questionnaire and identify poorly tolerated foods.
	Consider speech pathology evaluation.
	Evaluate cooking methods patient and family may use. Encourage moist techniques and not overcooking meats.
	Refer for dental consult if the fitting of dentures is an issue.
	Refer annually for dental exam and restoration.
	Don't:
	Don't serve foods that will present a choking hazard: • Tough meats or stringy proteins • Seeds and tough skins of fruits • Nuts • Stringy vegetables such as celery and pea pods
	Don't eliminate food groups or foods without taking into consideration how it will affect blood sugar control or insulin requirements.
Exercise	**Do:**
	Encourage patient to check with the PMD prior to beginning an exercise program.
	Ask for a detailed medical evaluation prior to beginning an exercise program that should include: • Evaluation of an ECG or workload capacity with stress • Evaluation of retinopathy to prevent vitreous hemorrhage with straining or lifting • Evaluation of neuropathy

Problem	*Do's and Don'ts*
Exercise	Ideal exercise programs should contain warm up, aerobic period, and cool-down period. Refer patients to qualified exercise physiologist or personal trainer to help determine exercise programs that are appropriate for them. Start the patient's exercise slowly. Encourage patient to wear a medic alert bracelet at all times. Have patient carry a readily available source of glucose. Encourage the patient to wear comfortable, well-fitting shoes and cotton socks. Check blood sugar before and after exercise. Adjust food intake for exercise accordingly: • 30 min or less, moderate activity Less than 100 = 30 gm extra carbohydrate 100–180 = 15 gm extra carbohydrate Greater than 180, no snack needed • 30–60 minutes, moderate activity Less than 100 = 30 gm extra carbohydrate 100–200 = 15 gm extra carbohydrate 200–250 = 15 gm extra carbohydrate Greater than 250, no snack needed • 60-plus minutes, moderate or 30-min, high-intensity Consider a lower insulin dose to promote weight loss or add 30 gm carbohydrates per hour. **Don't:** Don't recommend intensive exercise without a medical evaluation or taking medications into consideration. Don't recommend an unqualified personal trainer or exercise physiologist who is not familiar with diabetes. Don't continue exercising if experiencing leg pains or chest pains while exercising. Don't have the patient exercise if blood sugar is greater than 300 mg/dl or less than 70 mg/dl. Don't forget to tell the patient not to leave the house without a readily available form of absorbable glucose, identification, and a medic alert bracelet. Don't assume that the patient needs only one postexercise blood sugar check. The effects of exercise may continue for several hours following exercise.

Problem	*Do's and Don'ts*
Prediabetes (Fasting Glucose 110–125 mg/dl) *Impaired Fasting Glucose Tolerance (IFG) Impaired Fasting Glucose (IFG)*	**Do:** Do try to lower fasting and post-prandial glucose. Better control is associated with reduced incidence of cardiovascular disease (CVD) and death. Evaluate caloric intake and recent weight patterns. Evaluate places of weight gain on the body because abdominal fat is associated with diabetes and heart disease. Decrease calorie intake using smaller, more frequent meals. Even without decreased caloric intake, smaller boluses of food can equal a reduced postprandial glucose. Ask patient to keep a food history to determine foods that are overeaten. Identify carbohydrate sources in the diet and educate the patient on calorie-dense foods. Reduce portion sizes. Consider using the plate method to help patient understand the balance of the meal: • Half the plate is nonstarchy vegetables. • A quarter of the plate is protein. • A quarter of the plate is starch. • One serving of fruit. • One serving of milk. Encourage whole-grain starches (whole wheat, oats, and barley) along with reducing portions. Encourage liberal consumption of vegetables that are not starchy (corn, peas, legumes). Reduce consumption of beverages containing carbohydrates and fats. Try drinking all diet beverages, 1% milk, and sugar-free soft drinks. Encourage and facilitate weight loss with diet and exercise. Encourage the patient to enroll in a weight-loss program that encompasses behavior modification, exercise, and monitoring. Reduce dietary cholesterol and fat intake to lower risk of premature cardiovascular disease. Identify sources of trans fat (read labels) and saturated fat (animal fats) in the diet. Avoid cooking methods that may add additional fat calories to foods.

Problem	*Do's and Don'ts*
Impaired Fasting Glucose Tolerance (IFG) Impaired Fasting Glucose (IFG)	**Don't:** Don't ignore these metabolic symptoms: • HDL greater than 40 mg/dl for men and greater than 50 mg/dl for women • Elevated LDL • Elevated triglycerides • Waist circumference greater than 38 inches for men and greater than 32 inches for women Don't provide a meal plan if that will discourage patient from weight loss or if it is too restrictive. Don't recommend a general whole wheat to patients. Educate the patient on fiber content and whole-grain considerations. Educate the patient on reading labels.
Constipation	**Do:** Increase water or low-calorie soft drinks by at least 16 ounces per day, if not medically contraindicated. Increase consumption of vegetables high in fiber (that is, cabbage, carrots, broccoli, and potato with skin). Substitute high-fiber cereals (greater than 2–3 gm fiber per serving) and grains for refined cereals and grains. Substitute fresh fruits with skins for canned fruit products. Encourage increased exercise if safe to do so. **Don't:** Don't use laxatives without trying increased fluids and fiber first. Don't advocate exercise without evaluating safety. Don't recommend medications or laxatives that may cause electrolyte imbalances in conjunction with other medications.
Sick Day Guidelines for Patients on Insulin	**Do:** Treat the illness by giving prescribed and recommended medicines. Prevent dehydration by giving 8 fluid ounces every half hour to 1 hour, if not medically contraindicated. Use low-calorie beverages if the meal plan is to be followed. Alternate between diet and regular, sugar-containing fluids if the meal plan is not followed. Test blood every 2–3 hours, using a correction factor (if you have one) to correct high blood sugar every 3–4 hours.

Problem	*Do's and Don'ts*
	Substitute 1 of the 15 g carbohydrate suggestions for each serving of breads, cereals, fruit, and milk in the meal plan if vomiting.
	Check urine for ketones if blood glucose is greater than 240 mg/dl.
	Ketosis can precipitate inappropriate insulin dosage, illness, or other causes. One sign of ketosis is sweet acetone breath.
	Contact PMD if ketosis is present.
	Don't:
	Don't stop giving the patient insulin because he/she is not able to eat.
	Don't exercise when sick because exercise raises the blood sugar.

Sources

Beaser, R. S., & Hill, J. V. "The Joslin Guide to Diabetes." *Managing Diabetes and Its Complications-A Guide for Health Care Providers*. New York: Simon and Schuster. Lifescan, Inc. 1999.

Bode, B., Davidson, P., Steed, R., Robertson, D., Greenlee, C., & Welch, N. "Diabetes Dek: How to Control and Manage Diabetes." *Mellitus Infodek*. 2004.

American Diabetes Association. "Choose to Live: Your Diabetes Survival Guide." 2003.

Table 2-1 Table of 15 Grams Carbohydrate

4 oz orange juice or apple juice
3 oz cranberry or grape juice
6 oz regular ginger ale
5 oz regular colas
4 teaspoons sugar dissolved in water
8 Lifesavers
6 regular or 10 small jelly beans
3 glucose tablets
1 cup creamed soup
1 twin-pop Popsicle
¼ cup sweetened pudding
½ cup sugar-free pudding
6 saltines
½ cup cooked cereal
½ cup regular ice cream

Clinical Practice Recommendations 2005, American Diabetes Association, *Diabetes Care,* Volume 27, Number 1, Supplement 1.

Table 2-2 Insulin Commonly Used in the United States

Generic Name/Form	Onset	Peak	Duration	Clear/Cloudy
Lispro/Analog	<15 min	0.5–1.5 h	3–4 h	Clear
Aspart	<15 min	0.5–1.5 h	3–4 h	Clear
Regular	0.5–1.0 h	2–3 h	3–6 h	Clear
NPH	2–4 h	6–10 h	10–16 h	Cloudy
Glargine	2–4 h	peakless	18–24 h	Clear

min = minutes, h = hours

Clinical Practice Recommendations 2005, American Diabetes Association, *Diabetes Care,* Volume 27, Number 1, Supplement 1.

Table 2-3 Glycated Hemoglobin Levels and Glucose Levels

A1c %	Average Whole Blood Glucose	Average Plasma Glucose
13	330	370
12	300	335
11	270	300
10	240	270
9	210	235
8	180	200
7	150	170
6	120	135
5	90	100

7% or less is recommended

Clinical Practice Recommendations 2005, American Diabetes Association, *Diabetes Care,* Volume 27, Number 1, Supplement 1.

Table 2-4 Self-Management Blood Sugar Testing Goals

Testing Time	Goal for People with Diabetes	Take Action If
Before meals	80–120 mg/dl	<80 or >140
Blood sugar 2 hours after meals	140–180 mg/dl	<100 or >200

Clinical Practice Recommendations 2005, American Diabetes Association, *Diabetes Care,* Volume 27, Number 1, Supplement 1.

Eating Disorders (Including Anorexia Nervosa, Bulimia Nervosa, and Eating Disorder Not Otherwise Specified [EDNOS])

Author: Kendrin Sonneville, MS, RD, LDN

This list will assist the dietitian in addressing problems seen in patients with eating disorders such as early satiety, constipation, amenorrhea, refeeding syndrome, osteopenia, fat deficiency, orthostasis, binge eating, tooth enamel erosion, and other general symptoms of malnutrition. Refer all patients with eating disorders for nutritional counseling, behavioral therapy, psychological/psychiatric consultation, and family therapy.

Problem	*Do's and Don'ts*
Early Satiety	Delayed gastric emptying related to malnutrition can lead to early satiety in patients who are in the early stages of refeeding. **Do:** Encourage frequent small meals and snacks. Encourage energy-dense foods to decrease volume of food intake. Encourage calorie-containing fluids, such as milk and juice, because these will decrease the volume of food needed. Withhold fluids until after meals. **Don't:** Don't decrease meal plan to alleviate discomfort; early satiety will subside. Don't offer large meals.
Constipation	Constipation may be due to dehydration, low fiber intake, or laxative withdrawal. **Do:** Encourage consumption of fluids and fiber-containing foods like legumes, whole grains, fruits, and vegetables. **Don't:** Don't encourage continued use of laxatives to manage constipation.
Amenorrhea	Amenorrhea can be caused by low weight and/or low dietary fat intake. **Do:** Promote weight gain.

Problem	Do's and Don'ts
	Encourage dietary fat consumption. Dietary fats perceived as "healthy" (for example, monounsaturated fats: olive, sesame, and canola oils, and nuts) may be more accepted than less-healthy fats (for example, trans fats). Encourage the patient to read product labels. Encourage safe choices (for example, nuts, peanut butter, olive oil, and salad dressing).
Lowered Testosterone Levels	Levels of testosterone may decrease in males with eating disorders. **Do:** Promote weight gain. Encourage dietary fat consumption.
Refeeding Syndrome	Refeeding syndrome describes the glucose, mineral, electrolyte, and fluid shifts that are seen in the malnourished patient who begins aggressive refeeding. Hypophosphatemia characterizes this shift that results from a sudden increase in phosphorus demands. **Do:** Make gradual increases in caloric intakes (achieve calorie intake goal by eating 250 calories per day) in patients who are severely malnourished and/or patients who have a very low calorie intake prior to refeeding. Monitor electrolytes, phosphorus, magnesium, calcium, and glucose daily during inpatient admissions until reaching calorie goal. Administer prophylactic supplementation of phosphorus and potassium to inpatients who are receiving aggressive caloric increases or will be prescribed as needed based on the degree of electrolyte instability. **Don't:** Don't advance patients with a very low-calorie intake immediately to goal calories.
Hypokalemia	Hypokalemia may be seen in patients who vomit regularly. **Do:** Encourage consumption of potassium-containing foods: fluids such as orange juice or Gatorade (particularly after vomiting episodes).
Osteopenia/Low Bone Density	Results from amenorrhea, low weight, and/or insufficient intake of calcium and vitamin D.

Problem	*Do's and Don'ts*
	Do: Encourage weight gain. Recommend increased intake of calcium and vitamin D (or supplementation) with the PMD's approval. Individuals between 9 and 18 years of age need 1300 mg of calcium. Individuals between 19 and 50 years of age need 1000 mg. Recommend between 5 and 10 micrograms (200–400 IU) of vitamin D for individuals below age 50 years. Encourage weight-bearing activity (if medically stable).
Inadequate Fat Intake	Symptoms may include cold intolerance or hair loss. **Do:** Encourage the inclusion of healthier dietary fat at all meals. Allow for a gradual increase in fat intake in patients who are fearful of dietary fat; healthier sources of fat (versus trans and saturated fats) will likely be preferred.
Orthostatic Hypertension/ Bradycardia	Orthostatic hypertension/bradycardia can be caused by low weight and decreased muscle mass. **Do:** Promote weight gain. **Don't:** Don't allow exercise, which can exacerbate orthostasis.
Binge Eating	Binge eating is seen in patients with bulimia nervosa and may be observed in malnourished patients when they begin the refeeding process. **Do:** Encourage meal plan adherence. Encourage utilization of distraction techniques, such as going for a walk, calling a friend, or journaling to minimize binge or delay/prevent compensatory behaviors, such as intentional vomiting. **Don't:** Don't allow consumption of trigger foods (usually high-calorie foods such as ice cream) that make the patient want to perform self-induced vomiting.
Erosion of Tooth Enamel	Erosion of tooth enamal is seen in patients who vomit intentionally. **Do:** Encourage use of baking soda toothpaste.

Problem	*Do's and Don'ts*
	Don't: Don't encourage teeth brushing immediately after vomiting. Brushing immediately after vomiting can increase the damage to the surface enamel layer of the teeth. The abrasive properties of the toothpaste and brush can be particularly damaging to teeth in a sensitive state (postvomit). Rinsing with water or milk is best. If someone insists on brushing, advise no toothpaste or baking soda toothpaste and a soft toothbrush.
Malnutrition/ Weight Loss	Symptoms of malnutrition include fatigue, poor concentration, and worsening of disordered thoughts and behaviors. **Do:** Promote increased caloric intake and weight gain.
Hyperexercise	Patients may use excessive exercise to purge calories. Hyperexercise behaviors are often secretive. **Do:** Restrict exercise, particularly for those patients with cardiac complications that exercise exacerbates. Allow moderate exercise for patients who are compliant with treatment and achieving weight goals.
Esophagitis	Inflammation or rupture of the esophagus can result from frequent vomiting. **Do:** Encourage the consumption of cold, bland, and nonacidic foods (for example, dairy products) to minimize discomfort. Encourage the patient to avoid foods that typically trigger vomiting to allow for esophageal healing. **Don't:** Don't encourage acidic foods and fluids, such as citrus foods, juice, and tomato products.
Abnormal Food-Related Behaviors	Patients with eating disorders may develop unusual food rituals (for example, cutting foods excessively), eating patterns (for example, extremely slow eating), or food rules (for example, following strict vegetarian diets or avoiding all foods with added preservatives). **Do:** Establish rules that limit disordered behaviors (for example, limiting meals to 30 minutes). Refer to behavioral therapy.

Insulin Manipulation	Individuals with type 1 diabetes may decide to withhold insulin to "purge" calories through urine losses of sugar. **Do:** Educate the patient on long-term complications of diabetes associated with chronic elevation in blood glucose. Monitor insulin injections and blood sugar checks. See the section on diabetes on page 92.

Sources

Becker, A. E., Grinspoon, S. K., Klibanski, A., & Herzog, D. B. "Eating Disorders." *New England J Med.* 1999. 340(14), 1092–1098.

Schebendach, J., & Reichert-Anderson, P. "Nutrition in Eating Disorders." *Kraus's Nutrition and Diet Therapy*. Mahan, K., & Escott-Stump, S. (Eds.). New York, NY: McGraw-Hill. 2000.

Garner, D. M., & Garfinkle, P. E. *Handbook of Treatment of Eating Disorders* (2nd ed.). New York, NY: Guilford Press. 1997.

"Nutrition Intervention in the Treatment of Anorexia Nervosa, Bulimia Nervosa, and Eating Disorder Not Otherwise Specified" (EDNOS). *J Am Diet Assoc.* 2001. 101, 810.

Dysphagia

Author: Nicola O'Brien, MS, RD, LDN

Dysphagia can describe the loss of skills involved in swallowing food and/or fluids. The reasons for dysphagia can vary from medical conditions and medication side effects to cognition deficits. The following information will assist the dietitian in diminishing the development of choking and aspiration that could lead to malnutrition and/or dehydration.

Problem	***Do's and Don'ts***
Dysphagia	**Do:**
	Assess patients at all times for coughing or choking when eating or drinking.
	Watch for patients who are avoiding certain foods because of choking or coughing.
	Assess the mouth and teeth and whether there is a need for a dental consult.
	Evaluate the dentures and their fit and determine if there is a need for a dental consult or dental adhesive.
	Observe whether a patient is drooling.
	Monitor if patient has "pocketed" food (food left in the mouth after meals).
	Assess the patient's weight record for recent unexplained weight loss.
	Review the patient's medical records for a history of pneumonia that may have not been noted to be aspiration pneumonia.
	Determine whether the patient has had an elevated temperature and/or questionable lung sounds.
	Ask for a speech language pathologist (SLP) consult if the patient is at risk for the consequences of dysphasia. The SLP can either perform a chairside swallow evaluation or recommend a barium swallow.
	Ask the SLP to recommend texture modification of solid food served to the patient based on the swallow evaluation.
	Encourage the SLP to review the facility's current texture modifications outlined in the facility's current authorized diet manual.
	Encourage the SLP to utilize the accepted name for each texture modification to assure conformity of texture modification.

Problem	*Do's and Don'ts*
Dysphagia	Determine the safest environment for the patient to take his/her meals—a dining room with continuous supervision, one-on-one supervision, or dependent feeding. Minimize consequences of dysphagia by incorporating the following strategies in the patient's daily routine as recommended by the SLP: • Eat meals at a table in a chair at a 90° angle. • Encourage chin on chest swallowing. • Have the patient consume small amounts—½ teaspoon to 1 teaspoon of food at a time—and eat slowly. Determine whether liquids can be taken via a straw, a teaspoon, a cup, or a sippy cup. Observe the patient swallow before taking another bite or sip. Assess whether a double swallow is necessary for each swallow. Ask the patient to cough or clear the throat if the patient's voice sounds "gurgly" or "wet." Check the patient's mouth for food after the completion of meals. Stay upright for about 30 minutes after eating or drinking. Avoid tight-fitting waistbands or belts. Monitor weight status to avoid weight loss; weekly weight checks are recommended. Initiate use of nutrient-dense or fortified foods (for example, Super Cereal, Super Pudding, Super Spuds, Super Muffins, and Super Soup—recipes are available in the appendix on pages 459–460) as permitted by texture modification if the patient begins to lose weight. Monitor the patient's temperature and lung sounds. Ask for SLP evaluation should the patient show improvement in swallowing ability, with the intent to have the patient be provided with meals that are safe but also least restrictive. Give the patient ample time to eat. Avoid gelatin, ice cream, sherbet, and ice if SLP recommends thickened liquids; these items are thin liquids at body temperature. Thicken *all* liquids given to the patient at all times should this be recommended.

Problem	*Do's and Don'ts*
	Don't:
	Don't overlook completing a dental assessment.
	Don't avoid use of adhesive if it improves fit of dentures.
	Don't forget to examine the patient's mouth after meals.
	Don't ignore the possibility of aspiration.
	Don't overlook the possibility of an unsafe dining choice, such as eating in bed, eating quickly, consuming large amounts of food, or lying flat in bed after eating or drinking.
	Don't overlook the importance of keeping weekly weight records.
	Don't overlook the patient's progression of improvement in swallowing ability.
	Don't rush the patient at mealtime.
	Don't forget to thicken between-meal drinks or water at the bedside.

Sources

New England Diet Manual for Extended Care. Boston, MA. 2003.

National Dysphagia Diet. http://www.asha.org.

Human Immunodeficiency Virus (HIV) and Acquired Immunodeficiency Syndrome (AIDS)

Author: Kimberly Dong, MS, RD, LDN

This list will assist the dietitian in answering food tolerance questions and serve as a guide to assist patients who are experiencing symptoms of HIV/AIDS infection. The side effects of HIV/AIDS and/or complications associated with HIV/AIDS medications may include nausea, vomiting, diarrhea, decreased appetite, oral thrush, dysphagia, weight loss, weight gain, dyslipidemia, insulin resistance, fat accumulation, opportunistic infections, dehydration, micronutrient deficiencies, malabsorption, and taste changes.

Problem	*Do's and Don'ts*
Nausea	**Do:** Recommend small, frequent meals. Try bland foods (for example, potatoes, rice, canned fruits, dry crackers, or toast). Notice patterns of when nausea occurs and avoid offering food at these times. Position the patient at meals sitting up instead of lying down. Suggest eating in a cool environment, eating slower, and providing foods at room temperature. **Don't:** Don't provide drinks during mealtime; separate liquids from solids. Don't serve high-fat, greasy foods or strong-odor foods, such as ripe cheese and fish.
Vomiting	**Do:** Suggest small, frequent meals. Provide clear, cool liquids between meals. Try bland foods (for example, potatoes, rice, canned fruits). Patients should eat slowly. **Don't:** Don't serve high-fat, greasy foods or strong-odor foods, such as ripe cheese and fish.
Diarrhea	**Do:** Provide high soluble fiber (for example, rice, oatmeal, white bread, potatoes without skin, bananas, peeled apples/applesauce, and mangoes). Eliminate foods that exacerbate these symptoms, such as high-fat dairy.

Problem	*Do's and Don'ts*
	Provide electrolyte-replacing fluids (for example, broths, fruit juices, and oral hydration drinks). Suggest small, frequent meals. Try offering yogurt with active cultures or acidophilus capsules. **Don't:** Don't give high-dose vitamin C supplements, laxative teas, foods containing sorbitol (sugar-free candy and gums), lactose-rich dairy, caffeine, and high-fat foods.
Decreased Appetite	**Do:** Suggest small, frequent meals. Provide nutrient-dense foods (for example, milk shakes, lean meats/poultry/fish, eggs, nut butters, vegetables, fruits, and whole grains). **Don't:** Don't recommend large meals.
Oral Thrush	**Do:** Serve softer, colder foods and fluids with meals. Encourage good oral hygiene. **Don't:** Don't serve salty, hot, spicy, or acidic foods (citrus fruits, tomato-based products, vinegar/vinegar-based products).
Dysphagia	**Do:** Moisten foods with sauces and serve softer foods (for example, oatmeal, mashed potatoes, pudding, scrambled eggs, milk shakes, and yogurt). Provide liquids with meals. Try dry foods (for example, toast, crackers, and chips). **Don't:** Don't provide sticky foods that are difficult to swallow (for example, peanut butter).
Weight Loss	**Do:** Provide small, frequent nutrient-dense meals. Serve high-protein foods (for example, lean meats, poultry, fish, eggs, milk, yogurt, cheese, legumes, tofu, and nut butters like peanut butter). Serve high-calorie foods such as milk shakes, trail mixes with fruit and nuts, and cheese and crackers.

Problem	*Do's and Don'ts*
Weight Loss	Add rice, barley, and legumes to soups. Add dry milk powder or protein powder to casseroles, hot cereals, milk shakes, etc. to increase calories and protein content. Use oral supplements such as Carnation Instant Breakfast, Boost, and Ensure. If a patient infected with HIV has a decreased dietary intake, assess if nutrition supplements are appropriate. **Don't:** Don't allow "diet foods" or low-calorie foods.
Weight Gain	**Do:** Use traditional dietary approaches to weight management to achieve healthy weight, including adequate caloric intake, warranted caloric reduction, adequate protein intake, or low/moderate fat intake. Prepare food with less fat by steaming, grilling, baking, broiling, or microwaving instead of frying. Incorporate physical activity. See the table on weight control. **Don't:** Don't serve simple sugars such as candy, soda, Popsicles, jelly or other high-sugar foods such as cookies. Don't provide excessive dietary fat, especially trans and saturated.
Dyslipidemia	**Do:** Follow diet recommendations of the National Cholesterol Education Program (NCEP): • Try low/moderate fat diets (about 30% or less of total calories from fat). • Decrease saturated and trans fat intake (to less than 10% of total calorie intake). • Increase monounsaturated fats (for example, olive, sesame, and canola oils, and nuts) to 10–15% of total calorie intake. • Incorporate omega-3 fatty acids, such as fatty fish (for example, salmon, sardines, and mackerel) and certain nuts/seeds (for example, walnuts, flaxseeds). Prepare food with less fat by steaming, grilling, baking, broiling, or microwaving instead of frying. Incorporate physical activity. See the appendix on page 281 for figuring fat intake.

Problem	Do's and Don'ts
	Don't:
	Don't serve simple sugars (for example, candy, soda, and other high-sugar foods such as cookies).
Insulin Resistance	**Do:**
	Serve high-fiber foods (fruits, vegetables, legumes, and whole grains).
	Provide low glycemic index foods (for example, whole grains, fruits, vegetables, and legumes). See appendix on page 375 for glycemic index of some foods.
	Don't:
	Don't prepare a low-fiber diet.
Fat Accumulation	**Do:**
	Recommend adequate fiber (20–35 gm per day), adequate calories, and adequate protein. See Dietary Reference Intakes (DRI) in appendix on pages 301–308.
	Don't:
	Don't provide a low-fiber diet.
Opportunistic Infections	**Do:**
	Wash hands with soap and warm water often.
	Wash all fresh fruits and vegetables.
	Avoid cross contamination of raw and cooked foods.
	Refrigerate foods to less than 41°F.
	Don't:
	Don't serve raw or undercooked meats, poultry, fish, shellfish, and eggs.
	Don't purchase unpasteurized dairy products.
Dehydration	**Do:**
	Suggest electrolyte-repleting fluids (for example, broths, fruit juices, and oral hydration drinks).
	Limit foods high in sodium.
	Limit caffeine.
Micronutrient/ Trace Element Deficiencies	**Do:**
	Recommend an appropriate daily multivitamin after checking with a PMD.
Malabsorption	**Do:**
	Suggest a low-fat diet with medium-chain triglyceride (MCT) oils. Obtain MCT oil with a PMD recommendation.

Problem	*Do's and Don'ts*
Taste Changes	**Do:** Separate medications that cause taste changes from mealtime (if possible). Add spices and herbs to foods. **Don't:** Don't use oral supplements in metallic cans.

Sources

Batterham, M., Garsia, R., & Greendip, P. "Dietary Intake, Serum Lipids, Insulin Resistance and Body Composition in the Era of Highly Active Antiretroviral Therapy 'Diet FRS Study'." *AIDS*. 2000. 14, 1839–1843.

Bell, S. J., Swails, W. S., Bistrian, B. R., Wanke, C., Burke, P., & Forse, R. A. HIV–AIDS–AIDS. *Quick Reference to Clinical Dietetics*. Florida: ASPEN Publication. 1997.

Dong, K. R., & Hendricks, K. M. "The Role of Nutrition in Fat Deposition and Fat Atrophy in Patients with HIV–AIDS." *Nutrition in Clinical Care*. 2005. 8, 31–36.

Dube, M., Sprecher, D., Henry, W. K., et al. "Preliminary Guidelines for the Evaluation and Management of Dyslipidemia in Adults Infected with Human Immunodeficiency Virus and Receiving Antiretroviral Therapy: Recommendations of the Adult AIDS Clinical Trial Group Cardiovascular Disease Focus Group." *Clin Infect Dis*. 2000. 31, 1216–1224.

Gerrior, J., & Neff, L. M. "Nutrition Assessment in HIV–AIDS Infection." *Nutrition in Clinical Care*. 2005. 8, 6–15.

Hadigan, C., Jeste, S., Anderson, E., et al. "Modifiable Dietary Habits and Their Relation to Metabolic Abnormalities in Men and Women with Human Immunodeficiency Virus Infection and Fat Redistribution." *Clin Infect Dis*. 2001. 33, 710–717.

Hendricks, K. M., Dong, K. R., Tang, A., et al. "High-Fiber Diet in HIV–AIDS-Positive Men is Associated with Lower Risk of Developing Fat Deposition." *Am J Clin Nutr*. 2003. 78, 790–795.

Highleyman, L. "Managing Nausea, Vomiting, and Diarrhea. Bulletin of Experimental Treatments for AIDS." *San Francisco AIDS Foundation*. 2002. 29–39.

Moyle, G., Baldwin, C., & Phillpot, M. "Managing Metabolic Disturbances and Lipodystrophy: Diet, Exercise, and Smoking Advice." *AIDS Read*. 2001. 11, 589–592.

Position of the American Dietetic Association and Dietitians of Canada. "Nutrition Intervention in the Care of Persons with Human Immunodeficiency Virus Infection." *J Am Diet Assoc*. 2004. 104, 1425–1441.

Shevitz, A., & Knox, T. "Nutrition in the era of highly active antiretroviral therapy." *Clin Infect Dis*. 2001. 32, 1769–1775.

Woods, M. N. "Role of N-3 Fatty Acids in Prevention of Disease Complications in Patients with HIV–AIDS." *Nutrition in Clinical Care*. 2005. 8, 24–30.

Malnutrition

Author: Nicola O'Brien, MS, RD, LDN

Malnutrition—or undernutrition—is a common problem due to myriad factors, from illness to depression, cognitive impairment, or dementia. The following information will facilitate identifying those patients with malnutrition and steps to promote adequate nutrition.

Problem	*Do's and Don'ts*
Malnutrition	**Do:**
	Assess the patient's current weight status and weight history.
	Determine the patient's ideal body weight (IBW) range, using the patient's height.[a]
	Calculate the patient's daily estimated needs, based on actual current weight and height, using the Harris Benedict formula to determine basal energy expenditure (BEE).[b]
	Determine the patient's activity level.[c]
	Estimate protein needs based on kg of IBW.[d]
	Establish daily fluid needs.[e]
	Review the patient's meal completion record; attempt to determine whether there are meals more readily consumed than others, such as breakfast versus lunch.
	Interview the patient to identify why the patient is not eating.
	Attempt to identify what the patient feels like eating.
	Interview the nurse or nursing assistant for their observations regarding the patient at mealtimes.
	Assess the patient for depression with a psychiatric consult as an option.
	Evaluate the patient's medications to determine whether medications could be causing lack of appetite, GI upset, nausea, etc. Identify any medications that have a side effect of weight loss or anorexia.
	Initiate daily multivitamins, with the PMD's input.
	Look at patient's dentition for poor condition of own teeth, ill-fitting old dentures, or edentulousness. Consider dental consult if needed.
	Determine whether texture modification would improve the patient's meal completion. Ask an SLP to evaluate patient for chewing or swallowing concerns.

Problem	*Do's and Don'ts*
	Assess whether the patient's current diet order is necessary, ultimately determining the least restrictive diet to improve meal completion.
	Evaluate portion size and even the number of meals per day; the three meals a day of standard portion size may prove overwhelming. Small, more frequent meals may be called for. Review what foods the patient readily eats, with the intent of incorporating nutrient-dense or fortified foods (for example, Super Cereal, Super Pudding, Super Spuds, Super Muffins, and Super Soup—see appendix on pages 459–460 for recipes).
	Determine the degree of assistance the patient needs at mealtime and provide it. Have occupational therapy (OT) evaluate the patient for the use of adaptive equipment.
	Assess whether the patient is having meals in the correct dining area for their situation—from an independent situation to a supervised setting.
	Investigate whether the patient complains about the taste of foods—tasteless, metallic, etc.—or has a diminished sense of taste.
	Conduct a medication review to see whether this could be a cause.
	Encourage use of seasonings and condiments at meals as appropriate.
	Involve family and friends to encourage patient to eat or bring in favorite foods.
	Consider medications for PMD recommendation that stimulate appetite (for example, Remeron, Megace, or Periactin).
	Notify family and PMD of weight loss status.
	Review advance care directives (that is, feeding tube option).
	Don't:
	Don't ignore recording meal completion record.
	Don't ignore patient's food likes and dislikes.
	Don't skip weigh-ins. Don't ignore weight loss.
	Don't overly restrict diet. Encourage diet as orders tolerate.
	Don't ignore the possibility of the need to be fed.
	Don't hesitate to inform family of feeding options.

[a]IBW:
Male: 106 lbs for the first 60 inches of height + 6 lbs for each additional inch of height.
If the patient's height is less than 60 inches, subtract 3 lbs for each inch less than 60 inches.
Female: 100 lbs for the first 60 inches of height + 5 lbs for each additional inch of height.
If the patient's height is less than 60 inches, subtract 2.5 lbs for each inch less than 60 inches.

Convert pounds to kg (weight divided by 2.2).

[b]BEE: See energy equations.

[c]Physical activity factor: BEE × the following factor
Bedfast/bedrest = 1.2, Wheelchair/ambulatory = 1.3, Active = 1.5.

[d]Protein needs: kg of IBW × the following factor
Normal = 0.8–1.0 per kg
Decubitus = 1.2–1.5 per kg
Fracture/surgery = 1.0–2.0 per kg
Burns/multiple fractures = 2.0–2.5 per kg

[e]Fluid needs:
Weight in kg × 30 ml = daily fluid needs under normal metabolic conditions.

Sources

American Dietetic Association (ADA). *Liberalized Diets for Older Adults in Long-Term Care*. http://www.eatright.org/member/policyinitiatives/index_21039.cfm.

Initial Nutritional History–Assessment Form. Briggs Corporation. 1992.

New England Diet Manual for Extended Care. Boston, MA. 2003.

Robinson, G. E., Edge, M. S., Evans, W. J., & Morley, J. E. *Recent Advances in Managing Malnutrition and Weight Loss in the Elderly*. 2003.

Antianxiety Agents

Author: Mary Emerson, MS, RD, LD

This list will assist the dietitian in answering questions about common side effects encountered with medications prescribed in the treatment of anxiety disorders. One component of an anxiety disorder is either heightened or dampened response to thirst and hunger leading to either overeating or undereating. It is important that the dietitian assess lifestyle to determine if patient is overusing or avoiding food and beverages due to anxiety symptoms. Very often not eating throughout the day can heighten anxiety symptoms, and healthy meal patterning should be encouraged. Investigate the role of caffeine due to caffeine's effect in intensifying anxiety.

Problem	***Do's and Don'ts***
Jitteriness	**Do:** Assess daily caffeine intake. Look for all sources of caffeine, including soda, energy drinks, teas, etc. Realize that caffeine has a half-life of 5 hours and may intensify anxiety. Assess food intake structure—encourage healthy meal patterning. **Don't:** Don't allow patients to go more than 5 hours during the day without eating or more than 15 hours from night to morning without eating.
Weight Loss	**Do:** Evaluate current intake to ensure adequacy; if patient is anorexic or suffers from weight loss, encourage caloric density. Evaluate use of antianxiety agents for appetite-dampening effect.
Weight Gain	**Do:** Evaluate eating behaviors and if eating when emotional, suggest nutrition counseling. Encourage increasing low-calorie fluid intake. Suggest a food journal listing the foods eaten, time, and emotions at the time. This can be valuable in development of behavioral treatment plan. **Don't:** Don't encourage using food to soothe the patient.

Commonly used antianxiety drugs:
Lorazepam/Ativan
Diazepam/Valium
Alprazolam/Xanax
See the appendix on pages 309–319 for diet/drug interactions.

ADHD Medications

Author: Mary Emerson, MS, RD, LD

This list will assist the dietitian in answering questions about potential side effects of medications used to treat attention deficient hyperactivity disorder (ADHD). These medications are divided into groups based on their length of action. Typically taken once a day, long-acting stimulants (for example, Adderall XR, Concerta, Metadate CD, and Ritalin LA) last between 8–12 hours. The short-acting stimulants (for example, Ritalin, Ritalin SR, Metadate ER, Metadate CD, Methylin, Methylin ER, Focalin, Dexedrine, Dextrostat, and Adderall) range from 3–8 hours. The most common side effects of the stimulant medications are decreased appetite, weight loss, stomachaches, headaches, trouble getting to sleep, jitteriness, and social withdrawal. Manage these side effects by adjusting the dosage or time of day when the medication is given. Other side effects may occur in children on too high a dosage or those that are overly sensitive to stimulants, which might cause them to be overfocused while on the medication or appear dull or overly restricted. Another medication used for the treatment of ADHD is Strattera, which is not a stimulant and has not been shown to have the appetite-dampening effect.

If two or three stimulants do not work, the PMD may try second-line treatments, including tricyclic antidepressants (imipramine or desipramine) or bupropion (Wellbutrin). PMDs sometimes use clonidine for children who have ADHD and a coexisting condition.

Problem	*Do's and Don'ts*
Decreased Appetite and Weight Loss	**Do:**
	Give the medication with the meal rather than prior to the meal.
	Make sure that high-calorie items are offered to children if they are at risk of losing weight.
	Encourage healthy snacks, such as cereal and milk, energy bars, healthy shakes, etc. Encourage an evening snack when appetites are often maximized.
	Change dinnertime to a later time so the effects of the stimulant have worn off.
	Promote a consistent meal schedule.
	Monitor growth.
	Don't:
	Don't assume it is the medication only; children's appetites often vary due to changes in caloric needs with variations in growth.

Problem	*Do's and Don'ts*
Stomachaches	**Do:** Take with food.
Insomnia	**Do:** Establish a bedtime routine, including relaxation techniques. Avoid caffeine. Caffeine has a 5-hour half-life. Cocoa and many teas contain caffeine.
Jitteriness	**Do:** Avoid caffeine. Counsel with the client and/or family about caffeine content in many sodas and energy drinks that children consume.

Antidepressant Medications

Author: Mary Emerson, MS, RD, LD

This list will assist the dietitian in answering questions about potential side effects of antidepressant medications. Low appetite is a common component of anhedonia typically seen in major depressive disorder. Depression by itself takes a significant toll on nutritional status with diminished intake in most people. Antidepressant medications can be divided into different categories; each category has common side effects. Common goals of improving nutrition during treatment for depression are described in the following table:

Problem	***Do's and Don'ts***
(Category of Antidepressant)	
MAOIs (*Monoamine Oxidase Inhibitors*) *Parnate* *Nardil*	**Do:**
	Watch for side effects of MAOIs, including the following: decrease or increase in blood pressure, light-headedness, trouble sleeping, sleepiness, dry mouth, drowsiness, fainting, sexual dysfunction, weight gain, and reduced tolerance for alcohol.
	Encourage dietary adherence. If a severe reaction to food occurs, blood pressure may raise so high that it is life threatening, causing a hypertensive crisis. This extremely dangerous scenario has caused many deaths.
	Suggest lower-calorie meals and snacks if weight gain is a problem.
	If the patient eats prohibited foods or medications, recognize the signs of high blood pressure as stiff neck, headache, palpitations, chest pain, nausea or vomiting, flushing or chills, fear, pallor or sweating. *Caution:* Taking an MAOI requires that the patient adhere to a specific diet. Failure to do this can cause a heart attack, adverse reaction, or death.
	Tell patients that MAOIs react adversely with hundreds of other prescription medications. Make sure to obtain a list of these medications and have the patient avoid them.
	Don't:
	Don't allow the patient to consume all aged and fermented foods, cheeses (limited amounts of American may be okay), sour cream, yogurt, beef or chicken liver, tenderized meats, game meat, avocadoes, bananas, figs, raisins, soy sauce, fava beans, ginseng, Chianti wine, malt beverages.

Problem	*Do's and Don'ts*
Lithium Carbonate Carbolith, Cibalith-S, Duralith, Eskalith, Lithane, Lithizine, Lithobid, Lithonate, Lithotabs	**Do:** Maintain consistent fluid and sodium intake. Counsel the patient to salt food to taste to maintain consistent intake of daily salt and fluid. Encourage good oral hygiene. If experiencing dry mouth, encourage sugarless gum, moist foods, and low-calorie beverages. Monitor weight and adjust calories if weight gain occurs. Suggest small frequent feedings and fluid and electrolyte replacement if nausea and vomiting are a problem. Adjust fiber intake if diarrhea is an issue and monitor hydration. **Don't:** Don't over- or underhydrate. Lithium is a salt easily affected by the hydration balance of the body. It is important to have consistent intake of both fluids and salt from food when one is on lithium to help maintain a consistent level of lithium in the blood.
Tricyclics Amitryptyline Imipramine Nortriptyline Desipramine	**Do:** Reinforce measures for control for dry mouth: low-calorie fluids, moist foods, sugarless gum. Encourage adequate fluid intake and fiber (for example, beans, lentils, whole grains, legumes, and fresh fruits and vegetables). Reinforce healthy lifestyle measures to minimize weight gain.
SSRI (Selective Serotonin Reuptake Inhibitors) Fluoxetine Prozac Citalopram Celexa Sertraline Zoloft Paroxetine Paxil Fluvoxamine Luvox	**Do:** Advocate taking medication the same time every day. Counsel the patient about the role of healthy lifestyle habits, eating, exercise, and low-calorie fluids in their lives. **Don't:** Don't allow medications, such as St. John's Wort or SAM-e, to be taken with an SSRI.

SECTION 2

Problem	*Do's and Don'ts*
Bupropion *Wellbutrin*	**Do:** Reinforce techniques for dealing with dry mouth, such as low calorie fluids, sugarless gum, and use of moist foods.
Venlafaxine *Effexor*	**Do:** Monitor weight and medications. Encourage a healthy lifestyle to minimize weight gain.
Mirtazapine *Remeron*	**Do:** Emphasize importance of healthy eating, particularly fruits, vegetables, and diet or low-calorie beverages. Advise patients that while somnolence at the start of therapy may be "overwhelming," it usually lasts only 2–3 days. Monitor an increase in appetite and weight gain; however, this is time limited and should plateau after 2–3 months. Adjust calories accordingly.
Nefazodone *Serzone*	**Do:** Advise patients that the most common side effects—nausea, sedation, and dizziness—generally diminish after a week. Advise small frequent meals and sipping fluids.
Duloxetine *Cymbalta*	**Do:** Reinforce need for adequate fluid intake, as well as good fiber sources. Advise patients that the most common side effect is nausea. Recommend small frequent meals, low in fat. For most people, the nausea is mild to moderate and goes away within 1–2 weeks. Recommend moist foods, tart foods such as sugar-free lemonade, water with lemon, and sugarless gum if dry mouth is a problem. Recommend high-fiber foods (for example, whole-grain cereal, bread, fruits, and vegetables) for constipation. Suggest small frequent meals for decreased appetite. Advise patient that other side effects may include fatigue, sleepiness, and increased sweating. **Don't:** Don't serve spicy, high-fat foods; they may cause gastrointestinal distress.

Sources

Nursing 2004 Drug Handbook. Philadelphia, PA: Lippincott, Williams & Wilkins. 2004.

Walker, S. E., Shulman, K. I., Tailor, S. A. N., & Gardner, D. "Tyramine Content of Previously Restricted Foods in Monoamine Oxidase Inhibitor Diets." *J Clin Psychopharm*. 1996. 16(5), 383–388.

Common Issues with Mood Stabilizing Agents

Author: Mary Emerson, MS, RD, LD

This list will assist the dietitian in answering questions about common side effects encountered with the typical medications prescribed in the treatment of bipolar disease.

Problem	*Do's and Don'ts*
Medication Name	
Lithium Carbonate *Carbolith* *Cibalith-S* *Duralith* *Eskalith* *Lithane* *Lithizine* *Lithobid* *Lithonate* *Lithotabs*	**Do:** Maintain consistent fluid and sodium intake. Counsel the patient to salt food to taste to maintain consistent intake of daily salt and fluid. Encourage good oral hygiene. Encourage sugarless gum, moist foods, and low-calorie beverages for dry mouth. Monitor weight and adjust calories if weight gain occurs. Suggest small frequent feedings, fluid, and electrolyte replacement for nausea and vomiting. Adjust fiber intake if diarrhea is an issue and monitor hydration. **Don't:** Don't over- or underhydrate because this may lead to either lithium toxicity or dilution. A metallic taste is a sign of lithium toxicity. Don't provide high-fat foods.
Carbamazepine *Tegretol*	**Do:** Encourage adequate fluid intake. Be aware of moderate risk of weight gain, as well as diarrhea. See dietary suggestions previously listed. Advise patient that if constipation is a problem, increase fiber with foods (for example, whole-grain cereals, whole-grain bread, fruits, and vegetables). **Don't:** Don't give this medication with grapefruit juice.
Valproic Acid *Depacon* *Depakote*	**Do:** Give with food or milk to decrease GI symptoms. Monitor weight and adjust calories if weight gain occurs.

Problem	*Do's and Don'ts*
	Counsel the patient on dietary recommendations if nausea, vomiting, constipation, or diarrhea occur. (See section on pages 33 and 208 on nausea and vomiting on the pregnancy and cancer tables.) Do suggest small frequent meals, low in fat and spices, if heartburn becomes a problem.
Gabapentin *Neurontin*	**Do:** Be aware of risk of dizziness, nausea, and vomiting. (See section on pages 33 and 208 on nausea and vomiting in the pregnancy and cancer tables.) Encourage low-calorie beverages. Encourage tart beverages (for example, sugarless lemonade, lemon water, and citrus juices) if dry mouth occurs. Also, suggest moist food and sugarless gum. **Don't:** Don't use supplements or teas of chamomile, hops, kava, skullcap, and valerian.
Lamotrigine *Lamictal*	**Do:** Take recommended dose with or after meals to decrease adverse events, such as nausea, vomiting, and abdominal pain. (See section on pages 33 and 208 on nausea and vomiting in the pregnancy and cancer tables.)
Topiramate *Topamax*	**Do:** Take with food. Encourage patients who experience undesired weight loss to eat high-calorie snacks (for example, nuts, seeds, sandwiches, milkshakes, granola, and cheese and crackers); also maximize caloric content of foods and beverages by encouraging use of butter/margarine on foods, peanut butter on toast, shredded cheese on potatoes and vegetables, and by emphasizing caloric beverages over low-calorie beverages. Provide dietary advice if nausea, diarrhea, constipation, or dry mouth occur. (See section on pages 33 and 208 on nausea and vomiting in the pregnancy and cancer tables.) **Don't:** Don't encourage high-calorie foods if prescribed for binge eating disorder.

Sources

Nursing 2004 Drug Handbook. Philadelphia, PA: Lippincott, Williams & Wilkins. 2004.

Hasrallah, H. A., & Korn, M. L. "Metabolic Issues in the Management of Bipolar Disorder: Focus on Weight Gain." *Medscape*. August 31, 2005.

Abbott Laboratories. Depakote. http://www.abbott.com.

Ortho-McNeil. Neurologics. http://www.ortho-mcneil.com.

Antipsychotic Drugs and Diet Interaction

Author: Mary Emerson, MS, RD, LD

This list will assist the dietitian in answering questions about potential side effects of antipsychotic medications.

Antipsychotics are divided into the older medications used to treat schizophrenia, known as the typical antipsychotics (for example, Haldol, Mellaril, Thorazine, and Stelazine). The newer line of "atypical" antipsychotic medications are known to be equally effective in treating psychotic disorders but with a lower incidence of negative symptoms, such as anhedonia, withdrawal/lack of energy, and lower risk of extra-pyramidal side effects of involuntary movements (EPS). There is some experimentation with treating EPS with high-dose vitamin E; however, this is still in the experimental stages.

The atypical antipsychotic medications (for example, Clozaril or clonazepine, Zyprexa or olanzapine, Risperdal or risperidone, Seroquel or quetiapine, Abilify or aripiprazole, and Geodon or ziprasidone) are more prone toward weight gain (listed in descending order of tendency toward weight gain). The most common side effects of the antipsychotics include dry mouth, weight gain, photosensitivity, and constipation. Other side effects that are less common include diarrhea, nausea, headache, weakness, and sleeplessness. Patients are encouraged to avoid alcohol while taking any of the atypical antipsychotics. Another important concern with the atypical antipsychotics is the potential for metabolic syndrome (centralized obesity, insulin resistance, atherogenic dyslipidemia, and raised blood pressure). It is important to screen patients for several risk factors (for example, elevated blood pressure, abnormal lipid panel, elevated fasting blood glucose, elevated BMI, smoking, and a family history of cardiovascular disease) and discuss positive lifestyle changes to lower risk.

SECTION 2

Problem	***Do's and Don'ts***
Dry Mouth	**Do:**
	Encourage adequate water or noncaloric beverage intake. Not treating dry mouth can cause the patient to consume greater amounts of foods and caloric beverages than needed, leading to weight gain.
	Suggest use of sugarless gum.
	Encourage moist foods, such as fruits, casseroles, etc.
	Encourage tart foods, such as sugar-free lemonade, lemon water, and citrus fruits.
	Don't:
	Don't serve regular soda on a daily basis; this can lead to undesired weight gain.

Problem	*Do's and Don'ts*
Weight Gain	**Do:** Advise patients that certain drugs may increase tendency toward weight gain. It is important to evaluate the appetite-stimulating effect of any new medication early in the course of treatment to halt weight gain. Olanzapine tends to cause weight gain early in the course of treatment, with half of all weight gain occurring in the first 6 weeks and the second half occurring from 6 weeks to 6 months of treatment. Abilify has the lowest incidence of weight gain. Evaluate beverage consumption. Evaluate feelings of satiety. Discuss normal portions of food. Encourage consumption of low-calorie foods, such as nutrient-rich fruits and vegetables. Suggest use of frozen vegetables and fruits, as well as produce on special at the grocery store. Suggest that the patient drink a large glass of water prior to each meal to increase satiety effect with the meal. Increase fiber in the diet to increase satiety. Have client utilize relaxation techniques to slow down food consumption at mealtimes. Encourage family members who are involved in meal preparation to join in developing an intervention plan. See the table on weight control on page 42. **Don't:** Don't assume if the client has gained weight the medication needs to be changed. First, find out what the client is drinking and eating, and then make modifications as needed to achieve weight stabilization. Don't assume the client will feel full at the end of a meal; many times the feelings of satiety are diminished. Don't use negative words such as "Don't eat ice cream." Emphasize what the client should eat more of instead. Don't say "diet." Discuss instead a lifestyle change. Don't set unrealistic goals for weight loss. Aim for 10% and break that down to more meaningful amounts.
Constipation	**Do:** Advise patient that drug therapy may cause constipation due to inadequate fluid or food intake. If the patient suffers

Problem	*Do's and Don'ts*
	from constipation, try increasing the amount of fluid intake if medically appropriate. Recommend hot beverages. Suggest high-fiber foods (for example, raw fruits and vegetables—especially with the skins—whole-wheat bread, cereals, and dried fruits). Add unprocessed bran to casseroles and other foods normally eaten. Encourage movement or light exercise when possible to induce bowel movements. Emphasize positive benefits of exercise in stress management. **Don't:** Don't use laxatives, unless under the supervision of the PMD.
Nausea	**Do:** Nausea may occur for 2–3 days. Encourage small, frequent meals using blander foods. Contact healthcare provider if it continues more than 3 days. Avoid strong odors. **Don't:** Don't serve high-fat foods.
Diarrhea	**Do:** Advise patient that diarrhea may be transient, lasting less than 1 week. Contact PMD if it continues more than 1 week. Encourage the patient to avoid milk in quantities greater than four ounces and to consume more-binding foods (for example, bananas, rice, applesauce, and yogurt). **Don't:** Don't allow sugar-free hard candy containing sorbitol, which can cause diarrhea.
Sleeplessness	**Do:** Help the patient establish a sleep/wake cycle and stay active during the day. Establish a quiet sleep area. Caffeine-containing beverages should be avoided for 10 hours prior to sleeping. This includes regular tea, coffee, and caffeinated soda. **Don't:** Don't suggest daytime naps.

Chronic Renal Insufficiency

Author: Sandra Allonen, MEd, RD, LDN

This list will assist the dietitian in answering nutrition questions and serve as a guide to assist patients who have chronic renal insufficiency (CRI). Unlike acute renal failure (ARF), which develops quickly and is usually reversible, chronic renal failure (CRF) is slow progressing, gradually destroying kidney function. It may be caused by several reasons, such as diabetes, hypertension, polycystic kidney disease, lupus, HIV/AIDS, illicit drug use, IgA neuropathy, renal calculi, and obstructions of the urinary tract, to name a few. The disease advancement will differ between individuals. However, certain medications, as well as nutrition and lifestyle interventions, may help slow the progression of CRI. Some of the symptoms are similar to those patients on dialysis (especially as the disease progresses).

Problem	*Do's and Don'ts*
Nausea—Especially as Blood Urea Nitrogen (BUN) Levels Begin to Rise	**Do:**
	Have patients eat small meals more frequently.
	Drink small amounts of liquids throughout the day.
	Eat or drink when least nauseous.
	Eat foods low in fat (for example, sherbet, Popsicles, vanilla wafers, graham crackers, angel food cake, toast, cold foods), canned low-potassium fruits (for example, applesauce, blueberries, and canned pears), renal supplements (Nepro), or protein foods (for example, roasted skinless chicken, turkey). See Appendix FF on pages 446–457.
	Advise CRI patients that they may need to limit their protein to 0.6–0.8 grams per kg of body weight per day.
	Try chilled beverages.
	Don't:
	Don't serve foods that are high in potassium (that is, avocados, bananas, dried fruits, kiwi, melons, oranges, pomegranates, artichokes, dried peas and beans, beets, mushrooms, parsnips, rutabagas, potatoes, sweet potatoes, spinach, tomatoes and tomato products, winter squash, wax beans, chocolate and chocolate candy, bran cereals—Bran Flakes, Raisin Bran—All Bran, Bran Buds, Bran Chex, Raisin Nut Bran, and any other bran cereal or bran product (such as bran muffins). See Appendix FF on pages 446–457. Evaluate patient's lab values to make this assessment.
	Don't allow salt substitutes, low-sodium baking powder, Brewer's yeast, wheat bran, or wheat germ.

Problem	*Do's and Don'ts*
	Don't provide nuts (that is, almonds, pistachios, chestnuts, peanuts, cashews, pecans, walnuts, pine nuts, soy nuts, hazelnuts, and macadamia nuts). Don't serve beverages that are high in potassium and phosphorus (that is, apricot nectar, guava juice, orange juice, papaya juice, passion fruit juice, prune juice, tangerine juice, and tomato juice). Don't serve foods that are high in phosphorus because they may need to be avoided, depending on patient's lab values. Foods to avoid include: milk and other dairy products like cheese and ice cream, nuts, seeds, peanut butter, whole grains, and cola beverages; beverages that are high in phosphorus including cola beverages, milk and any beverages made from milk or milk products, such as frappes, milkshakes, and smoothies. Don't suggest fried foods. Don't serve hot beverages; they may not be well tolerated.
Vomiting	**Do:** Report repeated vomiting to the PMD. When vomiting is under control, try small amounts of clear liquids before moving on to solid food. Clear liquids include flat soda, water, broth, gelatin, juices without pulp, decaffeinated tea, decaffeinated coffee, and fruit ice. Patients may graduate to cold solid foods after a short time on clear liquids. **Don't:** Don't maintain patients on clear liquids for more than a day, unless directed by the PMD. Don't serve solid food until vomiting has subsided. Don't allow foods or beverages high in potassium and phosphorus. This would include coffee, both brewed and instant, cola beverage—both regular and sugar-free—Mountain Dew, tea, and chocolate—especially semisweet.
Diarrhea	**Do:** Avoid fatty and fried foods, raw fruit, and vegetables. Foods and beverages that are high in potassium and phosphorus may need to be avoided, depending on patient's lab values. See Appendix FF on pages 446–457. **Don't:** Don't allow excessive fluid intake.

Problem	*Do's and Don'ts*
Weight Gain Due to Edema	**Do:** Limit intake of fluids and food that are liquid at room temperature (that is, gelatin, Popsicles, soups, broths, fruit ices) between treatments. Limit sodium intake. Use low-salt foods. **Don't:** Don't allow excessive fluid intake. Don't provide foods high in salt and sodium, which may cause excessive thirst. These foods include: bacon, bologna, cold cuts, chipped beef, corned beef, franks, ham, salt pork, canned, smoked, and salted meats, bouillon, canned soups, frozen soups, frozen dinners, salted snack foods (potato chips, pretzels, and others), and seasonings such as salt, ketchup, celery salt, garlic salt, onion salt, chili sauce, monosodium glutamate, olives, pickles, mustard, soy sauce, and steak sauces.
Weight Gain from Excessive Caloric Intake	**Do:** Restrict caloric intake, making sure to provide the appropriate amount of protein in diet. CRI patients need to consume between 0.6–0.8 grams of protein per kg of body weight per day. **Don't:** Don't provide high-protein diets.
Muscle Wasting	**Do:** Recommend high biological value protein foods such as beef, veal, lamb, pork, fish, poultry, eggs, and renal supplements. Muscle wasting may occur if appetite becomes diminished. **Don't:** Don't advocate low biological protein foods, such as legumes, peas, nuts, and peanut butter. Don't serve dairy products, which are high in phosphorus and possibly sodium (food sources of both are previously listed).
Pruritis	**Do:** Serve foods and beverages that are low in phosphorus. Pruritis may be caused by excessive phosphorus intake. As kidney function declines, the kidneys' ability to excrete excess phosphorus diminishes. Take phosphorus binders with meals and snacks.

Problem	*Do's and Don'ts*
	Don't: Don't allow foods and beverages high in phosphorus. (See list earlier on page 145.) Don't let patients forget to take binders with meals and snacks.
Constipation	**Do:** Ease constipation by increasing fiber intake through soluble fiber laxatives like Metamucil or Benefiber, increasing fruits and vegetable intake (either raw or lightly cooked), and getting adequate hydration. **Don't:** Don't serve fruit and vegetables high in potassium, depending on patient's lab values. (See the preceding list on page 145.) Don't give excessive fluid intake if patient is edematous. Don't suggest certain whole-grain foods, such as wheat bran, wheat germ, and whole-wheat products. These foods are high in phosphorus and may need to be avoided, depending on patient's lab values.
Weight Loss	**Do:** Provide foods that are high in calories. Such foods also should be offered to avoid weight loss as kidney function decreases because of rising BUN levels (diminished appetite, excessive fatigue, dysgeusia). Add butter and margarine to soups, grits, rice, noodles, and cooked vegetables. Combine butter with herbs and spices to add to cooked meats, fish, and egg dishes. Use melted butter as a dip for cooked seafood. Add sherbet to renal supplements. Prepare foods ahead of time so that patient can easily reheat foods during periods of fatigue. **Don't:** Don't serve foods and beverages that are high in potassium and phosphorus. (See preceding list on page 145.)
Dysgeusia	**Do:** Limit the amount of protein that a patient consumes because it may help slow down a rising BUN level. Have the patient rinse his or her mouth frequently with water to remove any bad taste.

Problem	*Do's and Don'ts*
Dysgeusia	**Don't:** Don't provide high-protein diets.
Hypoglycemia	**Do:** Offer carbohydrate-rich foods or beverages that are rapidly absorbed, such as hard candies, glucose tablets, sugar-sweetened sodas, apple juice, cranberry juice, fruit punches. As kidney function decreases, insulin is not excreted as well, requiring the blood sugar levels to be checked more regularly. **Don't:** Don't serve foods and beverages that are high in phosphorus, such as cola beverages and sweetened dairy products like milkshakes and smoothies. They may need to be avoided depending on patient's lab values. Don't provide foods and beverages that are high in potassium, such as bananas, melons, oranges, tangerines, orange juice, and tangerine juice, depending on patient's lab values.

Sources

Manual of Clinical Dietetics. Chicago, IL: American Dietetic Association. 2005.

Mahon, L. K., & Escott-Stump, S. *Krause's Food, Nutrition, and Diet Therapy*. (11th ed.). Philadelphia, PA: W.B. Saunders Co. 2004.

2004 Physicians' Desk Reference. Montvale, NJ: Thomson Healthcare Co. 2004.

Pocket Guide to Nutritional Assessment of the Patient with Chronic Kidney Disease. (3rd ed.). New York: National Kidney Foundation.

http://www.kidney.org.

http://www.ikidney.com.

Table 2-5 Renal Medications Often Administered to Patients with CRI

Medication	Action
Phosphorus binders Include: Calcium acetate—PhosLo Calcium carbonate—Tums Lanthanum carbonate—Fosrenol	Phosphorus binders bind with the phosphorus in consumed foods and are eliminated through the large intestines.
Sevelamer hydrochloride–Renagel	Take with meals.
Vitamin D analogs Include: Calcitriol–Rocaltrol	Administer vitamin D analogs either orally or intravenously (IV). CRI patients receive these medications orally. Give them to help maintain bone health and suppress secondary hyperparathyroidism.
Parathyroid hormone (PTH) suppressor Includes: Cinacalet hydrochloride—Sensipar	Cinacalet hydrochloride suppresses secondary hyperparathyroidism by lowering the PTH produced by the parathyroid gland. This may help to prevent bone loss and calcification of soft tissues.
Anemia management Include: Epoetin alfa—Epogen Darbepoetin alfa—Aranesp	Give recombinant human erythropoietin, administered through IV, to dialysis patients to stimulate the red cell production.

Patients are usually prescribed a renal multivitamin supplement, such as Nephrocaps or Nephrovites. These supplements contain vitamin B complex and vitamin C. They do not contain any fat-soluble vitamins or minerals because of the possibility of these compounds having a nephrotoxic effect on the kidneys.

End Stage Renal Disease with Dialysis

Author: Sandra Allonen, MEd, RD, LDN

This list will assist the dietitian in answering nutrition questions and serve as a guide to assist patients who are undergoing dialysis, both hemo- and peritoneal. Some of the side effects of dialysis are nausea, vomiting, diarrhea, weight gain, muscle wasting, pruritis, dry mouth, constipation, weight loss, and dysgeusia.

Problem	***Do's and Don'ts***
Nausea	**Do:**
	Provide small meals more frequently.
	Suggest small amounts of liquids throughout day.
	Recommend that the patient eat or drink when least nauseous.
	Serve foods low in fat (for example, sherbet, Popsicles, vanilla wafers, graham crackers, angel food cake, toast, cold foods), canned low-potassium fruits (for example, applesauce, blueberries, and canned pears), renal supplements (Nepro), or protein foods (for example, roasted skinless chicken or turkey).
	Try chilled beverages. Avoid hot beverages, which may not be well tolerated.
	Don't:
	Don't provide foods high in potassium. Foods to avoid include: avocados, bananas, dried fruits, kiwi, melons, oranges, pomegranates, artichokes, dried peas and beans, beets, mushrooms, parsnips, rutabagas, potatoes, sweet potatoes, spinach, tomatoes and tomato products, winter squash, and wax beans. Other foods that are high in potassium include chocolate and chocolate candy, bran cereals, including Bran Flakes, Raisin Bran, All Bran, Bran Buds, Bran Chex, Raisin Nut Bran, and any other bran cereal or bran product, such as bran muffins.
	Don't serve salt substitutes, low-sodium baking powder, Brewer's yeast, wheat bran, or wheat germ.
	Don't provide nuts (that is, almonds, pistachios, chestnuts, peanuts, cashews, pecans, walnuts, pine nuts, soy nuts, hazelnuts, and macadamia nuts).
	Don't serve foods high in phosphorus. Foods to avoid include: milk and other dairy products like cheese and ice cream, nuts, seeds, peanut butter, whole grains, and cola beverages.

Problem	*Do's and Don'ts*
	Don't suggest foods high in phosphorus. Foods to avoid include: milk and other dairy products like cheese and ice cream, nuts, seeds, peanut butter, and whole grains. Beverages that are high in phosphorus include cola beverages, milk and any beverages made from milk or milk products, such as frappes, milkshakes, and smoothies. Don't recommend beverages that are high in potassium and phosphorus. Beverages high in potassium include apricot nectar, guava juice, orange juice, papaya juice, passion fruit juice, prune juice, tangerine juice, and tomato juice. Don't serve fried foods or those high in potassium or phosphorus. (See preceding list of foods to avoid on page 145.) Don't allow prolonged time on clear liquids. (See preceding list of clear liquids on page 145.) Don't serve caffeine (coffee, most teas, and soft drinks).
Vomiting	**Do:** Report repeated vomiting to the PMD. When vomiting is under control, try small amounts of clear liquids before moving on to solid food. Clear liquids include flat soda, water, broth, gelatin, juices without pulp, decaffeinated tea, decaffeinated coffee, and fruit ice. Patients may graduate to cold solid foods after a short time on clear liquids. Do not maintain clear liquids for more than a day unless directed by the PMD. **Don't:** Don't recommend foods or beverages high in potassium and phosphorus, which are listed earlier.
Diarrhea	**Do:** Advise patient that diarrhea causes both the malabsorption of food and electrolyte loss. Some renal medications and binders may cause diarrhea. The diet used for diarrhea is similar to that found in the vomiting section. Advance the diet to soft, low-fiber foods as the diarrhea subsides. Low-fiber foods include baked fish and chicken, ground beef, eggs, pureed low-potassium vegetables (such as frozen green beans), canned low-potassium fruit (such as applesauce and pears), rice, and white bread. Have the patient drink clear fluids.

Problem	*Do's and Don'ts*
Diarrhea	**Don't:** Don't serve fatty and fried foods, raw fruit, and vegetables. Don't provide foods and beverages high in potassium and phosphorus. See foods in the nausea section of this table on page 150.
Weight Gain Between Treatments	**Do:** Limit fluid and foods that are liquid at room temperature (gelatin, Popsicles, soups, broths, fruit ices) between treatments because the kidneys are no longer functioning normally. Limit sodium intake (see page 461). Use low-salt foods. **Don't:** Don't provide excessive fluids. Don't serve foods high in salt and sodium that may cause excessive thirst. These foods include: bacon, bologna, cold cuts, chipped beef, corned beef, franks, ham, salt pork, canned, smoked, and salted meats, bouillon, canned soups, frozen soups, frozen dinners, salted snack foods (potato chips, pretzels, and others); seasonings such as salt, ketchup, celery salt, garlic salt, onion salt, chili sauce, monosodium glutamate, olives, pickles, mustard, soy sauce, and steak sauces.
Weight Gain from Excessive Caloric Intake	**Do:** Restrict caloric intake, making sure to provide ample protein in diet (1.0–1.4 grams per kilogram of body weight determined by the PMD). **Don't:** Don't provide low-protein diets.
Muscle Wasting	**Do:** Advocate high biological value protein foods (for example, beef, veal, lamb, pork, fish, poultry, eggs), and renal supplements (Nepro). Diminished appetite could cause muscle wasting. **Don't:** Don't serve low biological value foods (for example, legumes, peas, nuts, and peanut butter).

Problem	*Do's and Don'ts*
	Don't serve dairy products that are high in phosphorus and possibly sodium.
Pruritis	**Do:**
	Advise patient that excessive phosphorus intake may cause pruritis.
	Provide foods and beverages that are low in phosphorus.
	Give phosphorus binders with meals and snacks.
	Don't:
	Don't serve foods and beverages high in phosphorus. (See foods in the nausea section of this table on page 150.)
	Don't forget to give binders with meals and snacks.
Dry Mouth	**Do:**
	Advise patient that with a limited fluid intake, patients often experience symptoms of dry mouth. Some suggestions to help better cope with dry mouth and not exceed their daily fluid allowance are: • Spray the patient's mouth with a water mister or spray bottle. • Provide hard candies (especially sour ones) or gum (regular). • Try ice chips. • Use low-sodium sauces, gravies, and dressing to moisten foods.
	Don't:
	Don't give excessive fluids.
	Don't provide fluids high in potassium and phosphorus.
	Don't buy sugarless products containing sugar alcohols (mannitol and sorbitol especially). These foods may cause bloating, flatulence, and diarrhea if eaten in large quantities. Included are sugar-free candies, chewing gums, frozen desserts, and baked goods.
Constipation	**Do:**
	Advise patient that some renal medications, phosphorus binders, restricted fluid intake, and a low-fiber diet may cause constipation.
	Ease constipation by increasing fiber intake through soluble fiber laxatives (Metamucil or Benefiber), increasing low-potassium fruit and vegetable intake (either raw or

Problem	*Do's and Don'ts*
Constipation	lightly cooked), and getting adequate hydration without exceeding fluid restrictions. **Don't:** Don't serve fruits and vegetables that are high in potassium. Don't give excessive fluids. Don't provide certain whole-grain foods, such as wheat bran, wheat germ, and whole-wheat products. These foods are high in phosphorus. (See foods in the nausea section of this table on page 150.)
Weight Loss	**Do:** Avoid patient weight loss while he or she is undergoing dialysis, which may cause diminished appetite and/or excessive fatigue. Offer foods that are high in calories and protein (for example, sauces, custards, puddings made with nondairy creamer). Modifications that can be made follow: • Add butter/margarine to soups, grits, rice, noodles, and cooked vegetables. Combine butter with herbs and spices to add to cooked meats, fish, and egg dishes. Use melted butter as a dip for cooked seafood. • Add eggs to casseroles, soups, and sauce to increase protein content. • Add whey or egg protein powder to casseroles, custards, gravies, puddings, sauces, soups. • Add sherbet to renal supplements. • Prepare foods ahead of time so that the patient can easily reheat foods during periods of fatigue. **Don't:** Don't give foods and beverages that are high in potassium and phosphorus. (See foods in the nausea section of this table on page 150.)
Dysgeusia	**Do:** Advise the patient that often when dialysis is first initiated, he or she may experience dysgeusia. An elevated level of BUN causes dysgeusia and usually dissipates as the treatment progresses. Some of the following suggestions may help, depending on how the individual's taste has been affected: • Offer bland foods (for example, rice, white toast, applesauce, or custard made with nondairy creamer).

Problem	*Do's and Don'ts*
	• Select cold-temperature foods (for example, gelatin, lemon pie, or sherbet). • Select foods that smell appealing to the patient. • Marinate meats in a small amount of fruit juice or sweet and sour sauces. • Use low-sodium seasonings, such as herbs or Mrs. Dash. • Rinse mouth out frequently with water to remove any bad taste. **Don't:** Don't provide foods that are salty or spicy. Some higher-sodium foods include: • Bacon, bologna, cold cuts, chipped beef, corned beef, franks, ham, salt pork, canned, smoked, and salted meats • Bouillon, canned soups, frozen soups, frozen dinners, salted snack foods (potato chips, pretzels, and others) • Seasonings such as salt, ketchup, celery salt, garlic salt, onion salt, chili sauce, monosodium glutamate, olives, pickles, mustard, soy sauce, and steak sauces Spicy foods include chili peppers, hot pepper sauces, black pepper, crushed pepper, cinnamon, ginger, and foods made from these ingredients. Don't cook foods with strong odors (for example, some meats, fish, and members of the cabbage family). Don't provide foods high in potassium and phosphorus. (See foods in the nausea section of this table on page 150.)
Hypoglycemia	**Do:** Advise patient that insulin is not excreted as well when kidney function decreases, requiring the blood sugar levels to be checked more regularly. Offer rich carbohydrate foods or beverages that are rapidly absorbed (for example, hard candies, glucose tablets, sugar-sweetened sodas, apple juice, cranberry juice, and fruit punches). **Don't:** Don't serve foods and beverages that are high in phosphorus, such as cola beverages and sweetened dairy products such as milkshakes and smoothies. Don't provide foods and beverages that are high in potassium (for example, bananas, melons, oranges, tangerines, orange juice, and tangerine juice).

Sources

Manual of Clinical Dietetics. Chicago, IL: American Dietetic Association. 2005.

Mahon, L. K., & Escott-Stump, S. *Krause's Food, Nutrition, and Diet Therapy*. (11th ed.). Philadelphia, PA: W.B. Saunders Co. 2003.

2004 Physicians' Desk Reference. Montvale, NJ: Thomson Healthcare Co. 2004.

National Kidney Foundation. *Pocket Guide to Nutritional Assessment of the Patient with Chronic Kidney Disease*. (3rd ed.). New York, NY.

http://www.kidney.org.

http://www.ikidney.com.

Table 2-6 Renal Laboratory Values

	Adult	Pediatric
BUN	Pre 21–101 Post 6–20 mg/dl	Pre 19–101 Post 5–18 mg/dl
Creatinine	2.5–14.2 mg/dl	0.3–0.7 mg/dl
Potassium	3.5–5.0 mEq/L	3.5–5.0 mEq/L
Sodium	135–145 mEq/L	135–145 mEq/L
CO_2	20–30 mEq/L	0.22 mEq/L
Calcium	8.4–10.2 mg/dl	8.4–10.2 mg/dl
Phosphorus	3.5–5.5 mg/dl	4.5–6.5 mg/dl
Calcium/phosphorus product	22–55 calculated	22–55 calculated
Alkaline phosphatase	47–265 U/L	65–210 U/L
PTH (3rd generation)	75–150 pgm/L	75–150 pgm/L
Albumin	3.5–5.0 gm/dl	4–5.9 gm/dl

Remember, these ranges may vary in different facilities depending on the particular samples.

Table 2-7 Renal Medications Often Administered to Patients on Dialysis

Medication	Action
Phosphorus binders Include: Calcium acetate—PhosLo Calcium carbonate–Tums Lanthanum carbonate—Fosrenol Sevelamer hydrochloride—Renagel	Phosphorus binders bind with the phosphorus in the foods and are eliminated through the large intestines. Take with meals.
Vitamin D analogs Include: Calcitriol injection—Calcijex Paracalcitriol injection—Zemplar Doxercalciferol—Hectorol	Administer vitamin D analogs either orally or intravenously (IV). Dialysis patients receive these medications through IV. Give them to help maintain bone health and suppress secondary hyperparathyroidism.
Parathyroid Hormone (PTH) suppressor Includes: Cinacalet hydrochloride—Sensipar	Cinacalet hydrochloride suppresses secondary hyperparathyroidism by lowering the PTH produced by the parathyroid gland. This may help to prevent bone loss and calcification of soft tissues.
Anemia management Include: Epoetin alfa—Epogen or Procrit	Give recombinant human erythropoietin, administered through IV, to dialysis patients to stimulate the red cell production.
Iron dextrans Include: Sodium ferric gluconate complex—Ferrlecit Iron saccharate—Venofer	Give iron dextrans to help maintain the body's iron stores.

Patients are usually prescribed a renal multivitamin supplement such as Nephrocaps or Nephrovites. These supplements contain vitamin B complex and vitamin C. They do not contain any fat-soluble vitamins or minerals because of the possibility of these compounds having a nephrotoxic effect on the kidneys.

Weight Management

Author: Deborah Shields, MS, RD, LDN

This section will assist the dietitian in providing information on weight loss to overweight and obese patients.

Problem	*Do's and Don'ts*
Overweight or Obesity	**Do:**
	Assess the patient's readiness for weight loss.
	Advise the patient that long-term weight loss usually requires gradual lifestyle changes of diet and increasing exercise.
	Decrease calorie intake gradually while choosing nutrient-dense foods. Reduce caloric intake by substituting healthier food choices for higher calorie items, reducing intake of added sugars, fats, and alcohol, reducing portion sizes, and increasing exercise.
	Begin regular activity. Aim for 30–60 minutes of moderate- to vigorous-intensity exercise most days of the week. Try enjoyable activities. Include more cardiovascular exercise to help burn calories. Exercises for flexibility and strength training are also important to help maintain/increase muscle mass and to prevent injury.
	Encourage a balanced diet, which includes three meals per day and a variety of nutrient-dense foods and beverages from each food group. Nutrient-dense foods include foods high in vitamins and minerals and low in calories (for example, vegetables, fruits, whole grains, low-sodium, broth-based soups, and low-fat versions of foods without added sugar or salt).
	Recommend six to eight 8-ounce glasses of water each day. For other beverages, select skim or 1% milk and diet drinks instead of regular soda, juice, or alcohol.
	Suggest a variety of fruits and vegetables, aiming for approximately 2 cups of fruit and 2.5 cups of vegetables every day. Choose fruit over fruit juices. Include more nonstarchy dark green and orange vegetables and legumes. Nonstarchy vegetables are very low in calories if not prepared with a lot of fat.
	Advocate a variety of grains daily and focus on eating more whole grains. Approximately 50% or more of the daily intake should include whole grains, such as whole-wheat bread, whole-grain cereal, oatmeal, whole-wheat pasta, or

Problem	*Do's and Don'ts*
	brown rice. Look for the first ingredient on the food label to say 100% whole grain. Help the patient select nonfat or low-fat dairy products and aim for about 3 cups per day. Include skim or 1% milk, nonfat/low-fat yogurt, and non-fat/low-fat cheeses. Total fat should comprise between 20–35% of calories: • Decrease the amount of saturated and trans fat in the diet. Mainly found in animal products, saturated fat should be less than 10% of total calories. Found in many processed foods, trans fats are indicated by the term "partially hydrogenated" oil on the ingredient list. • Aim for the majority of fats in the diet to come from monounsaturated or polyunsaturated sources (for example, fish, vegetable oils, and nuts). However, watch the portion sizes because these items are still high in calories. • When selecting protein sources, aim for more fish, skinless chicken breasts, lean cuts of meat (loin, round, and chuck), egg whites, and beans. Beans and legumes are also a good source of fiber. • Trim the fat off meat and use seasonings and herbs for flavor, instead of gravies, cream sauces, butter, or salt. • Bake, broil, grill, roast, steam, or poach instead of frying or sautéing in large amounts of oil. • Use low-fat products instead of the full-fat counterparts for items like sauces, mayonnaise, salad dressings, and cheese. Decrease patient portion sizes. For lunch and/or dinner follow these guidelines: 1/2 plate = nonstarchy vegetables, 1/4 plate = lean protein, and 1/4 plate = starch, and then round the meal out with a piece of fruit and a low-calorie beverage such as skim or 1% milk. Recommend a decrease in the frequency of eating out. Encourage smaller portion sizes at restaurants and choosing cooking methods that contain less fat, like grilling, broiling, poaching, and steaming. Place dressings and sauces on the side. Suggest substitutions for high-fat items with lower-fat items, such as steamed vegetables instead of french fries. Ask the patient to create more structure around meals and plan ahead. They should tune into their body and become

Problem	*Do's and Don'ts*
Overweight or Obesity	aware of internal cues of physical hunger instead of external hunger. Eating should be done in a relaxed environment. Take 25–30 minutes to eat meals to allow the body to register being full. Filling up on lower calorie items at the beginning of a meal, such as a tossed salad or broth-based soup, is a good idea. **Don't:** Don't promote quick fixes or short-term diets because this usually leads to regaining of the weight when the program is stopped. Don't restrict caloric intake below 1200 calories per day without medical supervision. It is difficult to obtain adequate nutrition much below this calorie amount. Don't have the patient spend most of the day sitting. Don't allow the patient to skip meals; this can lead to overeating. Don't allow beverages high in calories, sugar, and even fat. Don't prepare vegetables with lots of fat. Instead, serve them raw, steamed, or sautéed in less than 1 tsp of oil. Don't serve unrefined grains (for example, white bread, bagels, sugar cereals, chips, and baked goods). Don't serve high-fat meats, such as bacon, ribs, sausages, and salami. Don't serve cream, butter, high-fat cheeses, whole or 2% milk, ice cream, cotton and palm oils, and many baked goods. Don't serve fried foods, stick margarines, and baked or other products containing trans fats. Don't recommend eating at a restaurant or party when overly hungry. Don't grocery shop when overly hungry. This can make it harder to make healthy food choices and may lead to overeating.

Source

Dietary Guidelines for Americans 2005. http://www.health.gov/dietaryguidelines/dga2005/document/html/executivesummary.htm.

SECTION 3

Childhood Nutrition

Chronic Nutrition Care Problems

Overweight/Obese in Children and Adolescents (Ages 2–20) . . . 162
Type 1 Diabetes in Childhood . . . 169
Type 2 Diabetes in Childhood . . . 181

SECTION 3

Overweight/Obese in Children and Adolescents (Ages 2–20)

Author: Michael Mansueto Leidig, RD, LDN

Similar to other pediatric medical issues, weight loss in children and teens is a specialty. With the rise in pediatric obesity, dietitians are increasingly asked to provide compassionate and sound care to overweight patients. Quite often, weight-loss-related issues pertain to more than food alone. Therefore, to effectively address weight loss with children/teens, a comprehensive approach is required. This list provides dietitians with information organized in the following five categories: counseling, food, physical activity, behavioral concerns, and the emotional aspects of weight loss. The suggestions in the counseling category are more clinically oriented. The remaining categories, from food to emotional aspects, are framed as suggestions for the child/teen and/or the parent, guardian, or caregiver.

Problem	*Do's and Don'ts*
Counseling	**Do:**
	Calculate BMI for children and teens using the following formula: $\frac{\text{Weight (kg)}}{\text{Height (m)}^2}$
	Plot BMI annually for children ages 2 to 20 using age- and gender-appropriate growth charts available in the appendix on page 376. Identify patients with BMI percentile greater than or equal to the 85th to less than the 95th as "at risk for overweight" and those with BMI percentile greater than 95th as "overweight."
	Discuss any upward shifts in BMI percentile with parents, guardians, or caregivers to understand potential causes and formulate a treatment plan with the healthcare team.
	Begin the PMD's sanctioned treatment immediately for children older than 2 years of age that are overweight or at risk of overweight.
	Assess "readiness" by asking, "How important is it to you to lose weight right now on a scale of 1 to 10, with 1 being not at all important and 10 being very important?" If the answer is less than 7, then now might not be the right time to begin weight-loss counseling.

Problem	*Do's and Don'ts*
	Provide patient-centered counseling to achieve a partnership with each patient, allowing him or her to express, explore, and negotiate the next steps. Listen before speaking. Ask open-ended questions to increase dialogue. Keep size-friendly and age-appropriate reading materials in the waiting room. Refer parents to an RD specializing in childhood weight management for regular interaction. Patients can locate an RD in their vicinity by visiting www.eatright.org and click on "Find a Nutrition Professional." Provide acceptable macronutrient distribution ranges according to the 2002 Institute of Medicine's recommendations: • Carbohydrate - 45–65% of total calories • Protein - 5–20% for young children - 10–30% for older children • Fat - 30–40% of energy for children aged 1–3 years - 25–35% for children aged 4–18 years
	Don't:
	Don't simply measure weight. Don't simply calculate BMI. Don't label patients as "obese." Don't adopt a wait and see approach to excessive weight gain relative to linear growth or presume that a child will simply grow out of his or her overweight. Don't commence treatment in children less than 2 years old due to the critical development that occurs during this time. Don't assume everyone who is overweight wants to lose weight. Don't fall into advice giving. Don't judge. Don't ask closed-ended questions that elicit a "yes" or "no" response.

Problem	*Do's and Don'ts*
Counseling	Don't have inappropriate magazines in the waiting room.
	Don't provide extremely high or low macronutrient recommendations for carbohydrate, protein, or fat.
Food	**Do:**
	Think of food as fuel that is consumed throughout the day.
	Encourage healthful eating from all food groups.
	Plan meals with the child and shop on a weekly basis.
	Stock the refrigerator with healthful beverages (for example, plain water, flavored water, and reduced-fat milk/soy milk).
	Ensure 100% juice consumption is within the American Academy of Pediatrics recommended range: 4–6 ounces per day for children aged 1–6 years, 8–12 ounces per day for children aged 7–18 years.
	Provide a variety of foods for healthful snacks.
	Have nutrient-dense snacks readily available, such as chopped vegetables, fresh fruit, reduced-fat yogurt or cheese, and whole-grain crackers.
	Often bake, broil, and grill lean protein foods, such as chicken, fish, and seafood.
	Eat together as a family without the TV.
	Prepare one dinner for everyone in the family containing a nonstarchy vegetable, lean protein, and whole grain.
	Serve plate meals (as opposed to family style dining), but allow the child to decide how much of the meal he or she wants to eat.
	Require that breakfast be consumed within 1 hour of waking. For nonbreakfast eaters, encourage starting the day with light choices, such as fruit or reduced-fat yogurt.
	Consider fast food for special meals only (if at all).
	Evaluate the school lunch menu and help the child select healthful choices, or pack lunch for school if healthful choices are not consistently available. Work with school food service to provide healthful options. Suggest vegetable, fruit, or non–food-related fund-raising campaigns.
	Ask children for help in the garden so they see how vegetables are grown.

Problem	*Do's and Don'ts*
	Continue to offer foods that children say they don't like. (It takes 8–10 samples before they know if they do like it.)
	Encourage visiting www.mypyramid.gov for additional information on healthful food choices for children. While there, enter the child's age, gender, and activity level for specific information.
	Don't:
	Don't think of food as "good" or "bad."
	Don't allow the skipping of meals.
	Don't eliminate any one food group.
	Don't shop on a daily basis without a grocery list.
	Don't stock the refrigerator with caloric beverages, including soda, punch, or juice drinks. In addition, don't allow excessive 100% juice consumption.
	Don't give only one snack food choice.
	Don't fill cabinets with high-fat foods (for example, sugar crackers, cookies, candy, cakes, muffins, cereals, etc.).
	Don't prepare fried or breaded protein choices.
	Don't allow the child to eat in front of the TV.
	Don't take individual food orders from family members.
	Don't override child's internal hunger/satiety cues by adhering to the "clean plate club" mentality.
	Don't allow children to leave the house in the morning without eating breakfast.
	Don't make regular use of the drive through.
	Don't presume that school lunch will consist of healthful options.
	Don't assume all school meals contain healthful (and palatable) vegetables, fruits, lean protein, healthful fats, and whole grains.
	Don't support the sale of candy and donuts to raise money for school functions.
	Don't presuppose that children will dislike all vegetables.
	Don't assume a child will permanently dislike a food after trying it only a few times.

Problem	*Do's and Don'ts*
Physical Activity	**Do:** Encourage 30–60 minutes of physical activity most days. Make physical activity fun by encouraging team sports, active play, dancing, etc. Be physically active as a family. Plan active weekends, such as going to the park, playing sports, walking, biking, in-line skating, yard work, etc. Limit TV/video time to 2 hours per day as recommended by the American Academy of Pediatrics. Keep the TV in the family room. Encourage adequate sleep: • 12–14 hours for 1–3 year olds • 11–13 hours for 3–5 year olds • 10–11 hours for 5–12 year olds • 8.5–10 hours for 12–18 year olds **Don't:** Don't allow more than 2 hours of sedentary activity, such as television viewing or video game use. Don't make physical activity about winning, exercise, or redundant activities. Don't be a drill sergeant yelling on the sidelines. Don't plan weekend activities that involve food and/or inactivity, such as movies, video games, watching televised sporting events, etc. Don't allow unrestricted freedom with TV use. Don't keep the TV in the bedroom. Don't overstress the child with unmanageable extracurricular activities.
Behavioral	**Do:** Eat healthfully together as a family. Focus on healthful eating for life. Model healthful eating. Allow child to set, in writing, realistic goals related to healthful eating and physical activity. Meet with the child weekly or daily for check-ins regarding successes and challenges. Acknowledge positive changes with verbal praise and non–food-related rewards focusing on privileges and activities.

Problem	*Do's and Don'ts*
	Plan for setbacks. Discuss challenges/barriers and brainstorm possible solutions. Encourage self-monitoring, such as keeping food diaries as a way of journaling the experience. Make the social aspect the focus of celebrations.
	Don't: Don't alienate the overweight child by having him or her eat one way and the family another. Don't make the focus on dieting, restriction, or weight loss only. Don't play food police, commenting on every food as a "good" or "bad" choice. Don't establish broad, unattainable goals for the child. Don't assume goals will always be met. Don't presuppose the child is doing fine with his or her goal. Don't criticize shortcomings or use food as an incentive or threat. Don't ignore realities of problem situations. Don't use food diaries as punishment or a means to criticize failures. Don't make food the focus of celebrations. Don't assume that the only reason a child wants to change his or her eating habits is to be healthier.
Emotional	**Do:** Talk about what is motivating a child to change his or her eating habits. Discuss coping skills for dealing with feelings of unfairness about not eating like friends. Open up dialogue on the sensitive subject of self-esteem by asking what the child/teen likes about him- or herself. Ask if teasing is occurring at school. Adopt a no-tolerance policy for teasing in the household. Speak up for overweight individuals when they are ridiculed in conversations, jokes, or on TV programs. Address the beauty of all body types. Speak positively about physical appearance.

Problem	*Do's and Don'ts*
Emotional	**Don't:**
	Don't respond, "life isn't always fair."
	Don't ignore the sensitive issue of self-esteem.
	Don't be afraid to ask about teasing.
	Don't be silent when teasing occurs or inappropriate references regarding body size/shape occur in the media.
	Don't assume children know that extremely thin cartoon characters, movie stars, fashion models, and musicians do not possess the ideal body frame.
	Don't talk disparagingly about one's own or another's body.

Recommended Reading

American Academy of Pediatrics, Policy Statement. "Prevention of Pediatric Overweight and Obesity." *Pediatrics*. 2003. 112, 424–430.

"Position of the American Dietetic Association: Dietary Guidance for Healthy Children Ages 2 to 11 Years." *J Am Diet Assoc*. 2004. 104, 660–677.

Kirk, S., Scott, B. J., & Daniels, S. R. "Pediatric Obesity Epidemic: Treatment Options." *J Am Diet Assoc*. 2005. 105, S44–S51.

Sources

American Academy of Pediatrics, Committee on Nutrition. "The Use and Misuse of Fruit Juice in Pediatrics." *Pediatrics*. 2001. 107, 1210–1213.

American Academy of Pediatrics, Committee on Public Education. "Children, Adolescents, and Television." *Pediatrics*. 2001. 107, 423–426.

Kavey, R. E., Daniels, S. R., Lauer, R. M., Atkins, D. L., Hayman, L. L., & Taubert, K. "American Heart Association Guidelines for Primary Prevention of Atherosclerotic Cardiovascular Disease Beginning in Childhood." *Circulation*. 2003. 107, 1562–1566.

Kirk, S., Scott, B. J., & Daniels, S. R. "Pediatric Obesity Epidemic: Treatment Options." *J Am Diet Assoc*. 2005. 105, S44–S51.

Panel on Macronutrients. National Academy of Sciences. Institute of Medicine of the National Academies. *Dietary Reference Intakes for Energy, Carbohydrate, Fiber, Fat, Fatty Acids, Cholesterol, Protein, and Amino Acids*. Washington, DC: National Academy Press. 2002.

Type 1 Diabetes in Childhood

Author: Kattia M. Corrales-Yauckoes, MS, RD, LDN

This list will assist the dietitian in answering food-related questions for the child with type 1 diabetes. (Refer to Table 3-1 in Type 2 Diabetes in Childhood, titled "Diagnostic Criteria for Impaired Glucose Tolerance and Diabetes" and Table 3-2 "Plasma Blood Glucose Goal Range in Pediatric Diabetes" on page 188.)

Problem	*Do's and Don'ts*
Dietary Carbohydrate	**Do:**
	(Note that due to the complexity of a diabetic diet, an RD should provide consultation to the healthcare team.)
	Instruct the patient on which foods contain carbohydrate.
	Count the total carbohydrates of meals and snacks.
	Suggest distributing carbohydrate grams over a variety of foods (for example, fruits, vegetables, grains, milk, and other). See the food exchange list in the appendix on page 345.
	Measure and weigh food for more precise counting of carbohydrates.
	Read food labels to determine carbohydrate content of meals. For foods without food labels, use a reference book that contains carbohydrate values of foods.
	Substitute juices and caloric beverages with calorie-free beverages.
	If on an intermediate-acting insulin (for example, NPH human insulin isophane suspension) and sliding scale rapid-acting insulin (Humalog or NovoLog or regular), provide carbohydrate gram goals for each meal and snack. See the appendix on page 394 to learn more about insulin types.
	Adjust carbohydrate goals based on hunger/appetite and growth.
	If on insulin pump or on a nonpeaking basal insulin (for example, glargine–Lantus or detemir–Levemir) and fast-acting insulin, educate family on how to use an insulin-to-carbohydrate ratio and a sensitivity/correction factor.
	Use an insulin-to-carbohydrate ratio to dose insulin to the carbohydrate grams in food. For example, the ratio may be 1 unit of insulin for every 30 grams of carbohydrate. However, this ratio is determined individually for each child based on his or her total insulin usage.

Problem	*Do's and Don'ts*
Dietary Carbohydrate	Use a sensitivity/correction factor to treat the blood glucose. For example, the factor may be 1 unit of insulin drops blood glucose 50 mg/dl. However, this factor is determined individually for each child based on his or her total insulin usage. When working with carbohydrate choices or exchanges (see the food exchange list in the appendix on page 345), 1 carbohydrate choice or exchange = 15 grams of carbohydrate. **Don't:** Don't eliminate sugar from the diet. Foods with sugar and other sweeteners (for example, honey, corn syrup) can be included in the diet as long as they are offered occasionally and counted as part of the carbohydrate allotment. Don't forget that protein and fat affect caloric intake and should not be consumed in excess. Don't use the term "serving" when referring to choices/exchanges because one serving of a food on the food label could be more or less than 15 grams of carbohydrate.
Protein	**Do:** Instruct on choosing protein-rich foods that are low in fat (for example, poultry without skin, fish, pork, and lean beef). Provide guidelines for appropriate portions of protein-rich foods. Recommended amounts of meat or legumes (beans) per day based on age and moderate activity: 2–3 years of age: 2–4 oz. meat or beans per day 4–8 years of age: 4–5 oz. meat or beans per day 9–13 years of age: 5–6 oz. meat or beans per day 14–18 years of age: 6.5–7 oz. meat or beans per day **Don't:** Don't use protein-rich foods as free foods. Although protein does not raise blood glucose, consumption should be limited to avoid excess fat and caloric intake. Don't recommend protein at every meal and snack. If snacks and meals are close together, protein could lead to excess caloric intake.
Fat	**Do:** Instruct patient to choose healthier versions of fat: • Replace saturated fat (for example, butter, creams, whole milk, cheese, fat in meat) with monounsaturated (for

Problem	*Do's and Don'ts*
	example, olive, canola, and peanut oil; peanuts; hazelnuts; cashews; almonds; avocado; and seeds) and polyunsaturated fats (safflower, sunflower, corn, or soybean oils; walnuts; seeds; fish). • Avoid trans fat (margarines, foods made with hydrogenated fat, such as crackers and cookies). Look for products marked "trans-fatty acid free" or "trans fat free." • Choose lean meats, poultry, and fish. Consider that foods rich in fat may delay the blood glucose response. **Don't:** Don't use fat as a free food. Although fat does not raise blood glucose, consumption should be limited to avoid excess caloric intake.
Fiber	**Do:** Encourage foods rich in fiber, such as fruit, vegetables, legumes (for example, beans, chickpeas, lentils) and whole grains (for example, whole-wheat bread, bran flakes, whole-grain cereal, and whole grain pasta). Look for the word "whole" in the ingredient list. A food rich in fiber has 3 grams per serving or more. Fiber goals: Males aged 9–18 years: 31–38 grams per day Females aged 9–18 years: 26 grams per day **Don't:** Don't rely on fiber supplements as the main source of fiber. Don't increase fiber intake too quickly because it can cause intestinal upset; aim for a gradual increase in fiber.
Meal Planning	**Do:** Instruct on which foods make up the different food groups and instruct on use of exchange lists. See the appendix on page 328. Develop a personalized meal plan that takes into account age and development, food likes/dislikes, and family food choices. Provide suggestions for the number of servings of each food group to consume at meals and snacks. Recommend a regular eating schedule separating meals and snacks by 2 and 3 hours.

Problem	*Do's and Don'ts*
Meal Planning	Adjust meal plan periodically based on hunger/appetite and growth. Meal plan adjustments may need to occur as early as a few weeks after diagnosis because hunger/appetite may change with initiation of insulin and weight regulation. Instruct on carbohydrate counting (see sections on protein and fiber intake and the appendix on pages 170–171 and 345) because this method is often used in conjunction with or in place of exchanges. Consult an RD/CDE for teaching of exchanges and/or carbohydrate counting and development of personalized meal plan. Guidelines for distribution of calories: Carbohydrate: 45–65% of calories Fat: 1–3 years: 30–40% of calories 4–18 years: 25–35% of calories Protein: 1–3 years: 5–20% of calories 4–18 years: 10–30% of calories **Don't:** Don't give a standard meal plan that does not take into account the child's and family's food choices and eating pattern. Don't be too restrictive on the timing or quantity of meals and snacks, which may change frequently after diagnosis. Aim to change the insulin as much as possible according to the child's and family's eating pattern.
Free Foods	**Do:** Advise the patient that the term "free foods" refers to foods or beverages that have little impact on blood glucose. By definition, a free food is less than 5 grams of carbohydrate *and* less than 25 calories per serving: • Nonstarchy vegetables (for example, asparagus, bok choy, broccoli, cabbage, cauliflower, celery, cucumber slices, eggplant, green beans, kale, lettuce and other salad greens, mushrooms, onions, peppers, spinach, tomatoes, watercress, and zucchini) • Sugar-free, calorie-free beverages • Sugar-free gelatin • Sugar-free Popsicles • Sugar-free gum Keep in mind that some nonstarchy vegetables in larger portions may contribute more than 5 grams of carbohydrate.

Problem	***Do's and Don'ts***

Dyslipidemia

Do:

Do optimize glycemic control screening with the PMD's order. Obtain lipid profile at diagnosis and then, if normal, every 5 years. Begin screening at aged 12 years, unless the patient has reached puberty or has a positive family history.

Goals:
LDL less than 100 mg/dl
HDL greater than 35 mg/dl
Triglycerides less than 150 mg/dl

If elevated LDL:

- Improve glycemic control.
- Implement the American Heart Association TLC diet.
  - Less than 200 mg cholesterol per day.
  - Less than 7% of calories from saturated fat.
  - Instruct on lowering trans fat.
  - Aim for normalization of weight, if needed.
  - Consider use of a plant sterol or plant stanol esters (2 g per day used in adults) found in products such as Benecol and Take Control.
  - Increase fiber intake (see fiber section on page 171), in particular soluble fiber (oat/oat bran, beans, peas, barley, flaxseed, apples, oranges, and vegetables) to meet the DRI.
  - Repeat a fasting lipid profile 3 months and 6 months after dietary intervention and optimization of blood glucose control. If lipids normalize, repeat lipid profile annually thereafter.

If LDL is not improved:

- LDL = 100–129 mg/dl
  - Maximize nonpharmacologic treatment.
- LDL = 130–159 mg/dl
  - Consider pharmacological treatment if child is older than 10 years of age.
- LDL ≥ 160 mg/dl
  - Initiate pharmacological treatment (bile acid sequestrants or statin drugs) if child is older than 10 years of age. Monitor liver function.

For triglyceride greater than or equal to 150 mg/dl, improve glycemic control and weight management.

Blood Glucose Goals

Do:

Refer to Table 3-2: Plasma Blood Glucose Goal Range in Pediatric Diabetes.

Problem	*Do's and Don'ts*
Blood Glucose Goals	**Don't:** Don't allow extreme fluctuations in blood glucose levels.
Hypoglycemia (defined as blood glucose below 80 mg/dl)	**Do:** Advise patient of the typical symptoms of hypoglycemia including: Sweatiness Shakiness Weakness Dizziness Headache Irritability Difficulty concentrating Confusion Changes in vision Increased hunger Behavioral changes Dilated pupils Treat using a carbohydrate-rich food that does not contain fat or protein: ≤5 years of age = 5–10 grams carbohydrate 6–10 years of age = 10–15 grams carbohydrate 10 years of age = 15–20 grams carbohydrate Inform patient of carbohydrate sources for treating a low blood glucose: Glucose tablets: 4–5 grams carbohydrate each Insta-glucose: 24 grams carbohydrate per tube Soda or juice: 3–4 grams of carbohydrate per 1 oz Table sugar, honey, syrup: 4–5 grams carbohydrate per teaspoon Cake icing: 4 grams of carbohydrate per teaspoon Life Savers: 3 grams of carbohydrate each Check blood glucose every 15 minutes and treat with an additional dose of carbohydrate (see previous age-based guidelines) until blood glucose normalizes (above 80 mg/dl). Give glucagon injection per directions if patient is unresponsive or unconscious. Give a food containing carbohydrate (see previous list) when the person regains consciousness. Carry at all times a fast-acting carbohydrate. Teach caregivers how to recognize signs of hypoglycemia and how to treat with food and/or glucagon.

Problem	*Do's and Don'ts*
	Don't: Don't treat low-blood glucose with foods that contain fat or protein because they may slow down the glycemic response. Do not overtreat low-blood glucose. Using too much carbohydrate to treat low-blood glucose can lead to rebound hyperglycemia. Do not give anything by mouth due to increased risk of choking if patient is unresponsive or unconscious.
Hyperglycemia	**Do:** Advise patient of the typical symptoms of hyperglycemia including: Increased thirst Increased urination Fatigue Blurred vision Increased frequency of infections Dry mouth Delayed healing Weight loss Treat with insulin according to the child's sliding scale or insulin instructions given by the PMD. Check for ketones if blood glucose is 250 mg/dl or greater. Assess possible reasons for high blood glucose: Too little insulin or improper dosing of insulin Too much food Increased exercise Expired insulin Illness, injury, infection, surgery **Don't:** Don't always attribute a high blood glucose to overconsumption of food. Blood glucose can increase due to stress, exercise, and poor insulin dosing.
Sick Day Nutrition Guidelines	**Do:** Provide plenty of fluids. Encourage 6 to 8 ounces of fluid (sugar-free soda, sugar-free flavored drinks, water, sugar-free gelatin) every 1 to 2 hours to prevent dehydration. Patients may tolerate clear liquids better than creamier foods.

Problem	*Do's and Don'ts*
Sick Day Nutrition Guidelines	Encourage food consumption. If the patient's appetite is decreased, try to replace the carbohydrate portions of the meal plan as much as possible. Alternatively, offer 10–30 grams of carbohydrate every 1 to 2 hours. Examples (confirm carbohydrate content via food label): 1/2 cup applesauce 1/2 cup juice 1/2 cup baby cereal 3–4 oz pureed fruit 1 small banana 1 cup Gatorade 1/3 cup fruited yogurt 1 Tbsp honey 1/2 cup hot cereal 1 lollipop 1/4 cup milkshake 1/2 cup regular gelatin 1/2 cup regular ice cream 1/4 cup sherbet 1/4 cup regular pudding 1 slice toast Tomato juice and broth are low in carbohydrate. Consider using a pediatric rehydration solution if child is unable to keep solids down. Example: Enfamil Enfalyte (Mead Johnson) 4 oz = 3.8 grams of carbohydrate Pedialyte (Abbott) 4 oz = 3 grams of carbohydrate Pedialyte Freezer Pops (Abbott) 2.1 fl oz (1 pop) = 1.5 grams of carbohydrate
Exercise and Physical Activity	**Do:** Encourage daily physical activity. Ideally do at least 60 minutes of physical activity daily. Instruct patient to monitor blood glucose before, during, and after exercise. Give a snack of 15–30 grams of carbohydrate plus 1–2 oz of protein before exercise. **Don't:** Don't forget that blood glucose may increase during or immediately after exercise, but insulin sensitivity (and potentially low blood glucose) may occur hours after physical activity.

Problem	*Do's and Don'ts*
Sugar Substitutes	**Do:** Counsel the patient that the Food and Drug Administration and the World Health Organization established an acceptable daily intake for high-intensity noncaloric sweeteners that includes a 100-fold safety factor: Aspartame (Equal, NutraSweet, SweetMate): 50 mg/kg body weight Saccharine (Sweet'N Low, SugarTwin): 5 mg/kg body weight Acesulfame-K (Sweet One, Sunett): 15 mg/kg body weight Sucralose (Splenda): 5 mg/kg body weight Discuss polyols (sugar alcohols) often found in diet or sugar-free products (for example, sorbitol, mannitol, xylitol, erythritol, isomalt, lactitol, maltitol, maltitol syrup, and hydrogenated starch). They contain anywhere from 0.2 kcal/g (erythritol) to 2.6 kcal/g (sorbitol) as compared to 4 kcal/g from sugar. Maltitol syrup and hydrogenated starch hydrolysates contain about 3 kcal/g. Due to their lower caloric value, polyols exhibit a lower glycemic response than sugar. Subtract half of the grams of sugar alcohol out of the total carbohydrates in the food if counting carbohydrates. Example: Product contains 20 grams of total carbohydrate and 6 grams of sugar alcohol. Subtract 3 grams from the total and count product as 17 grams of total carbohydrate. **Don't:** Don't encourage consumption of diet or sugar-free cookies or bread products; these products may contain equal amounts of carbohydrate as compared to their regular food counterparts due to the use of flour and starch in the product. However, diet or sugar-free versions of beverages, Popsicles, and gelatin are often truly carbohydrate free. Don't allow excessive consumption of sugar alcohols (polyols), which can have a laxative effect.
Behavioral and Psychosocial	**Do:** Include the child in meal planning. Encourage dietary changes at the family level, which may enhance adherence and prevent the child from feeling different. Consider meeting with prepubertal or adolescent child separately from parents to stimulate self-management.

Problem	*Do's and Don'ts*
Behavioral and Psychosocial	Inquire about favorite foods and foods consumed on special occasions, such as parties, holidays, etc. Many foods can be included as part of a healthy diet if planned in advance. Identify cultural and religious beliefs related to food and dietary patterns. Understand that food struggles may arise after diagnosis related to: • Parental fears of low blood glucose if given insulin before a meal • Child's response to increased attention to food and eating Share techniques for avoiding food struggles: Offer a range of food choices at meals, particularly with young children. Example: 15–20 grams of carbohydrate or 0.5–1 starch. Consider giving the insulin 15–20 minutes into the meal, and adjust the dose according to food consumed. Allow the child to contribute to meal planning. Be flexible with food choices. All children eat high-calorie, high-fat and/or high-sugar foods occasionally. Share diabetes care: Instruct parents to share the responsibilities of care to avoid burnout. Instruct parents to negotiate diabetes care responsibilities with the child, particularly in the older child. Provide positive reinforcement for the child's cooperation with the regimen. Be sensitive to a child's difficulties with insulin injections and blood glucose checks. Reassure the child that diabetes is no one's fault. Adjust diabetes care regimen to accommodate participation in school/peer activities. Be sensitive to the interaction between self-esteem, peer influence, and diabetes care. Monitor for signs of depression, eating disorders, and risky behaviors. Consult a therapist with experience in pediatric diabetes if the child and family are having a difficult time adapting to diabetes.

Problem	*Do's and Don'ts*
	Don't:
	Don't refer to the child as a "diabetic." Use the term "child with diabetes."
	Don't refer to meal plan as a "diet." Likewise, avoid negative words, such as "never," "do not," "bad," and "cheating" when referring to food or meal planning.
	Don't allow the child or adolescent to take on all or most of diabetes care. Encourage parental involvement in diabetes care throughout adolescence.

Sources

American Diabetes Association. "Management of Dyslipidemia in Children and Adolescents with Diabetes." *Diabetes Care*. Vol. 26, 2003. 2194–2197.

American Diabetes Association. "American Diabetes Association Position Statement: Evidence-Based Nutrition Principles and Recommendations for the Treatment and Prevention of Diabetes and Related Complications." *J Am Diet Assoc.* 2002. 102, 109–118.

American Dietetic Association. "Position of the American Dietetic Association: Use of Nutritive and Nonnutritive Sweeteners." *J Am Diet Assoc.* 2004. 104, 255–275.

American Heart Association. Step I , Step II and TLC Diets. http://www.americanheart.org/presenter.jhtml?identifier=4764.

Food and Nutrition Board. Institute of Medicine, The National Academies of Science. *Dietary Reference Intakes for Energy, Carbohydrate, Fiber, Fat, Fatty Acids, Cholesterol, Protein and Amino Acids*. Washington, DC: National Academy Press. 2002.

Higgins, L. A., & Chalmers, K. H. "Diabetes." *Handbook of Pediatric Nutrition.* Samour, P. Q., & King, K. (Eds.). (3rd ed.). Sudbury, MA: Jones and Bartlett Publishers. 2005. 421–448.

Joslin Diabetes Center. High Blood Glucose: Hyperglycemia. 2002. http://www.joslin.org. All rights reserved. Adapted with permission.

——— Low Blood Glucose Hypoglycemia / Insulin Reaction. 2002. http://www.joslin.org. High Blood Glucose: Hyperglycemia. Copyright © 2002 by Joslin Diabetes Center. (www.joslin.org) All rights reserved. Adapted with permission.

——— Sick Day Nutrition Guidelines for Children. 2002. http://www.joslin.org.

Krauss, R. M. et al. (2000). "AHA Dietary Guidelines: revision 2000: A Statement for Healthcare Professionals from The Nutrition Committee of the American Heart Association." *Stroke.* 31, 2751–2766.

Powers, M., Franz, I. M., & Bantle, J. (Eds.). "Sugar Alternatives and Fat Replacers." *American Diabetes Association Guide to Medical Nutrition Therapy for Diabetes.* American Diabetes Association. 1999. 148–164.

Silverstein, J., et al. "Care of Children and Adolescents with Type 1 Diabetes: A Statement of the American Diabetes Association." *Diabetes Care*. 2005. 28, 186–212.

U.S. Department of Health and Human Services. Sick Day Nutrition Guidelines for Children. Copyright © 2002 by Joslin Diabetes Center. (www.joslin.org) All rights reserved. Adapted with permission. Dietary Guidelines for Americans 2005. U.S. Department of Agriculture. http://www.healthierus.gov/dietaryguidelines.

http://www.mypyramid.gov/downloads/MyPyramid_Food_Intake_Patterns.pdf/

http://www.mypyramid.gov/downloads/MyPyramid_Calorie_Levels.pdf.

Type 2 Diabetes in Childhood

Author: Kattia M. Corrales-Yauckoes, MS, RD, LDN

This list will assist the dietitian in answering food-related questions for the child with type 2 diabetes. Included are Tables 3-1 and 3-2, Diagnostic Criteria for Impaired Glucose Tolerance and Diabetes and Plasma Blood Glucose Goal Range in Pediatric Diabetes.

Problem	*Do's and Don'ts*
Weight Management	**Do:**
	Share that children/adolescents with type 2 diabetes (DM) are often overweight. A component of treatment is to normalize body weight. Assess level of overweight using BMI percentiles. The patient is at risk for overweight if BMI is between 85–94th percentile. The patient is overweight if BMI is greater than or equal to the 95th percentile.
	Weight goals 2–7 years of age: — If BMI is in the 85–94th percentile, aim for weight maintenance. — If BMI is greater than the 95th percentile and the patient has no complications, aim for weight maintenance. See the following sections. — If BMI is greater than the 95th percentile and the patient has complications, aim for a weight loss. A weight loss of 1 lb per month is reasonable and realistic. See the following sections.
	Weight goals if older than 7 years of age: — If the BMI is in the 85–94th percentile and the patient has no complications, aim for weight maintenance. See the following sections. — If the BMI is in the 85–94th percentile *and* the patient has complications, aim for weight loss. A weight loss of 1 lb per month is reasonable and realistic. See the following sections. — If the BMI is greater than the 95th percentile, aim for weight loss. A weight loss of 1 pound per month is reasonable and realistic. See the following sections.
	Complications include mild hypertension, dyslipidemias, and insulin resistance. Refer children with acute complications, such as sleep apnea, obesity hypoventilation syndrome, orthopedic problems, and pseudotumor cerebri, to an obesity center. Schedule regular nutrition visits.

Problem	*Do's and Don'ts*
	Don't:
	Don't use the term "obese." The term "overweight" is preferred.
	Don't expect rapid weight loss. Weight maintenance, depending on age and complications, is often a reasonable goal. Otherwise, a weight loss of 1 lb per month is realistic and does not put undue pressure on the child and family.
Dietary Assessment	**Do:**
	Assess the child's usual food and beverage intake, frequency of eating, and location of meals. Include foods consumed at home, school, after-school programs, and with friends or other caregivers.
	Inquire about favorite foods and foods consumed on special occasions, such as parties, holidays, etc. With advance planning, many foods can be included as part of a healthy diet.
	Assess the family's food and eating habits. Look at food purchases (frequency, types of foods, budget), food preparation (for example, method and by whom), and dietary philosophies (special diets, dietary restrictions or dieting behavior among family members, beliefs about what constitutes good or bad foods, beliefs about how to feed children). Identify cultural and religious beliefs related to food and dietary patterns.
	Assess parental opinion about the child's eating behavior (for example, "picky eater" or "lack of self-control").
	Assess frequency of eating out or ordering delivery of food (take out).
Lifestyle Modification (general)	**Do:**
	Assess child and family's readiness for change.
	Consider meeting with prepubertal or adolescent child separately from parents to stimulate self-management.
	Include the child in meal planning.
	Encourage dietary and physical activity changes at the family level, which may enhance adherence to changes and prevent child from feeling different. Discuss relationship between eating and activity habits and diabetes and weight management.
	Help the child and family identify problem behaviors. Guide the child and family in creating small and achievable goals. Examples: Increase physical activity from 10 minutes to

Problem	*Do's and Don'ts*
	15 minutes per day; eat one more fruit per day; and decrease frequency of eating out from twice a week to once a week. Involve a multidisciplinary team that includes an endocrinologist, nurse, RD, and, if possible, a mental health practitioner and an exercise physiologist for best treatment modality. Provide frequent follow-up (every 2 to 4 weeks) for continued goal setting. **Don't:** Don't use judgmental language and reactions. Don't use negative terms, such as "bad," "never," "do not."
Meal Planning	**Do:** Offer a meal plan if it will provide the child and family with structure and guidance on food choices. However, a meal plan is not always necessary if the aim is to help the child and family make small and achievable changes to current eating and activity habits. If a meal plan is given, instruct or have an RD instruct on which foods make up the different food groups and instruct on use of exchange lists. See the appendix on page 328. Develop a personalized meal plan that takes into account age and development, food likes/dislikes, and family food choices. Provide suggestions for the number of servings of each food group to consume at meals and snacks. Recommend a regular eating schedule. Adjust meal plan periodically based on hunger/appetite and growth. Share guidelines for distribution of calories. Carbohydrate: 45–65% of calories Fat: 1–3 years: 30–40% of calories 4–18 years: 25–35% of calories Protein: 1–3 years: 5–20% of calories 4–18 years: 10–30% of calories Focus on increasing consumption of fruits and vegetables and whole grains, as well as limiting high-fat foods. Develop small and achievable goals with the child and family. Examples include increasing intake of fruit (vegetable) from one to two servings per day, switching to whole grain breads, and drinking skim milk versus soda during lunch.

Problem	*Do's and Don'ts*
	Don't:
	Don't give a standard meal plan that does not take into account the child's and family's food choices and eating pattern.
	Don't be too restrictive on the timing or quantity of meals and snacks, which may change frequently after diagnosis.
	Don't refer to a meal plan as a "diet."
	Don't use negative words such as "never," "do not," "bad," and "cheating" when referring to food or meal planning.
Dietary Carbohydrate	**Do:**
	Instruct on carbohydrate counting if child is on insulin. See the section on dietary carbohydrate in Type 1 Diabetes in Childhood on page 170. While allowing sugar and other caloric sweeteners in the diet of the child with diabetes, foods containing added sugars (for example, table sugar, honey, corn syrup) should be consumed in moderation due to the often high-caloric content of these foods.
Protein	See protein section in Type 1 Diabetes in Childhood on page 170.
Fat	See fat section in Type 1 Diabetes in Childhood on pages 170–171.
Fiber	See fiber section in Type 1 Diabetes in Childhood on page 171.
Free Foods	See free food section in Type 1 Diabetes in Childhood on page 172.
Dyslipidemia	See dyslipidemia section in Type 1 Diabetes in Childhood on page 173.
Hypoglycemia	See hypoglycemia section in Type 1 Diabetes in Childhood on pages 174–175.
Hyperglycemia	See hyperglycemia section in Type 1 Diabetes in Childhood on page 175.
Exercise and Physical Activity	**Do:**
	Encourage daily physical activity. Ideally, do at least 60 minutes of physical activity daily. However, aim for a

Problem	*Do's and Don'ts*
	slow progression toward this goal. Structure exercise guidelines based on extent of overweight: • If the BMI is in the 85–94th percentile, recommend weight-bearing exercise (walking, field sports, skating or in-line skating, jumping rope, indoor sports, swimming, dancing, playing, etc.). • If the BMI is greater than or equal to the 95th percentile, recommend primarily non–weight-bearing exercise (swimming, cycling, strength training, or short walks). • If the BMI is greater than or equal to the 97th percentile, do only non–weight-bearing activities. Consider referring to a trained exercise professional for regular monitoring. Monitor blood glucose before, during, and after exercise. Give a snack of 15–30 grams of carbohydrate plus 1–2 oz of protein before prolonged (greater than 1 hour) exercise. **Don't:** Don't forget that blood glucose may increase during or immediately after exercise, but insulin sensitivity (and potentially low blood glucose) may occur hours after physical activity.
Sugar Substitutes	See sugar substitutes section in Type 1 Diabetes in Childhood on page 177.
Medications	**Do:** Advise the patient that initial treatment may only involve oral medication advised by the physician and therapeutic lifestyle modifications aiming for weight loss and glycemic control. Use insulin in the case of ketosis or if glucose control is not achieved after 3 to 6 months of treatment with lifestyle modification and medication. Advise the patient of the side effects of medications used for type 2 DM: • Sulfonylureas (glimepiride, glyburide, and glipizide): Hypoglycemia and weight gain • Meglitinides (repaglinide and nateglinide): Hypoglycemia and weight gain • Thiazolidinediones (rosiglitazone and pioglitazone): Edema, weight gain, anemia, and possibly liver damage (Monitor liver functions. Watch for symptoms of hepatic dysfunction: nausea, vomiting, abdominal pain.)

Problem	*Do's and Don'ts*
Medications	• Glucosidase inhibitors (acarbose): Gastrointestinal upset • Metformin: Gastrointestinal disturbances and lactic acidosis (Currently, metformin is the only drug approved by the Food and Drug Administration in pediatric type 2 diabetes.)
Behavioral and Psychosocial	**Do:** Understand food struggles that may arise after diagnosis related to: increased focus on child's eating habits, extensive dietary restrictions, parental fears of low blood glucose if insulin is given before a meal, and child's response to increased attention to food and eating. Share the following techniques for avoiding food struggles: • Allow the child to contribute to meal planning and goal setting. • Avoid placing too many dietary restrictions. • Create small, achievable goals with the child and family. • Focus on dietary and activity changes at the family level. • Be flexible with food choices. All children eat high-calorie, high-fat, and/or high-sugar foods occasionally. Instruct parents to share the responsibilities of care to avoid burnout. Instruct parents to negotiate diabetes care responsibilities with the child, particularly in the older child. Provide positive reinforcement for the child's cooperation with the regimen. Be sensitive to the child's difficulties with insulin injections and blood sugar checks. Reassure the child that diabetes is no one's fault. Adjust the diabetes care regimen to accommodate participation in school/peer activities. Be sensitive to the interaction between self-esteem, peer influence, and diabetes care. Monitor for signs of depression, disordered eating, and risky behaviors. Consult a therapist with experience in pediatric diabetes if the child and family are having a difficult time adapting to diabetes. Encourage parental involvement in diabetes care throughout adolescence.

Problem	*Do's and Don'ts*
	Don't:
	Don't refer to the child as "diabetic." Use the term "child with diabetes."
	Don't have the child or adolescent take on all or most of diabetes care.

Sources

American Diabetes Association. "American Diabetes Association Position Statement: Evidence-Based Nutrition Principles and Recommendations for the Treatment and Prevention of Diabetes and Related Complications." *J Am Diet Assoc*. 2002. 102, 109–118.

Barlow, S. E., & Dietz, W. H. "Obesity Evaluation and Treatment: Expert Committee Recommendations." The Maternal and Child Health Bureau, Health Resources and Services Administration and the Department of Health and Human Services. *Pediatrics*. 1998. 102, E29.

BMI - Body Mass Index: BMI for Children and Teens. Centers for Disease Control and Prevention. http://www.cdc.gov/nccdphp/dnpa/bmi/bmi-for-age.htm.

Corrales-Yauckoes, K. M., & Higgins, L. A. "Nutritional Management of the Overweight Child with Type 2 Diabetes." *Pediatric Annals*. 2005. 34, 701–709.

Food and Nutrition Board. Institute of Medicine, The National Academies of Science. *Dietary Reference Intakes for Energy, Carbohydrate, Fiber, Fat, Fatty Acids, Cholesterol, Protein and Amino Acids*. Washington, DC: National Academy Press, 2002.

Hannon, T. S., Rao, G., & Arslanian, S. A. "Childhood Obesity and Type 2 Diabetes Mellitus." *Pediatrics*. 2005. 116, 473–480.

Higgins, L. A., & Chalmers, K. H. "Diabetes." *Handbook of Pediatric Nutrition*. Samour, P. Q., & King, K. (Eds.). (3rd ed.). Sudbury, MA: Jones and Bartlett Publishers. 2005. 421–448.

Sothern, M. S. "Exercise as a Modality in the Treatment of Childhood Obesity." *Pediatr Clin North Am*. 2001. 48, 995–1015.

Silverstein, J., et al. "Care of Children and Adolescents with Type 1 Diabetes: A Statement of the American Diabetes Association." *Diabetes Care*. 2005. 28, 186–212.

U.S. Department of Health and Human Services. Dietary Guidelines for Americans 2005. U.S. Department of Agriculture. http://www.healthierus.gov/dietaryguidelines.

Wrotniak, B. H., Epstein, L. H., Paluch, R. A., & Roemmich, J. N. "Parent Weight Change as a Predictor of Child Weight Change in Family-Based Behavioral Obesity Treatment." *Arch Pediatr Adolesc Med*. 2004. 158, 342–347.

Table 3-1 Diagnostic Criteria for Impaired Glucose Tolerance and Diabetes

	Plasma Glucose
Normal	Fasting Blood Glucose (BG): 100 mg/dl OGTT (oral glucose tolerance test) 2 hours postprandial: < 140 mg/dl Casual BG
Impaired glucose tolerance	Fasting BG: 100–125 mg/dl OGTT 2 hours postprandial: 140–199 mg/dl Casual BG
Diabetes	Fasting BG: >126 mg/dl OGTT 2 hours postprandial: ≥200 mg/dl Casual BG ≥200 mg/dl + symptoms (polyuria [increased urination], polydipsia [increased thirst], weight loss)

Source: Expert Committee on the Diagnosis and Classification of Diabetes Mellitus. Report of the expert committee on the diagnosis and classification of diabetes mellitus (2003). *Diabetes Care*, 26 (suppl 1), S5–S20.

Table 3-2 Plasma Blood Glucose Goal Range in Pediatric Diabetes

Age Group	Before Meals	Bedtime/ Overnight	A1C[a]
Toddlers and preschoolers (< 6 years)[b]	100–180	110–200	< 8.5% (but > 7.5%)
School age (6–12 years)	90–180	100–180	< 8%
Adolescents and young adults (13–19 years)	90–130	90–150	< 7.5%[c]

Other considerations:

- Goals should be individualized, and lower goals may be reasonable based on benefit–risk assessment.
- Postprandial blood glucose values should be measured when there is a disparity between preprandial blood glucose values and A1C levels.
- Blood glucose goals should be higher than those listed in children with frequent hypoglycemia or hypoglycemia unawareness.

[a]A1C: Glycosylated hemoglobin or hemoglobin A1C

[b]Blood glucose targets are set higher due to the high risk and vulnerability to hypoglycemia.

[c]A lower goal (7.0%) is reasonable if it can be achieved without excessive hypoglycemia.

SECTION 4

Adult Nutrition

Acute Nutrition Care Problems

Aspiration Pneumonia 190
Gastric Bypass Surgery 193
Cancer (Nutrition During Chemotherapy and Radiation) 208
Adult Parenteral Nutrition (PN) Guide 215
Troubleshooting with Parenteral Nutrition (PN) 221
Adult Tube Feeding Guide 224
Troubleshooting with Adult Tube Feeding 232
Diverticulitis 238
Gastroesophageal Reflux Disease (GERD) 241
Lactose Intolerance 243
Inflammatory Bowel Disease (IBD) 245
Celiac Disease or Celiac Sprue
(Gluten Sensitive Enteropathy) 248
Cholecystitis (Inflammation of the Gallbladder) or
Cholecystectomy (Gallbladder Removed) 250
Colostomy/Ileostomy 253
Short-Bowel Syndrome 257
Liver Disease 260
Renal Calculi 266

Aspiration Pneumonia

Author: Nicola O'Brien, MS, RD, LDN

Aspiration pneumonia can develop due to dysphagia or decreased ability to swallow foods and/or fluids. Causes of dysphagia include medical conditions (Parkinson disease, CVA, etc.), neurological disorders, or side effects of medication. Symptoms include elevated temperature and suspicious lung sounds.

Problem	*Do's and Don'ts*
Aspiration Pneumonia	**Do:**
	Ask a speech language pathologist (SLP) to evaluate the patient's swallowing ability via a chairside swallow evaluation or barium swallow.
	Request an SLP to recommend appropriate texture modification. Refer to facility's current authorized diet manual to review the textures provided and use the proper vernacular when determining the texture desired.
	Ask an SLP to recommend whether thickened liquids are necessary and also the degree to which the liquids must be thickened (that is, nectar, honey, or pudding).
	Determine whether the patient has experienced a weight loss by reviewing the patient's weight record. Should there be weight loss, to recalculate the patient's estimated needs by using the Harris Benedict Basal Energy Expenditure (BEE) formula: Male: 66 + wt/kg × 13.7 + ht/cm × 5 − age × 6.8 Female: 655 + wt/kg × 9.6 + ht/cm × 1.8 − age × 4.7 Ascertain level of activity factor: Bedfast/bedrest = 1.2 Wheelchair/ambulates = 1.3 Active = 1.5
	Establish protein needs. Determine the patient's IBW range, using the patient's height. The following formula is routinely employed:
	Male: 106 pounds for the first 60 inches of height plus 6 pounds for each additional inch of height. If the patient's height is less than 60 inches, subtract 3 pounds for each inch less than 60 inches.
	Female: 100 pounds for the first 60 inches of height plus 5 pounds for each additional inch of height. If the patient's

Problem	*Do's and Don'ts*
	height is less than 60 inches, subtract 2.5 pounds for each inch less than 60 inches. Convert pounds to kilograms (weight divided by 2.2). This will be the base protein need in grams. Take into account protein factors: Normal = 0.8–1.0/kg of body weight Decubitus = 1.2–1.5/kg of body weight Surgery = 1.0–2.0/kg of body weight Burns/multiple fractures = 2.0–2.5/kg of body weight If serum albumin is depleted, protein needs may be even higher. Also, be aware that there are medical conditions that will alter protein needs—renal disease, for example. Ascertain daily fluid needs, using the following formula: Actual weight/kg × fluid factor = ml fluids Fluid factors: normal = 30 ml/kg of body weight CHF = 25 ml/kg of body weight UTI = 40 ml/kg of body weight Evaluate the safest environment for the patient to have meals; the choices may be continuous supervision in a specified dining area, one-on-one supervision, or have the staff feed the patient. Encourage the patient to have meals out of bed, sitting upright in a chair at a 90 degree angle. Encourage chin tuck or chin-on-chest when swallowing. Prompt the patient to eat slowly. Suggest putting the fork down on the table after every bite. Consume small amounts, one half to one teaspoon at a time. Give patient ample time at meals to eat. Alternate solids and liquids when eating. Have SLP determine safest strategy for liquids (that is, cup, sippy cup, with a straw, via spoon). Observe the patient swallowing before having him or her eat another bite or sip. Encourage a double swallow for each swallow. Check the patient's mouth for "pocketing" of food after the completion of a meal.

Problem	*Do's and Don'ts*
Nausea	Don't serve higher fat foods. Don't serve highly spiced, greasy, or overly processed foods.
Constipation	**Do:** Advise the patient that constipation commonly occurs following gastric bypass surgery due to limited hydration, lack of activity, lack of fiber, and the abundance of protein in the diet. Be sure to offer plenty of water: 48–56 ounces per day minimum for women, 56–64 ounces per day minimum for men. Encourage physical activity. Encourage short, frequent walks during the first months postsurgery for those with limited activity. Add fiber to the diet (for example, whole-wheat bread and cereal, fresh fruit and vegetables). Increase dietary intake of fruits and vegetables and choose whole grains when starches are permitted or approximately 2 months after surgery. Increase fruit with skin and raw vegetable consumption when advised by the surgeon or approximately 4 months after surgery. Check with the PMD prior to starting over-the-counter medications. Medications that might be considered include: one tablespoon Milk of Magnesia or mineral oil during the first few months postop; Benefiber or sugar-free Metamucil following the 2-month postoperative period. **Don't:** Don't offer sweetened drinks that could trigger dumping syndrome. Don't encourage too much fluid that will interfere with food intake. Don't forget to have the patient wait 30 minutes after eating. Don't suggest overexercising or overexerting to the point of the patient's dehydration. Don't let patients consume poorly tolerated fruits and vegetables that can potentially cause a blockage. These foods include: oranges, grapefruits, celery, pea pods, and grapes that are not thoroughly chewed.

Problem	*Do's and Don'ts*
Vomiting	**Do:** Counsel the patient that vomiting is a common issue during post-RNY gastric bypass surgery, given the decreased capacity of the pouch and the behavioral changes necessary in eating patterns. The most common causes of vomiting include the pace of eating and the type and amount of food consumed. Vomiting can signal more significant medical issues because it is associated with strictures and medical stenosis. With persistent intolerance to solid food, strongly consider an endoscopic evaluation. Measure portion sizes. Use sectioned or compartmentalized plates or plastic containers that hold a measured portion, such as a half cup. Ask the patient to chew foods thoroughly and be sure that all foods are moist and tender. Following a gastric bypass, the pouch size is smaller and diminishes the stomach's ability to grind food during digestion. It is important to chew food to almost liquid consistency. Ask the patient to document the amount of time it takes to consume a meal. Eating quickly may cause overfilling of the pouch and potentially vomiting. Prepare or cook foods in a moist fashion, such as bake, broil, and steam. Crock-Pots can help prepare foods in a moist method. Marinate foods in a low-sugar marinade prior to cooking to help tenderize the meat. Add broth to meats prior to reheating to provide moisture to the food. Keep a food record: type of food, preparation method, amount eaten, time of day, place, meal company, time meal started, and time meal ended. If the patient continues with vomiting difficulty, go back to the patient's prior diet stage, and slowly advance the diet again. Use a measuring cup or other visual aid to demonstrate the size of the pouch. Encourage the patient to keep this at the table during mealtime to help remind him or her of the pouch size. Call the PMD immediately if the patient is vomiting fluids that are bright red or brown in color. **Don't:** Don't ignore persistent vomiting because frequent vomiting can lead to hypokalemia and/or hypomagnesemia. Persistent vomiting can also potentially cause future food avoidance.

Problem	*Do's and Don'ts*
Vomiting	Don't fail to measure amounts eaten. Don't have the patient eat and drink at the same time. The patient should stop drinking 30 minutes before a meal and resume drinking 30 minutes following a meal. Remember, the pouch can usually hold a half cup or less in the initial stages of diet advancement. Don't allow the patient to consume meats or foods that are dry, chunky, or not well chewed. Don't allow the patient to eat quickly and not thoroughly chew foods. Don't cook foods in or on a dry heat; also, grilling and frying can denature protein that can make it tougher to digest. Don't use a microwave to reheat foods because it can dry the food from the inside out.
Stomach Bloating After Eating	**Do:** Advise the patient that bloating is typically a problem following the initial weeks of gastric bypass surgery. Swallowed air is the most common cause of bloating, and adjusting eating habits can help lessen bloating. Recommend that the patient eat small portions slowly and wait to drink fluids until after eating. The patient should avoid swallowing air when eating by limiting talking while eating, using a sippy cup, or by taking small sips. Remind the patient that chewing gum and eating hard candy can lead to swallowing air that can contribute to bloating. Serve only flat carbonated beverages (without any bubbles). Remind the patient of the importance of staying active! **Don't:** Don't allow the patient to eat large portions quickly and drink using a straw or take big gulps when drinking. Don't serve carbonated beverages unless they are flat. Don't chew gum or eat hard candy.
Diarrhea	**Do:** Advise the patient that the initial stages of the postgastric bypass diet include a significant amount of liquids, with limited fiber and solid foods. Many patients have a change

Problem	*Do's and Don'ts*
	in bowel habits during the first few weeks following surgery. Patients may have a different bowel elimination pattern than preoperatively. Softer, more liquid stools are common during the first few weeks.
	Limit foods that can contribute to diarrhea, including high-fat or spicy foods (for example, sausages, fried foods, cream sauces, ground beef, salami, pepperoni, regular cheeses, and fatty pork), seasonings (for example, pepper, hot sauce, garlic, onions), foods high in simple sugars that can cause dumping syndrome, sugar-free candies, cookies or ice cream, which contain sugar alcohols, and caffeine-containing beverages.
	Consider electrolyte replacement with frequent diarrhea using a diluted or low-sugar electrolyte replacement formula (for example, Pedialyte, diluted Gatorade, or Propel water).
	Consider that the patient may be lactose intolerant if diarrhea is associated with cramping gas pain following the consumption of lactose-containing foods (for example, milk, cheese, cottage cheese, and yogurt). See the following section on lactose intolerance.
	Don't:
	Don't serve fluids with meals or foods that can contribute to diarrhea.
	Don't provide a high-sugar electrolyte replacement drink that can cause dumping syndrome.
Lactose Intolerance	**Do:**
	Advise the patient that lactose is a natural sugar found mainly in dairy products. Lactose intolerance is caused by a decrease in the functionality of the lactase enzyme that aids in lactose digestion. Many RNY gastric bypass patients can develop a lactose intolerance following gastric bypass surgery, which diminishes their ability to tolerate lactose-containing products. This can be challenging to the patient if lactose intolerance goes undiagnosed or if the patient does not have sufficient guidance to make appropriate lactose-free food substitutions for the different diet progressions. In many cases, the patient is able to tolerate lactose further out from surgery.
	Try offering the patient chewable tablets, drops, or commercial products that assist in digesting lactose or provide predigested milk sugars, such as Dairy Ease or LACTAID.

Problem	*Do's and Don'ts*
Lactose Intolerance	Separate the difference between whey protein allergy and lactose intolerance with proper diagnostic tests if symptoms persist or become more severe. Consider soy-based proteins as an alternative. Offer the patient products that assist in lactose digestion. **Don't:** Don't avoid all lactose-containing products; try to find a lactose-free substitute. Don't prepare protein shakes with water instead of milk because many of the mixes can contain some milk-based powders.
Dizziness, Headaches, or Sudden Light-Headedness	**Do:** Advise the patient that lack of energy immediately following surgery can be a normal occurrence, however, some related symptoms are hydration and electrolytes and not the surgical procedure. Schedule a PMD visit close to surgery to help assess the continued need for medications or any dosage adjustments necessary. Some medications can cause electrolyte imbalance, while others may need to have the dosages adjusted with significant weight loss. Have the patient drink plenty of water, but include some higher-sodium or electrolyte-containing beverages (for example, tomato juice, chicken, beef, or vegetable broth, Pedialyte, diluted Gatorade, or Propel water). Add salt to the daily intake. Increased consumption of water with decreased intake of sodium due to the types of foods eaten can lead to low-serum sodium levels. Many gastric bypass patients are careful of their sodium intake preoperatively due to issues with fluid retention. After surgery, patients drastically reduce their sodium intake due to the limited intake of processed foods. Try a cup of bouillon daily to increase sodium intake. Have the patient eat on a regular schedule. Ask PMD to review medications and adjust as necessary with recent changes in weight and diet. **Don't:** Don't allow the patient to get dehydrated. Don't have the patient avoid sodium completely because this could lead to water toxicity. Don't let the patient skip meals.

Problem	*Do's and Don'ts*
Tiredness and Weakness	**Do:** Advise patients that fatigue is common immediately postop, as is weakness. Healing from gastric bypass surgery is not only the immediate postop period, but it extends for at least 6 months following surgery. The decreased food intake due to the smaller pouch can lead to fatigue and weakness. It is important to have the patient eat more frequently, make the calories more nutrient dense, eat regularly, limit caffeine-containing beverages to 4 ounces per day, and stay well hydrated and active. Evaluate sleep schedule. Check timing of vitamins, specifically B complex, because it may need to be taken earlier in the day. Ask the PMD to check laboratory values to evaluate any vitamin or mineral deficiencies that may cause tiredness, specifically, iron, B_{12}, and folate. Evaluate the need for fluids or hydration that can lead to fatigue. **Don't:** Don't allow the patient to skip meals or get dehydrated. Don't allow the patient to drink more than 4 ounces of caffeinated beverages near bedtime. Don't forget to encourage the patient to use the CPAP (continuous positive air pressure) mask if postoperative sleep apnea has been diagnosed. Many patients continue to need to use the mask for several weeks to months following surgery. Don't allow the patient to exercise close to bedtime. Try a relaxing schedule to help wind down prior to sleeping.
Heartburn	**Do:** Advise the patient that heartburn is common preoperatively and usually lessens following surgery with weight reduction. Ask the patient if he or she is taking the medications prescribed postoperatively to decrease acid production. The taste of the liquid medication often leads to avoidance. Consider asking for an alternative form of medication (melts) when not tolerating liquid medication. Limit caffeine and spicy, fatty foods (for example, sausages, fried foods, cream sauces, ground beef, salami, pepperoni, regular cheeses, fatty pork, and seasonings such as pepper, hot sauce, garlic, and onions).

Problem	***Do's and Don'ts***
Heartburn	Offer Tums. Avoid offering foods that are too hot or too cold. Check for the side effects of medications. Provide vitamins or mineral supplements, such as iron, before bedtime to lessen the heartburn. **Don't:** Don't serve salted crackers to help quell the heartburn. Don't add simple carbohydrates, such as crackers, breads, pretzels, and milk to the diet without planning or portioning because it can lead to grazing or slowed weight loss. Don't ignore persistent heartburn because the patient may need to be on different types or doses of medication. Don't add new foods all at once. Try one new food at a time to determine if the symptoms relate to a certain type of food.
Leg Cramps	**Do:** Provide vitamins that contain minerals to help lessen leg cramps. Have the patient stay active and eat a well-balanced diet. Have the PMD check electrolyte levels, including potassium and magnesium. **Don't:** Don't forget to offer vitamins. Don't provide a quinine-containing beverage that is carbonated without consulting with the PMD/RN because it may cause gastric distress. Don't allow the patient to overexercise leg muscles. In the initial stages of gastric bypass, avoid using the abdominal muscles to prevent hernias; the leg muscles often have to compensate. Leg cramps may result with overexerting exercises. Don't advance the diet without consulting the PMD/RN to determine if healing has progressed to allow a variety of foods to be included in the diet.
Excessive Hair Loss	**Do:** Provide adequate protein, a minimum of 60 grams per day. Suggest that the patient take chewable multivitamins.

Problem	*Do's and Don'ts*
	Consider adding a B vitamin supplement that contains biotin. Typically, a B complex vitamin providing about 50% of the recommended intake, or B50 once per day, is helpful.
	Evaluate fat intake and consider omega-3 fats found in the following fish: salmon, sardines in oil, pollack, bluefish, lake trout, flounder, canned tuna, and herring. Other sources include canola oil, flaxseed (ground) and flaxseed oil, wheat germ, soybean oil, and walnuts.
	Don't:
	Don't increase protein to excessive amounts due to potential kidney problems.
	Don't avoid protein if the patient is having difficulty tolerating it. Try a protein supplement (for example, whey, soy protein powder, or dry skim milk powder) to increase protein in the consumed amount.
	Don't provide a multivitamin that is not complete with 100% US Recommended Dietary Allowances (USRDA) for all vitamins and minerals. See the appendix on page 301.
	Don't offer a B vitamin supplement that is not chewable, liquid, or sublingual.
	Don't give more than 100% of USRDA of B complex daily. See the appendix on page 301.
	Don't completely avoid giving fat. Try to incorporate small amounts of heart-healthy fat in measured portions.
Very Slow Weight Loss	**Do:**
	Advise the patient that many gastric bypass patients reach plateaus where they have slowed weight loss at times during the postop course. Try to remember the weight loss patterns that happened prior to surgery (slow and steady or weight loss, plateau, weight loss, plateau); they would likely be similar after surgery.
	Have the patient keep a food record to document intake, including portions, intensity of hunger, and emotions. Also, record who they were with and what they were doing.
	Recommend slowing the pace of eating.
	Measure the portions of foods.
	Consider having the patient increase exercise and changing exercise routine.
	Suggest the entire hydration fluid needed daily.

Problem	*Do's and Don'ts*
Very Slow Weight Loss	Read labels; be aware of the fat calories of items that may not count as a fat serving.
	Don't:
	Don't forget to remind the patient to reread his or her diet education material. The postop portions often get magnified, even with a small stomach.
	Don't allow the skipping of meals. Long periods without eating can slow the metabolism and contribute to slow weight loss.
	Don't forget to remind the patient to eat protein first, fruit and vegetables second, and starches last.
	Don't take portioning for granted. Actually measuring food can help shed light on those extra calories that can sneak in and slow weight loss.
	Don't have the patient continue with the same old exercise routine. Consult with a trainer to help with several routines to work different muscle groups.
	Don't serve high-calorie beverages.
	Don't let hidden fat calories sneak in with starchy foods or high-fat meats.
	Don't allow caffeinated beverages (coffee and some soft drinks) because they may be a trigger to eat additional foods.
Extreme Hunger	**Do:**
	Advise the patient that gastric bypass patients have both physical hunger and mental hunger. Mental hunger refers to eating because of the surroundings or emotions, not in response to the need to eat. Oftentimes, mental hunger happens following surgery, and it is frustrating to the patient who does not understand why he or she is still hungry.
	Keep a food record for the patient and document surroundings.
	Consider journaling the patient's feelings and separate mental hunger from physical hunger.
	Discuss evaluating pouch size with the PMD.
	Refer to the PMD for other potential causes of extreme hunger, including low blood sugar, side effects of medications, or the need for psychiatric counseling.

Problem	Do's and Don'ts
	Don't:
	Don't allow grazing to quell hunger. This can work against the gastric bypass.
	Don't forget to schedule extra appointments with the therapist, psychologist, or social worker around the time of surgery to help the patient deal with some of the behavior changes and losses that occur after surgery.
	Don't ignore the patient's hunger. This could signal that the pouch has stretched and needs evaluation.
Excessive Weight Loss	**Do:**
	Advise the patient that excessive weight loss in a patient following gastric bypass surgery can occur and can result from several causes. The most common etiology of excessive weight loss is the anatomy of the surgery and issues with eating. Other etiologies include underlying eating disorders or psychological issues relating to the patient's new body and his or her self-image.
	Keep a food record or diary to document foods consumed. Look at the types of food eaten, paying close attention to the textures. Delineate tolerance of foods that are mushy and soft from those that may be chunky and poorly chewed.
	Evaluate exercise patterns, including type and amount.
	Consider decreasing exercise or changing the type and amount of exercise.
	Use prudence in adding snacks or protein drinks around exercise if needed.
	Seek the help of a trained mental health worker in disordered eating patterns.
	Don't:
	Don't forget to refer the patient back to the PMD to evaluate the potential anatomical issues and symptoms related to surgery.
	Don't try to make the patient eat more if it is a physical issue that is causing pain or discomfort when eating.
	Don't tell the patient not to exercise. Work on a schedule and provide them with calories burned with certain activities so they can help plan their intake and activity.

Problem	Do's and Don'ts
Excessive Weight Loss	Don't chalk up the symptoms to surgery. Be vigilant if you feel that the patient is having mental issues, such as underlying eating disorders or posttraumatic stress disorder, causing the excessive weight loss.
Reactive Hypoglycemia	**Do:** Advise the patient that reactive hypoglycemia sometimes occurs in patients following a gastric bypass because their blood sugar levels drop too low a few hours after eating. The symptoms are weakness, nausea, extreme hunger, headaches, dizziness, and sweating. It is important for the patient to eat regularly and have a balanced diet, which includes protein, carbohydrate, and some healthy fat. Include high-fiber carbohydrates in the patient's diet when serving carbohydrate. Typically, 3 or more grams of carbohydrate per serving are a good source of fiber. Offer five to six small meals per day. Suggest exercise. **Don't:** Don't allow the patient to skip meals or try to bring blood sugar up with simple sugars consistently without proper intervention. Don't recommend carbohydrates alone. Don't provide low-fiber, refined carbohydrates. Don't have the patient eat only once or twice per day. Don't recommend juice to consistently bring up blood sugar. Juice can provide additional calories as well as the potential for dumping. Consider glucose tablets or gels as a temporary solution. Don't have the patient exercise without a proper protein and carbohydrate snack if needed.
Gallstones	**Do:** Have an abdominal ultrasound done prior to surgery if the patient still has a gallbladder when presented for surgery. Ensure the patient has appropriate postoperative medications prescribed to avoid gallstones. **Don't:** Don't ignore right upper quadrant pain if the patient has been losing weight and their gallbladder is still intact.

Problem	*Do's and Don'ts*
B_{12} Deficiency	**Do:** Advise the patient that B_{12} deficiency is a concern in patients who are status post (s/p) RNY gastric bypass surgery because the pouch now bypasses the lower part of the stomach and makes B_{12} absorption more difficult with less intrinsic factor available. Check B_{12} levels every 3 months for the first year. Continue to check B_{12} levels yearly because the prevalence of B_{12} deficiency increases yearly. Try sublingual vitamin B_{12} supplements for those whose vitamin B_{12} levels are trending downward and close to low normal. If the PMD recommends a B_{12} supplement, look for a sublingual brand that has a minimum of 350 micrograms of B_{12} per tablet. If levels do not respond, a B_{12} shot may be necessary on a short-term or an ongoing basis. Consider increasing dietary sources of B_{12}, including salmon, tuna, lean beef, fortified breakfast cereals, milk, and yogurt. **Don't:** Don't avoid getting B_{12} levels checked following surgery. Don't ignore low normal vitamin levels. Though they are normal, if they are low normal they may need supplementation. Rely mainly on sublingual for patients who need repletion. Many patients require IM injections of B_{12}.
Iron Deficiency	**Do:** Advise female patients that typically menstruating women, or those who are anemic prior to surgery, are at risk for iron deficiency following gastric bypass surgery. Oral iron may be difficult to absorb due to the bypassing of the lower part of the stomach. In addition, red meat, a good source of heme iron in the diet, is often poorly tolerated, thus making dietary iron intake less than optimal. Monitor ferritin iron levels and erythrocytes. The PMD may recommend iron either in a preventative dosage or in a replenishment dose.

Iron Supplements	Preventative	Replenishment
Vitron C	1 tablet/day	3 tablets/day
Feosol	1 tablet/day	3 tablets/day
Ferro-Sequels	1 tablet/day	3 tablets/day
Slow FE	1 tablet/day	3 tablets/day
Fergon	2 tablets/day	4 tablets/day

Problem	*Do's and Don'ts*
Iron Deficiency	Consider trying better-tolerated foods that are higher in iron (for example, dark-meat poultry, beans, fortified oatmeal, beef, and raisins). Try adding sources of vitamin C with iron-containing foods to facilitate absorption. **Don't:** Don't recommend a poorly absorbed form of iron, such as a ferric form or one without fiber, for those who are easily constipated. Vitamin C with iron also assists in absorption.
Pregnancy after RNY Gastric Bypass Surgery	**Do:** Advise the patient that pregnancy after gastric bypass surgery can be a challenge depending on the patient's capacity to eat. Regular prenatal care is essential. Seek an obstetrician who is familiar with the gastric bypass surgery. If the patient is pregnant less than 6 months postop, slow down or minimize weight loss by increasing intake with calorie-dense foods to five to six meals per day. If the patient is pregnant more than 6 months following surgery, increase oral intake by 300 calories above the regular postoperative diet. Provide vitamin supplements prescribed by the obstetrician based on medical history. Typical recommendations include: Chewable vitamins: One to two tablets per day Chewable prenatal vitamins: One per day Calcium: 1200–1500 mg per day Choose beta-carotene as a source of vitamin A. Obtain a gestational diabetes test at 28 weeks. Some women who experience dumping syndrome may not be able to tolerate the glucola or other source of oral glucose. Discuss with the PMD if the patient has dumping syndrome; recommend a possible alternative test. Ask the patient to avoid caffeine consumption during pregnancy, less than 300 mg of caffeine daily if at all. **Don't:** Don't increase intake with nonnutritive foods to gain weight. Don't avoid weight gain postoperatively.

Problem	*Do's and Don'ts*
	Don't allow excessive vitamin supplements without consulting with the PMD or checking vitamin levels.
	Don't choose detrimental sources of vitamin A.
	Don't avoid the dumping syndrome test if it is suspected.
	Don't allow more than 10 ounces of caffeine-containing beverages per day.
	Don't delay the patient seeing an obstetrician for fear of weight gain.
	Don't refer the patient to an obstetrician who is not familiar with gastric bypass surgery.

Sources

Brigham and Women's Hospital Program for Weight Management. *Dietary Guidelines for Gastric Bypass*. July 2004.

Brigham and Women's Hospital Program for Weight Management. *Iron*. August 2004.

Fujioka, K. "Follow-up Nutritional and Metabolic Problems After Bariatric Surgery." *Diabetes Care*. 2005. 28, 481–484.

National Institutes of Health, National Institute of Diabetes and Digestive and Kidney Disease (NIDDK). Weight-Control Information Network (WIN). Gastrointestinal Surgery for Severe Obesity. NIH Publication number 01-4006, December 2001.

Cancer (Nutrition During Chemotherapy and Radiation)

Author: Stephanie Vangsness, MS, RD, LDN, CNSD

This list will assist the dietitian in answering food tolerance questions and serve as a guide to assist patients who are undergoing chemotherapy and radiation. The side effects of chemotherapy and/or radiation may include nausea, vomiting, diarrhea, constipation, dehydration, bloatedness, heartburn, mouth sores, taste changes, dry mouth, and weight loss or weight gain.

Problem	***Do's and Don'ts***
Nausea	**Do:**
	Recommend six to eight small meals a day instead of three large meals.
	Sip clear liquids, such as ginger tea, ginger ale, or lemonade frequently to prevent dehydration.
	Try homemade ginger root tea. Peel and slice fresh ginger root (about the size of a nickel). Add 8 oz boiling water and sip.
	Suck on crystallized ginger or ginger chews.
	Choose dry foods that do not have an odor (for example, crackers, toast, and dry cereals).
	Try low-fat, bland foods (for example, canned fruit, sherbet, fruit ice, pretzels, toast, crackers, graham crackers, cottage cheese, cheese and crackers, pudding, tapioca, and other cold foods) that may be better tolerated when nausea is a problem.
	Try chilled beverages. Freeze a favorite beverage into ice cubes.
	Don't:
	Don't suggest large meals.
	Don't provide foods that are overly greasy, fried, spicy, or sweet.
	Don't forget to offer fluids. Patient may not tolerate hot beverages.
Vomiting	**Do:**
	Report repeated vomiting to the PMD. When vomiting is under control, try small amounts of clear liquids before moving on to solid food. Clear liquids include sports drinks, such as Gatorade or Powerade, chicken or vegetable

Problem	Do's and Don'ts
	broth, fruit juices diluted 1:1 with water, flat ginger ale, gelatin, Pedialyte, and decaffeinated coffee or tea. Patients may graduate to solid foods after tolerating clear liquids. Clear liquids should not be maintained for more than a day unless directed by the physician. Suggest when vomiting subsides to start with soft bland foods, such as cream of rice cereal, chicken noodle/rice soup, and dry toast. **Don't:** Don't serve solid food until vomiting has subsided. Don't spend prolonged time on clear liquids.
Diarrhea	**Do:** Advise the patient that diarrhea causes the malabsorption of food and can result in the loss of electrolytes. The diet used for diarrhea is similar to that found in the vomiting section. Advance the diet to soft, low-fiber foods as the diarrhea subsides. Small, frequent meals are best. Drink clear fluids, such as Gatorade or Powerade, chicken or vegetable broth, fruit juices diluted 1:1 with water, flat ginger ale, gelatin, or Pedialyte. Introduce low-fiber foods (for example, baked fish and chicken, ground beef, eggs, pureed vegetables, canned fruit, ripe bananas, mashed potatoes, rice, and white bread) when diarrhea subsides. Canned fruits (apples/applesauce, peaches, pears) and ripe bananas are usually tolerated. Include certain cooked vegetables (for example, asparagus tips, carrots, sweet potatoes, green beans, and mushrooms). Limit milk and milk products if the patient is lactose intolerant. Try soy or Lactaid products as a substitute. **Don't:** Don't serve milk and lactose products until diarrhea subsides. Don't provide fried foods, poultry skin. Don't promote high-fiber foods, those that contain greater than 3 grams of fiber (for example, nuts, seeds, whole grains, dried and raw fruits, and vegetables).
Constipation	**Do:** Advise the patient that drug therapy or inadequate fluid or food intake may cause constipation. If the patient suffers from constipation, encourage adequate fluid intake. Hot

Problem	*Do's and Don'ts*
Constipation	beverages may be especially helpful to stimulate intestinal peristalsis. Increase fiber intake by choosing whole-grain crackers, cereals and breads, oatmeal, legumes (beans), fresh or frozen fruits, and vegetables. Try stewed prunes or prune juice heated in the microwave. Add lemon for taste. Encourage movement or light exercise whenever possible to facilitate bowel movements. Suggest supplements (Benefiber and senna tea, such as Smooth Move tea) that may help alleviate constipation with PMD's approval. • How to use Benefiber – Mix 1 tablespoon of Benefiber in 6 oz of any liquid, hot or cold. – Take one dose per day for 3 days unless otherwise advised by your PMD. – After 3 days, increase to 2 tablespoons per day if needed. The patient may increase by 1 tablespoon every 3 days as needed. Do not exceed 4 tablespoons per day. • Where to get Benefiber – Find it in drug stores. – Also, find it in local grocery markets near other anti-constipation medications. • How to use senna tea – Steep tea bag in one cup hot water for 10–15 minutes. – Drink before bedtime. – Take an additional cup of tea in the morning, if needed. – Do not drink more than two cups of tea per 24-hour period. – Senna tea is not intended for long-term use. • Where to get senna tea – Senna tea can be purchased in vitamin stores or health-food specialty stores (Whole Foods). **Don't:** Don't exercise and/or encourage movement to induce bowel movements if patient is unable due to pain.

Problem	Do's and Don'ts
Dehydration	**Do:**
	Advise the patient that diarrhea, severe vomiting, diminished fluid intake, and excessive sweating due to fever may cause dehydration or large losses of body fluids. Take fluids as directed in the sections on diarrhea and vomiting. The PMD will manage severe dehydration.
Bloatedness	**Do:**
	Advise the patient that certain foods may contribute to a bloated feeling.
	Recommend the patient try to eat slowly, eat low-fat foods, and eat soft, bland foods.
	Maintain some exercise or movement that may help clear gas or air in the intestines.
	Don't:
	Don't serve spicy, high-fat foods, chew gum, or drink carbonated beverages.
	Don't encourage movement if the patient is in pain.
Heartburn	**Do:**
	Some suggestions for the patient to prevent heartburn are:
	Sit upright for at least 30 minutes after eating.
	Speak with the PMD about the use of antacids after meals and before bedtime.
	Don't:
	Don't serve spicy foods and caffeine.
	Don't ask the patient to lie down within 30 minutes of eating.
Mouth Sores	**Do:**
	Advise the patient that drug therapy or radiation may cause mouth sores, tender gums, and inflammation of the throat and esophagus. Soft foods (for example, mashed potatoes, pudding, custard, ice cream, scrambled eggs, sherbet, fruit ice, milk shakes, cottage cheese, yogurt, watermelon, peach and pear nectars, overcooked, cooled angel hair pasta with cheese, cooled, cooked cereals, soups, gelatin, and canned fruit) may be more comfortable to eat if mouth sores persist.
	Use a straw with beverages to bypass the contact between the mouth and food. If this is successful, try high-calorie beverages.
	Use milk substitutes if diarrhea is present.

Problem	*Do's and Don'ts*
Mouth Sores	Add gravy and sauces to foods to aid in ease of swallowing. Try cold foods because they may be better tolerated than hot foods. Puree foods in a blender to make them easier to swallow. Ask the patient to rinse his or her mouth often with baking soda mouthwash (1 quart water and 1 tablespoon baking soda) to remove food and germs. **Don't:** Don't serve spicy foods, citrus and pineapple juice and fruits, rough coarse foods, and salty foods. Don't use straws with sharp edges or use more than one time. Don't provide products with lactose, such as pudding and cream soup, if diarrhea is present.
Taste Changes	**Do:** Advise the patient that chemotherapy or radiation treatments can cause foods to have a bitter taste or a taste that is different from usual. Drink fluids with meals to rinse away any bad taste in the mouth before eating. Select foods that smell appetizing to the patient; meats that are less odorous (chicken) may be accepted more easily than those with strong odors (beef and fish). Try cold foods without odors (for example, sliced deli turkey and sliced or cubed cheese). Marinate meats in fruit juices or sweet and sour sauce. Use herbal seasonings (for example, basil, oregano, rosemary, and lemon juice). Suggest for metallic tastes to try sips of cranberry juice and use plastic silverware rather than metal silverware. Maintain adequate hydration because dehydration makes taste changes worse. **Don't:** Don't offer foods too high in salt, such as bacon, hot dogs, canned soup, regular frozen dinners, and snack foods like potato chips and pretzels.
Dry Mouth	**Do:** Advise the patient that drugs and radiation may cause mouth dryness. This, in turn, may change the taste of food and make food difficult to swallow. Some suggestions for

Problem	*Do's and Don'ts*
	patients to combat mouth dryness are sipping fluids regularly or sucking on hard candy or Popsicles to stimulate the production of saliva. Recommend tart foods like lemon drops to stimulate the production of saliva. Add gravies, broth, sauces, and salad dressings to moisten foods and ease swallowing. **Don't:** Don't offer sugarless products with sugar substitutes; they may cause diarrhea or abdominal gas pain if eaten in medium to large quantities.
Weight Loss	**Do:** Suggest eating nutrient-dense foods that offer a high calorie level for combating weight loss during or after chemotherapy and radiation. The following may be some acceptable suggestions for high-protein, high-calorie food ideas: • Melt or grate cheese for use with sandwiches, potatoes, vegetables, casseroles, mashed potatoes, rice, grits, noodles, meat loaf, and bread. • Add cottage cheese to casseroles, pasta, scrambled eggs, and pudding desserts. • Add milk or cream, use milk substitutes if needed, instead of water to hot cereal, beverages, rice, grits, and soups. • Add powdered milk or milk (if tolerated) to casseroles, scrambled eggs, sauces, meat loaf, custards, pudding, and to milk shakes. • Add chopped, cooked egg to salads, vegetables, mashed potatoes, and meat purees. • Put ice cream between graham crackers or cookies and on cake or pie. • Eat peanut butter alone or on a favorite cracker or bread product. Add peanut butter to meat loaf and milkshakes for a delicious nutty flavor. • Add chopped nuts to cereals, yogurt, salads, casseroles, ice cream, and meat loaf. Try commercially prepared nutritional supplement drinks (Ensure, Boost, or Carnation Instant Breakfast), which are available in several brand names and flavors. To fortify calories of these drinks, further add one container of Benecalorie.

Problem	*Do's and Don'ts*
Weight Loss	Add 1 tablespoon olive oil or canola oil to vegetables, meat, chicken, or fish.
	Don't:
	Don't serve baby food because it is too low in calories for adults.
	Don't provide high-fat foods if bloatedness, diarrhea, or nausea is present.

Sources

Mahan, L. K., & Escott-Stump, S. (Eds.). *Krause's Food, Nutrition and Diet Therapy* (11th ed.). Philadelphia, PA: W. B. Saunders Co. 2004.

Nutritional Supplements. http://www.novartisnutrition.com/us/productDetail?id=233.

Adult Parenteral Nutrition (PN) Guide

Author: Teresa Fung, ScD, RD

Parenteral nutrition is a complex nutrition therapy and requires those who are highly trained and medically authorized to oversee the patient's care. The following table is a general guideline for parenteral nutrition, but note that individual requirements will be a part of every patient case.
Note: All parenteral nutrition should have the daily oversight of a dietitian and/or physician.

Problem	***Do's and Don'ts***
When to Use (Indication)	**Do:** Consider for patients who cannot absorb nutrients properly and cannot tolerate enteral (oral) feeding. **Don't:** Don't consider for patients who have a functional GI tract unless all other enteral access routes have been explored and are not feasible.
Choosing Total Parenteral Nutrition (TPN) Route/Site	**Do:** Consider the anticipated duration of TPN use. Take note of the characteristics of the different routes: Catheters for short-term TPN are inserted into the subclavian vein and then threaded through to the superior vena cava. Alternative routes to the superior vena cava are the internal or external jugular veins. Known as "tunneled" catheters for long-term TPN, surgically thread the catheter into the superior vena cava via the subclavian, cephalic, or internal jugular veins. Then create a tunnel below the surface of the skin to allow the catheter to exit the body a few inches away from the entry site. Note that the peripherally inserted central catheter (PICC) is threaded through the antecubital vein, into the subclavian vein, and finally into the superior vena cava. Properly trained individuals can perform this procedure.
Choosing Peripheral Parenteral Nutrition (PPN) Route/Site	**Do:** Consider the anticipated duration of PPN use. Consider if need is for shorter duration than for parenteral nutrition. Place catheters for PPN in any vein that is in good condition. Limit the formula concentration to 800–900 mOsm/L. The PMD should change the insertion site regularly unless using an extended dwell catheter. Insert extended dwell catheters into a vein 5 to 7 inches for 3 to 6 weeks.

Problem	*Do's and Don'ts*
Choosing Peripheral Parenteral Nutrition (PPN) Route/Site	**Don't:** Don't use if osmolarity of solution exceeds 900 mOsm/L. Don't use in patients who are fluid volume restricted. Don't use in patients with poor peripheral access. Don't use in patients with significant malnutrition and/or severe metabolic stress.
Understanding Stock Solution Characteristics	**Do:** Understand that standard parenteral nutrition solutions contain a mixture of water, amino acids, carbohydrates, fats, electrolytes, vitamins, and trace elements and minerals. Adjust specific amounts of each macronutrient to the patient's needs. • Glucose or dextrose monohydrate: Stock solution concentration ranges from 5% to 70% (weight by volume) total ml for 24 hours × percent dextrose in decimal form × 3.4 kcal = total dextrose calories • Lipids: Three concentrations are available: 10% (weight by volume), 1.1 kcal/ml; 20%, 2 kcal/ml and 30%, 3.0 kcal/ml • Amino acids: Stock solution concentration = range from 3.5% to 20% (weight by volume), 4 kcal/g
Understanding Admixture Type	**Do:** Select proper admixture according to patient characteristics. Note that there are three main types of admixtures available: • A traditional or two-in-one mixture contains a designated ratio of amino acids to dextrose, with the fat emulsion added separately. • Total nutrient admixture contains a three-in-one mixture of carbohydrates, fats, and amino acids. **Don't:** Don't omit lipids for long periods due to risk of essential fatty acid deficiency.
Storing Solution	**Do:** Keep solution refrigerated and away from light at all times until just prior to infusion. Infuse lipid-containing formulas within 24 hours. Keep fat emulsions separate from the rest of the solution using a dual-chamber administration bag. Remove the roll-bar between the chambers to combine the components just before use.

Problem	*Do's and Don'ts*
Calculating Osmolarity for PPN	**Do:** Note the upper limit of solution osmolarity is 900 mOsm/L. Note that dextrose has the greatest impact on osmolarity, amino acids, and electrolytes. Note that lipids have little effect. Calculate the osmolarity of a solution: • Multiply grams of dextrose per liter by 5 • Multiply grams of amino acids per liter by 10 • Multiply grams of lipids per liter by 1.5 • Multiply mEq/L of electrolytes by 2 • Add together the preceding products to obtain total osmolarity
Determining Maximum Macronutrients in PN Formulation	**Don't:** Don't exceed the following: • Glucose or dextrose: 5 mg/kg/min • Amino acids: 2 gm/kg body weight • Lipids: 2.0 g/kg/day or 60% of total kcals
Determining Fluid Needs	**Do:** Work up to 30–35 ml/kg body weight of fluid, with daily amounts totaling between 1.5 to 3 liters; make sure to account for all IVs in this figure. Adjust according to patient's physiological needs, such as cardiopulmonary, hepatic, or renal insufficiency or failure.
Determining Electrolyte Needs	**Do:** Advise the patient that normal electrolyte ranges are as follows: • Calcium: 10–15 mEq • Magnesium: 8–20 mEq • Phosphate: 20–40 mmol • Sodium: 60–150 mEq • Potassium: 60–120 mEq • Acetate: Amount needed to maintain acid-base balance • Chloride: Amount needed to maintain acid-base balance Adjust according to the patient's physiological needs.
Determining Vitamin and Trace Mineral Needs	**Do:** Note that RDA/DRI amounts for vitamins, minerals, and trace elements are usually added to PPN and TPN solutions. Add selenium to prevent cardiomyopathy if individuals are on long-term parenteral feeding. Note that iron is not included in solutions due to its incompatibility with lipids.

Problem	*Do's and Don'ts*
Choosing Administration Schedule	**Do:** Take note that there are two types of infusions: • Administer continuous infusion feeding over a 24-hour period. • Administer cyclic infusion feeding over a 12–18 hour period, often with the majority overnight, allowing the patient more flexibility during the daytime for normal activities. The goal rate is achieved by incremental advancements. Do continuous infusion. Initiate Total parenteral nutrition (TPN) with approximately half of the patient's calorie needs. Advance to goal calories as tolerated. If discontinuing TPN abruptly, contact the PMD to obtain dextrose IV orders unless the patient has already transitioned to oral POs. (Exception: PPN does not require any tapering or any dextrose IV if abruptly discontinued because it has a lower dextrose; use amino acid concentration.) Do cyclic infusion. Start and stop infusion gradually by using this pattern: • Start the infusion rate by half of the goal TPN rate for the first 1 to 2 hours. • Decrease the TPN rate by half 1 to 2 hours before turning the TPN off. **Don't:** Don't stop infusion suddenly for risk of hypoglycemia.
Monitoring	**Do:** Follow this schedule by monitoring the following: • Weight (daily) • Blood electrolyte levels (daily) • Blood glucose levels (daily); chemBG's three times daily unless otherwise indicated • Acid-base balance (daily) • Calcium, phosphorus, and magnesium levels (daily) • Plasma transaminases (three times per week) • Albumin (three times per week) • Ammonia level (two times per week) • Hemoglobin (weekly) • Prothrombin time (weekly) • Triglycerides (weekly) • Prealbumin (every 4 days)

Problem	Do's and Don'ts
Monitoring	• Monitor urine for glucose and ketones (four to six times per day) • Monitor urine for specific gravity or osmolarity (two to four times per day) • Urinary urea nitrogen (weekly) • Volume infusate (daily) • Oral intake (if applicable—daily) • Urinary output (daily) • Activity, temperature, and respiration (daily) • WBC and differential counts (as needed) • Cultures (as needed)
Caring for Insertion Sites	**Do:** Prevent infections at the catheter site by having medical personnel: Change dressings every 48–72 hours. Change tubing every 24–72 hours. Clean catheter site with chlorhexidine. Use dressings made of gauze and tape or a semipermeable membrane. Consider patient characteristics when choosing.
Transitioning to Enteral or Oral Feedings	**Do:** Attempt enteral or oral feedings if the patient's GI tract is functioning. Maintain nutritional needs continually throughout the transition. Use the following transition guidelines: Transitioning to enteral feeding: Begin enteral feeding slowly, 20 ml/hr, and decrease the TPN macronutrients by approximately one-fourth of the dextrose, lipid, and amino acid calories. If the patient continues to tolerate the enteral feeding, advance the enteral feeding 10 cc each 6 to 8 hours, as tolerated. If the patient has already reached goal enteral tube feeding (TF) rate, discontinue the TPN by the end of the second day; if tube feed goal rate has not been reached yet, then continue to decrease TPN calories. Transitioning to oral feeding: Administer the parenteral solution overnight and reduce the amount; also infuse at a slower rate, which will result in remaining TPN solution. (Discard all three-in-one mixtures after 24 hours.) Another option for weaning off TPN is to reduce the calories in the TPN

Problem	*Do's and Don'ts*
Transitioning to Enteral or Oral Feedings	admixture by one-forth to one-half the macronutrient calories. Initiate oral feedings during normal mealtimes and monitor intake. Meet nutrient requirements with a supplement as tapering off TPN. Having met 75% of nutrient needs orally, discontinue TPN. The length of transition time varies.
Oversights	**Do:** Maintain close communication with the healthcare team and the physician about any initiation or orders that include parenteral nutrition. Receive medical consultation from appropriate trained professionals. **Don't:** Don't proceed with parenteral nutrition changes without the oversight of the PMD/RD and other appropriate medical personnel.

Sources

Bloch, A. S., & Mueller, C. "Chapter 23: Enteral and Parenteral Nutrition Support." Mahan, L. K., & Escott-Stump, S. (Eds.). *Krause's Food, Nutrition and Diet Therapy* (11th ed.). Philadelphia, PA: W.B. Saunders. 2004. 533–553.

Matarese, L. E., & Gottschlich, M. M. *Contemporary Nutrition Support Practice: A Clinical Guide* (2nd ed.). Philadelphia, PA: W. B. Saunders. 2003.

Worthington, P. H. *Practical Aspects of Nutritional Support: An Advanced Practice Guide*. Philadelphia, PA: W. B. Saunders. 2004. 265–341.

Troubleshooting with Parenteral Nutrition (PN)

Author: Teresa Fung, ScD, RD

This guideline is only meant to educate the bedside staff. Those caring for patients with parenteral nutrition should be medically trained and able to handle the complications that may arise.
All parenteral nutrition should have the oversight of a PMD/RD.

Problem	*Do's and Don'ts*
Elevated Blood Glucose	**Do:** Control blood glucose from the onset of administering parenteral nutrition. Tight glycemic control is necessary with appropriate insulin coverage, if needed. Maintain a maximum dextrose infusion rate of 4 mg/kg/min in patients, who are at risk for hyperglycemia. **Don't:** Don't initiate dextrose at goal rate.
Elevated Blood Triglycerides	**Do:** Omit lipid emulsion if serum triglyceride levels exceed 400 mg/dl for adults.
Air Embolism	**Do:** Have the RN position patient flat during catheter insertion/change/removal; secure catheter and tube junctions with proper locking connectors; close clamps before moving catheter; apply ointment and proper dressing to catheter insertion site after removal.
Extravasation	**Do:** Elevate the limb where infiltrated tissues are and apply a cold compress; flush area with saline; administer subcutaneous hyaluronidase to absorb the solution.
Clogged Catheter	**Do:** • Have the PMD/RN make sure all clamps are open and there are no kinks in the tubing. • Have the PMD/RN determine if tip of catheter has migrated and is being obstructed by the wall of the vessel or by the clavicle and first rib. • Consider using radiographic contrast imaging to determine if thrombus is causing blockage. • Consider the contents of the used admixture—high amounts of lipids can cause a buildup over time. • Consider if a precipitate is causing the blockage; consult a pharmacist to determine the best method.

Problem	*Do's and Don'ts*
Catheter Infection	**Do:** Medical personnel should wash hands thoroughly before and after handling insertion site; use chlorhexidine to clean site; change dressings every 48–72 hours; change tubing every 24–72 hours; remove catheter and determine type and severity of infection before resuming infusion; determine what type of dressing best suits catheter type and insertion site. **Don't:** Don't replace catheter before infection type is determined and treatment has been administered.
Refeeding Syndrome	**Do:** • Correct any electrolyte imbalance first before initiating parenteral nutrition (PN). • Ensure feeding begins slowly at dextrose levels of 150 g/day and progress slowly (over 5 to 7 days) to goal rate; start at calorie levels below maintenance needs (15 kcal/kg). • Closely monitor serum potassium, magnesium, and phosphorus, as well as weight and insulin levels; monitor hemodynamic stability and metabolic indicators, such as serum glucose, triglycerides, and other electrolytes; correct any electrolyte imbalances before next PN; slowly add dextrose and calories as tolerated by the patient. **Don't:** Don't begin PN before establishing proper electrolyte levels; don't initiate dextrose levels at goal rate.
Dehydration	**Do:** Control/replace fluid losses through supplemental fluid and/or electrolyte infusions.
Fluid Overload	**Do:** Reduce fluid levels; concentrate PN formula; consult PMD or RD regarding administration of diuretics.
Hypersensitivity	**Do:** Stop lipids immediately if allergic symptoms present in the patient. Notify the pharmacist and PMD to treat the patient if needed; administer a trial of lipid-free PN solution when allergic conditions are gone. **Don't:** Don't continue with normal PN formulation administration. Don't discontinue TPN and not obtain the PMD's orders for supplemental IV dextrose solution.

Problem	*Do's and Don'ts*
Catheter Tip Displacement or Migration	**Do:** Determine location of catheter tip and reposition or replace as needed. Secure catheter tube with tape or a fastener; change tape/fastener every 2 to 3 days; ensure site is clean and sterile. **Don't:** Don't remove catheter without closing all clamps first; don't attempt to remove catheter without first determining where tip has become lodged.
Drug/Nutrient Interactions	**Do:** Permit very few medications in PN due to the limitations in PN compatibility. Because PN has very little medication added to it, check with the patient's pharmacist and/or physician to determine what type of interactions the patient's medication may have with other IVs the patient is receiving.
Sudden Weight Change	**Do:** Check weight again; check fluid intake from all IV and fluid sources and output; check for signs of edema; check infusion pump rate.
Oversight	**Do:** Receive proper training to calculate patient needs and make appropriate recommendations. Maintain close communication with the healthcare team and the physician about any initiation or orders that include parenteral nutrition. Receive medical consultation from appropriate trained professionals. **Don't:** Don't proceed with parenteral changes without the oversight of the physician and other appropriate medical personnel.

SECTION 4

Sources

Bloch, A. S., & Mueller, C. "Enteral and Parenteral Nutrition Support." Mahan, L. K., & Escott-Stump, S. (Eds.). *Krause's Food, Nutrition and Diet Therapy* (11th ed.). Philadelphia, PA: W. B. Saunders. 2004. 533–553.

Matarese, L. E., & Gottschlich, M. M. *Contemporary Nutrition Support Practice: A Clinical Guide* (2nd ed.). Philadelphia, PA: W. B. Saunders. 2003.

Worthington, P. H. *Practical Aspects of Nutritional Support: An Advanced Practice Guide.* Philadelphia, PA: W. B. Saunders. 2004. 265–341.

Adult Tube Feeding Guide

Author: Teresa Fung, ScD, RD

Enteral nutrition is a complex medical therapy and requires those who are highly trained and medically authorized to oversee the patient's care. The following table is a general guideline for enteral nutrition, but note that individual requirements will be a part of every patient's case.

Problem	*Do's and Don'ts*
When to Use (indication)	**Do:** Tube feeding is indicated for patients who have a functional GI tract (at least 100 cm small bowel; can sustain fluid/electrolyte balance; can absorb nutrients properly) but cannot nourish themselves adequately by mouth. Consider for patients who refuse to eat or should not eat (oral intake is unsafe or ineffective and/or oral intake is inadequate to meet needs). Consider for patients who have not ingested food orally for 5 to 7 days (and have a functioning gut), and there is no clear indication of when they will again be able to do so.
When Not to Use (contraindication)	**Don't:** Don't use with patients who have impaired GI function (less than 100 cm of small bowel; cannot sustain fluid/electrolyte balance; and cannot absorb nutrients properly). Don't use with patients with: • Complete obstruction of distal small bowel • Massive GI bleeding • Congenital anomalies of GI tract • Intractable diarrhea • Intestinal ischemia • Fistula or perforation
Choosing Types of Formula	**Do:** Choose formula based on: • Functional status of GI tract • Physical characteristics of formula—osmolality, fiber content, caloric density, viscosity • Macronutrient ratios and specific metabolic needs of patient • Digestion/absorption capability of patient • Contribution of formula to fluid/electrolyte needs • Cost effectiveness

Problem	*Do's and Don'ts*
	Consider the following formula class according to patient condition: General purpose–intact (polymeric): This is the most common type of formula. It is nutritionally complete and is best for patients who have normal/minimally impaired digestion; absorption of nutrients in GI tract is required. The formula contains intact protein, carbohydrate, and fat; 1–1.2 kcal/ml; osmolality range is 300–500 mOsm/kg. This formula is inexpensive. Fiber-enriched: This formula's nutrient composition is similar to general-purpose formula but contains fiber. It promotes normal bowel function; works well for long-term feeding; and requires the patient to have normal GI function and absorption. Defined–hydrolyzed (monomeric): This formula is for use with GI-compromised patients. It is nutritionally complete and usually lactose free. It has 1–1.2 kcal/ml; has higher osmolality than general formula; and is more expensive than general formula. Macronutrients can be partially hydrolyzed or completely hydrolyzed for easy absorption—also called semi-elemental and elemental, respectively. Disease specific: This formula is for specific organ dysfunction or metabolic abnormality (hepatic, renal, pulmonary diseases, glucose intolerance, and trauma); it is expensive. Modular: This formula provides protein, carbohydrate, or fat as single nutrients to alter nutrient composition of other formula or foods. Modular is more expensive than general purpose.
Determining Formula Rate/Volume	**Do:** Gradually increase full-strength formulas in rate or volume until goal rate/volume is achieved. See initiation and advancement on page 228. If enteral tolerance is questionable before initiation, start tube feeds at a very low rate (that is, 10–15 cc/hr) instead of diluting formula. **Don't:** Don't dilute formulas at initiation unless specifically ordered by the PMD.

Problem	*Do's and Don'ts*
Determine Delivery Route	**Do:** Determine if stomach or small intestine is appropriate delivery route. The stomach should be the first choice if not contraindicated. Use one of the following routes appropriate for patient condition: Nasogastric (NG) route: This route is for short-term feeding for 3 to 4 weeks. It allows for normal digestive, hormonal, and bactericidal processes in the stomach. Pass the tube through the nose and into the stomach. Nasoduodenal (ND) or nasojejunal (NJ) route: This route is for short-term feeding of 3 and 4 weeks in patients with gastric motility disorders, reflux, or persistent nausea and vomiting. Pass the tube through the nose to the stomach; it migrates into the small intestine via peristalsis. Percutaneous endoscopic gastrostomy (PEG): This route is for feeding longer than 3 to 4 weeks. Place the tube directly into the stomach through the abdominal wall using an endoscope. The tube can also be placed in the jejunum (percutaneous endoscopic jejunostomy/PEJ). Connect the formula tube through a stoma (opening) in the abdominal wall that connects with the tube inside the stomach or jejunum. Percutaneous gastrojejunostomy (PGJ): This route is for feeding longer than 3 to 4 weeks. Feeding is into the jejunum and allows for gastric decompression, which has the advantage of feeding earlier in postoperative patients or in patients who are at increased risk for aspiration and/or regurgitation.
Choosing Tube Size	**Do:** Note the two categories of tubes for short-term feeding use are small bore and large bore. Use a tube appropriate for the patient's condition. Small bore is the more common type of tube used. It is nasally placed. Because it is made of silicone or polyurethane, it is soft, flexible, and comfortable. Used largely in acute-care settings, this tube's size is 8–12 French. It is prone to clogging and slips out of position easily. The cost is six to seven times more than large bore. Large bore is an older-style tube that is made of PVC. With a wide diameter (12–18 French) and rigid body, it increases

Problem	Do's and Don'ts
	the risk for sinusitis, otitis media, mucosal ulceration, or necrosis. A large-bore tube allows for easier measurement of gastric residual volumes, is easy to insert, has less risk of clogging, requires changing often, and is inexpensive.
Choose Delivery Systems	**Do:**
	Note the three different systems that deliver formula to enterally fed patients: administration pumps, open systems, and closed systems.
	Use a system appropriate for the patient's condition.
	Administration pumps are simple devices that deliver the formula at a prescribed rate. They either attach to a pole near the patient or are portable (for home use). Pumps are equipped with alarms to alert staff of tube occlusion, empty container, or low battery. They can maintain constant flow of formula at very slow rate if needed and can reduce GI problems associated with enteral feeding.
	Open systems are traditional systems where formula is transferred from the original container to a refillable administration set to be connected to administration pumps. It can introduce bacteria and can contaminate formula. Formula must be changed every 8–12 hours of hang time to prevent spoilage; rinse bag and tube thoroughly with water; discard bag/set every 24 hours.
	Closed systems are designed to reduce the possibility of contamination to the formula. Formula comes in closed delivery containers that are ready to be connected to the enteral tube, and a sealed container eliminates the possibility of adding supplements to the patient's formula. The formula must be changed every 48 hours.
Determine Feeding Schedule	**Do:**
	Select schedule based on patient's clinical status. One method may also serve as an introduction to another method.
	Bolus feeding is the best method for stable patients with a functional GI tract, especially adequate stomach volume for the desired bolus volume and for patients who want to maximize the ease of mobility. Patients receive 240–400 ml of formula three to six times per day; the amount depends on the formula nutrient density (that is, 1.0, 1.2, 2.0 kcal/cc formula, etc.) and the patient's estimated calorie require-

Problem	*Do's and Don'ts*
	ments. Begin with 100–150 ml per feeding and increase incrementally as tolerated. Bolus feeding into the small intestine is not recommended because the small intestine does not have a reservoir as does the stomach.
Determine Feeding Schedule	Deliver formula by gravity drip from a syringe or feeding bag into the stomach; ingest full amount in 30–60 minutes. Bolus feeding may also be administered by a syringe injection directly into the stomach stoma, eliminating the gravity component; this process takes 10–15 minutes. Intermittent and continuous drip is best for patients who cannot tolerate a larger volume of formula administered through bolus feedings. Those with impaired GI function are best suited for this method. It requires a pump and is fed over 18–24 hours.
Initiate and Advance Feedings	**Do:** Start slowly and advance rate only as tolerated. Gradually increase full-strength formulas in rate or volume until goal rate/volume is achieved. Determine the rate of feeding advancement by the patient's clinical condition and the type of administered enteral feeding method. Consider the following: Bolus feeding: Initial feedings are 30–60 ml every 3 to 4 hours, with the volume increased every two to three feedings by 60–120 ml as tolerated until goal is reached. Bolus feeding usually reaches the goal within 48 hours. Pump-controlled feeding: The tube placement and patient's condition determines the rate of advancement. Begin continuous feedings at 10–40 ml/hr; advance in 10–25 ml/hr increments every 4 to 6 hours as tolerated. Pump-controlled feeding usually reaches goals within 48 hours. **Don't:** Don't use bolus for patients who cannot tolerate large volumes. Don't dilute formulas. Don't check small bowel residuals.
Monitoring	**Do:** Regularly monitor patients to prevent and correct complications and ensure proper amount of ingested formula to ensure meeting nutritional goals.

Problem	Do's and Don'ts
	Consider this monitoring schedule: • Weight (three times per week) • Signs/symptoms of edema (daily) • Signs/symptoms of dehydration (daily) • Fluid intake/output (daily) • Adequacy of enteral intake (two times per week) • Nitrogen balance (if appropriate, weekly) • Gastric residuals (if appropriate, every 4 hours—see measure gastric residual volume section) • Serum electrolytes, blood urea nitrogen, creatinine (two to three times per week) • Serum glucose, calcium, magnesium, phosphorus (weekly) • Stool output and consistency (daily) • Triglycerides level (weekly) • Blood glucose (daily)
Maintain Tube Patency	**Do:** Prevent tube clogging by: • Flush tube with 10–30 ml of warm water every 4 to 6 hours during continuous feeding and after every intermittent feeding. • Flush with same amount of water any time feeding is interrupted. • Use a larger diameter tube when possible if formula is concentrated. • Administer solid medications by crushing thoroughly and dissolving in water before putting in tube. • Flush tube with 5 ml warm water before and after medications. • Flush before and after checking residual volumes. **Don't:** Don't use acidic liquids (for example, juices or cola) to flush tube.
Measure Gastric Residual Volume	**Do:** Avoid having excessive residual volume because it can put the patient at risk for vomiting, aspiration pneumonia, and increased risk for mortality. Measure residual volume by aspirating fluid in stomach through 60 ml syringe, measure volume, and return fluid to stomach. Check levels every 4 to 5 hours immediately after tube has been placed in patient, until volume is consistently less than

Problem	Do's and Don'ts
	150 ml. When consistent, check residuals on a daily basis or whenever a sudden change in condition arises.
Prevent Aspiration	**Do:** Have the RN position the patient with head and shoulders above chest at all times during feedings and immediately following feedings (elevate bed 30 degrees; preferably 45 degrees in patients at increased aspiration risk). Have the RN check gastric residuals regularly for high-risk patients every 4 hours or as needed. Consider a prokinetic (that is, Reglan). Consider placing the tube transpylorically beyond the ligament of Treitz.
Caring for Insertion Sites	**Do:** Prevent skin irritation and dislodgement of tube. For patient comfort, do the following: Nasally placed tubes: These tubes should be secured with tape or a fastener; change tape/fastener every 2 to 3 days (sooner if needed). Remove old tape/fastener and cleanse the area with soap and water before applying new tape/fastener. Apply tape to new area of skin, and be sure that tube is not pulling up against nostril. Enterostomy tubes: Routine care involves removing old dressing that covers insertion site (stoma), cleansing area with soap and water, replacing the external ring in the proper position, and covering with clean dressing. Prevent excess motion of tube by taping to abdomen (in absence of sutures). If granulation builds up around stoma (usually due to leakage from site), apply silver nitrate to the area.
Transitioning to Oral Feedings	**Do:** Transition from enteral feeding to oral feeding gradually—from continuous feeding, to 12-hour feeding cycles, to 8-hour feeding cycles—all carried out at night to minimize discomfort from the change, and stimulate appetite during the waking hours. Patients should be encouraged to eat orally. Continue enteral supplementation simultaneously with oral intake, or administer oral supplements if adequate nutrition levels through oral intake cannot be maintained.

Problem	***Do's and Don'ts***
Oversight	**Do:** Receive proper training to calculate patient needs and make appropriate recommendations. Maintain close communication with the healthcare team and the PMD about any initiation or orders that include enteral nutrition. Receive medical consultation from appropriate trained professionals. **Don't:** Don't proceed with enteral nutrition changes without the oversight of the PMD and other appropriate medical personnel.

Sources

Bloch, A. S., & Mueller, C. "Chapter 23: Enteral and Parenteral Nutrition Support." Mahan, L. K., & Escott-Stump, S. (Eds.). *Krause's Food, Nutrition and Diet Therapy* (11th ed.). Philadelphia, PA: W. B. Saunders. 2004. 533–553.

Matarese, L. E., & Gottschlich, M. M. *Contemporary Nutrition Support Practice: A Clinical Guide* (2nd ed.). Philadelphia, PA: W. B. Saunders. 2003.

Parrish, C. R., & Malone, A. "Enteral Formula Selection: A Review of Selected Product Categories." *Practical Gastroenterology*. June 2005. 44–74. http://www.healthsystem.virginia.edu/internet/digestivehealth/nutritionarticles/MaloneArticle.pdf.

Parrish, C. R., & McCray, S. "Enteral Feeding: Dispelling Myths." *Practical Gastroenterology*. Sept 2003. 33–50. http://www.healthsystem.virginia.edu/internet/digestive-health/nutritionarticles/practicalgastrosept03.pdf.

Worthington, P. H. *Practical Aspects of Nutritional Support: An Advanced Practice Guide*. Philadelphia, PA: W. B. Saunders. 2004. 265–341.

Troubleshooting with Adult Tube Feeding

Author: Teresa Fung, ScD, RD, LDN

This is meant as a guideline to educate only the bedside staff. Those caring for patients with enteral nutrition should be medically trained and able to handle the complications that may arise.

Problem	*Do's and Don'ts*
Diarrhea	**Do:** Determine first the cause of the diarrhea; check for underlying medical condition (for example, Clostridium difficile infection), intolerance to osmolarity of formula, administration rate, other characteristics of the formula, bacterial contamination of tube, or complications of medications. Review medication list. Check if the medication is hyperosmolar (that is, containing sorbital). Check with the pharmacy if the medication can be diluted with water or given in a smaller, more frequent dose. Discontinue any stool softeners–laxatives, prokinetics, etc. Try fiber-containing formula, if not contraindicated, or add a soluble fiber (that is, guar gum or Benefiber diluted in water and bloused down the feeding tube). Continue to feed at a lower rate. **Don't:** Don't dilute the patient's formula. This reduces nutritional intake and can introduce bacteria, making diarrhea worse.
Constipation	**Do:** Assess GI motility. Consider changing the formula to a fiber-enriched formula. Increase volume of fluids with water flushes if medically appropriate. Encourage activity if possible. Evaluate medication profile. Consider administering laxative; monitor for diarrhea after treatment for constipation.
Abdominal Distention	**Do:** Check gastric residual. Reassess tube-feeding rate. Eliminate lactose if applicable. Evaluate medication profile. Check date of last bowel movement.

Problem	*Do's and Don'ts*
	Don't: Don't administer formula too quickly; continue to use hypertonic formula.
High Residual Volume	**Do:** Watch for other symptoms, such as nausea or abdominal distention. Monitor closely and check levels frequently (every 4 to 5 hours). Stop feeding only if two consecutive readings yield levels between 150–200 ml. Consider trying prokinetic agents to improve gastric emptying. Position patient on right side to facilitate stomach emptying. Reposition feeding tube beyond the ligament of Treitz and use parenteral nutrition to supplement feeding until tolerance is established. Continue to check levels every 4 to 5 hours until readings are consistent at less than 150–200 ml.
	Don't: Don't return residuals that exceed 150 ml in volume to the stomach.
Vomiting/Nausea	**Do:** Reassess tube-feeding regimen and adjust formula or feeding method if applicable. Maintain proper feeding rate. Have medical personnel anchor tube properly. Have medical personnel position patient on right side to facilitate stomach emptying. Have medical personnel administer prokinetic agents if necessary. Consider transpyloric access of feeding tube. Review medication profile.
	Don't: Don't continue to use hypertonic formula; don't ignore existing medical conditions that may impair gastric emptying.
Hyperglycemia	**Do:** Monitor patient closely, especially those with existing diabetes, sepsis, critical illness, or use of steroid therapy.

Problem	Do's and Don'ts
Hyperglycemia	Make sure calories and rate of administration are appropriate. Use insulin or oral hypoglycemic agents when necessary with PMD order; adjust timing of feedings with onset, peak, and duration of insulin. Consider use of a lower carbohydrate product.
Aspiration	**Do:** Make sure the following are observed by medical personnel: • Position patient with head and shoulders above chest at all times during feedings and immediately following feedings (elevate bed at least 30 degrees). • Check gastric residuals regularly for high-risk patients (every 4 hours or as needed). • Consider placing tube transpylorically (beyond the ligament of Treitz). • Consider using prokinetic agent. **Don't:** Don't use blue dye to tint formulas for detection of aspiration.
Clogged Tube	**Do:** Have medical personnel flush tube every 4 to 6 hours with 10–30 ml of warm water during continuous feeding and after each intermittent feeding. Have medical personnel flush tube before and after checking gastric residual volumes. Consider changing to a larger tube if possible for concentrated or fiber-rich formulas. For medication not available in liquid form, consider crushing solid medications and dissolving in water before administration if possible; flush tube with 30 ml of warm water before and after medication administration and between medications. Consider using enzymes such as activated Viokase mixed with sodium bicarbonate in a small amount of water for clogged tubes not cleared by water flushes. **Don't:** Don't use acidic liquids (for example, cranberry juice or colas) to flush tubes.

Problem	*Do's and Don'ts*
Microbial Contamination	**Do:**
	Use closed-system formulas when possible.
	Sanitize all preparation equipment and discard open containers after 24–48 hours. Wash hands thoroughly before administering feeding, and wear gloves. Wash top of formula container before opening. Administer only an 8–12 hour supply at one time. Make sure administration set has a drip chamber, rinse set prior to adding new formula, and change set every 24 hours.
	Don't:
	Don't add water, food dye, or medication to formula.
	Don't touch parts of feeding administration set that come in contact with formula.
	Don't add fresh formula to formula already in the administration set.
	Don't reuse disposable feeding sets.
	Don't open set unnecessarily.
Refeeding Syndrome	**Do:**
	Ensure feeding begins slowly at calorie levels below maintenance needs.
	Monitor closely weight, hemodynamic stability, and metabolic indicators, such as serum glucose, triglycerides, and electrolytes.
	Add calories slowly as tolerated by the patient.
	Don't:
	Don't overfeed a malnourished patient.
Dehydration	**Do:**
	Make sure the patient receives 30 ml/kg body weight of water (or 1 ml/kcal in formula) unless contraindicated due to the patient's physiological needs (that is, renal, CHF patients).
	Review the patient's intake–output (I–O); check if any free water is administered.
	Check the patient for hyperglycemia.
	Check the patient for fever.
	Assess the patient's activity level.
	Check the patient for diarrhea.

Problem	*Do's and Don'ts*
Dehydration	Make sure the patient receives the volume of formula prescribed. Check if free-water flushes are regularly done. **Don't:** Don't continue use of concentrated formula (1.5 kcal/ml or greater) unless indicated. Don't continue use of formulas with a high renal solute load.
Tube Displacement or Migration	**Do:** Have medical personnel secure tube with tape or a fastener. Have medical personnel change tape/fastener every 2 to 3 days. Have medical personnel ensure site is clean and sterile. Consider using a different type of tube.
Drug/Nutrient Interactions	**Do:** Check with the patient's pharmacist and/or PMD to determine what type of interactions the patient's medication may have with the type of formula being administered. Medication administration may require delaying the tube feeding to administer certain medications, resulting in an adjustment to the tube feeding rate to compensate for tube feeding interruption.
Sudden Weight Change	**Do:** Check weight again. Check fluid intake and output. Check for signs of edema. Check formula pump rate.
Oversight	**Do:** Maintain close communication with the healthcare team and the PMD about any initiation or orders that include enteral nutrition. Receive medical consultation from appropriate trained professionals. See the appendix for a list of tube feedings on page 430. **Don't:** Don't proceed with enteral changes without the oversight of the PMD and other appropriate medical personnel.

Sources

Bloch, A. S., & Mueller, C. "Chapter 23: Enteral and Parenteral Nutrition Support." Mahan, L. K., & Escott-Stump, S. (Eds.). *Krause's Food, Nutrition and Diet Therapy* (11th ed.). Philadelphia, PA: W. B. Saunders. 2004. 533–553.

Matarese, L. E., & Gottschlich, M. M. *Contemporary Nutrition Support Practice: A Clinical Guide* (2nd ed.). Philadelphia, PA: W. B. Saunders. 2003.

Parrish, C. R., & Malone, A. "Enteral Formula Selection: A Review of Selected Product Categories." *Practical Gastroenterology*. June 2005. 44–74. http://www.healthsystem.virginia.edu/internet/digestivehealth/nutritionarticles/MaloneArticle.pdf.

Parrish, C. R., & McCray, S. "Enteral Feeding: Dispelling Myths." *Practical Gastroenterology*. Sept 2003. 33–50. http://www.healthsystem.virginia.edu/internet/digestivehealth/nutritionarticles/practicalgastrosept03.pdf.

Worthington, P. H. *Practical Aspects of Nutritional Support: An Advanced Practice Guide*. Philadelphia, PA: W. B. Saunders. 2004. 265–341.

Diverticulitis

Author: Linda S. Cashman, MS, RD, CNSD

Diverticulitis is inflammation of the diverticula, which are tiny sacs or pouches in the intestinal wall. The colon is the most frequent site. Complications from diverticular disease, in which diverticula become inflamed or infected (diverticulitis), may result in severe lower abdominal pain and distention. Patients with diverticulosis (without the inflammation) usually have no symptoms.

Problem	*Do's and Don'ts*
Acute Abdominal Pain	**Do:** Require bed rest and maintain nothing by mouth (NPO) status for the first few days. The PMD will manage medications and intravenous fluids. Counsel the patient that surgery may be necessary, depending on the severity of the disease and/or if the bowel wall is perforated. **Don't:** Don't allow the patient to consume any food or beverage.
Slight Abdominal Pain	**Do:** Initiate a clear liquid diet after the acute phase has subsided. A trial with clear liquids (for example, water, apple or cranberry juice, tea, flat soda, gelatin, fruit ice, broth—beef, chicken, or vegetable) can be initiated by the PMD's order. Offer a clear liquid supplement for additional protein and carbohydrate calories if the patient has already been NPO for greater than 3 days and/or is below ideal body weight range. **Don't:** Don't have the patient consume any solid foods except those listed as clear liquid items. Don't have the patient consume any carbonated beverages because carbonation can cause abdominal gas/pain. Don't have the patient remain on a clear liquid diet greater than 5 days because the diet does not meet the recommended dietary requirements for calories, protein, vitamins, and minerals.
Minimal or No Abdominal Pain	**Do:** Transition the diet by the PMD to a low-fiber diet after the patient tolerates the clear liquid diet. This is a temporary

Problem	*Do's and Don'ts*
	diet, usually followed for approximately 2 weeks, to provide a minimum amount of fiber and residue in the intestinal tract. Low-fiber foods include white bread and low-fiber cereal (less than 2 gm/serving). Offer either canned fruits or fresh fruits without skins and seeds. Vegetables can either be frozen, canned, or fresh; however, remove the skins and seeds. Vegetables, such as carrots and green beans, are usually well tolerated. Meats do not contain fiber; however, low-fat items, such as lean beef, pork, chicken, and fish, are usually a better choice to reduce the risk of recurrence of abdominal pain. Add only small amounts of butter/margarine to food. Advise the patient that dairy may or may not cause abdominal distress, so patients might try Lactaid dairy (lactose-free) products instead. Advise patients to gradually transition to a high-fiber diet (after approximately 2 weeks or until the PMD's follow-up visit/advice). Advise the patient that high-fiber diets provide soft, bulky stools that pass more easily through the intestines, resulting in lower intracolonic pressure and fewer side effects and flare-ups of diverticulitis. However, it is important to continue drinking adequate fluids because higher fiber without added fluids can cause constipation. Add the fiber back into the diet slowly, otherwise bloating and flatulence can occur. The recommended dietary fiber intake is 20–35 grams per day depending on the patient's body size. Increasing the amount of fiber in patients with diverticulosis may prevent complications that result in diverticulitis. Counsel the patient that until more recently, patients were advised to avoid all seeds, nuts, and skins because they could get lodged in the tiny pouches of the colon and cause inflammation. Avoiding seeds, nuts, and skins does not appear to have any benefit in preventing diverticulitis; however, the issue whether to avoid these items remains unresolved. Eliminate from the diet some foods (for example, corn, popcorn, nuts, and seeds) that may cause distress for some patients.

Problem	*Do's and Don'ts*
Minimal or No Abdominal Pain	**Don't:**
	Don't have the patient consume high-fat foods; they can intensify colonic smooth muscle contractions. Therefore, avoid serving high-fat foods, such as fatty meats, fried foods, rich desserts, creamed soups, and sauces.
	Don't have the patient consume moderate to large amounts of either butter or margarine.

Source

Mahon, L. K., & Escott-Stump, S. (Eds.). "Medical Nutrition Therapy for Lower Gastrointestinal Tract Disorders." *Krause's Food, Nutrition & Diet Therapy* (11th ed.). Philadelphia, PA: W. B. Saunders. 2004. 728–729.

Gastroesophageal Reflux Disease (GERD)

Author: Linda S. Cashman, MS, RD, CNSD

GERD is a backward flow of gastric and/or duodenal secretions into the esophagus. The most common cause of GERD is the relaxation of the lower esophageal sphincter (LES). This list will assist the dietitian in guiding the patient to make some dietary and lifestyle modifications to help relieve the symptoms of esophageal burning and substernal pain, which is often associated with GERD or other problems involving the esophagus. Medications may also be necessary to control symptoms. Occasionally, surgery might be required.

Problem	***Do's and Don'ts***
Burning Sensation in Esophagus; Substernal Pain	**Do:** Offer small, frequent meals; have the patient sit up 1 hour before and after meals. Have the patient relax at mealtimes. Try offering a healthful diet, including whole-grain products (breads, cereals, pasta, fat-free crackers), fruits (for example, cantaloupe, strawberries, etc.), vegetables without added fat, lean beef, pork, chicken, dry beans, and low-fat dairy products. Use fats in limited quantities because they result in delayed gastric emptying. Recommend some lifestyle changes: • Achieve and maintain a healthy weight. • Elevate head of bed 6 to 8 inches when sleeping. • Reintroduce problem foods in small amounts. **Don't:** Don't allow foods that tend to lower the esophageal sphincter pressure or cause irritation to the esophagus (for example, chocolate, mint—spearmint and peppermint—carbonated beverages, citrus juices, tomato juices, tomato products, and coffee, with and without caffeine). Don't serve fermented alcoholic beverages (beer and wine) because they stimulate gastric acid. Don't allow eating a meal 3 hours before bedtime, particularly meat or cheese, which increase the likelihood of reflux. Don't serve certain citrus juices and fruits (for example, lemons, grapefruits, oranges, pineapples, and tangerines); they may not be tolerated.

Problem	*Do's and Don'ts*
Burning Sensation in Esophagus; Substernal Pain	Don't serve fried foods, fatty meats, large high-fat meals, high-fat dessert/bread items, such as croissants, muffins, and cakes. Don't allow spicy foods because they may also cause discomfort in certain esophageal disorders. Don't allow smoking because smoking is not only dangerous to one's health, but it also lowers the LES pressure. Don't encourage tight-fitting clothing around the stomach area.

Sources

American Dietetic Association. "Gastroesophageal Reflux Disease." *The Manual of Clinical Dietetics*. Chicago, IL: American Dietetic Association. 2000, 2005.

Mahan, L. K., & Escott-Stump, S. (Eds.). "Medical Nutrition Therapy for Upper Gastrointestinal Tract Disorders." *Krause's Food, Nutrition & Diet Therapy* (11th ed.). Philadelphia, PA: W. B. Saunders. 2004. 688–690.

Lactose Intolerance

Author: Linda S. Cashman, MS, RD, CNSD

Lactose intolerance occurs when the body doesn't produce enough of the lactase enzyme, which is needed to digest milk sugar (lactose). Lactose is typically found in milk and milk-containing products. Diet modification is the simplest way to control the symptoms of bloating, cramping, and/or diarrhea. This list will assist the dietitian in answering food-tolerance questions; however, because there are usually varying degrees of lactose intolerance, patients will need to find their own individual tolerance. If patients are lactose intolerant, when lactose is removed from the diet, the side effects of bloating, usually cramping and diarrhea, are alleviated within 3 to 5 days.

Problem	*Do's and Don'ts*
Gas, Bloating, Cramping, and/or Diarrhea	**Do:**
	Review carefully all nutrition labels and ingredients for milk products. Foods that do not contain lactose are the following: fresh fruits, fruit juices, fresh vegetables, all meats, poultry, fish, eggs, fats (for example, margarine and butter), nondairy creamer, whole grains or enriched breads, cereals, and pastas (provided they're not prepared with lactose/milk products).
	Avoiding all dairy products may result in insufficient amounts of calcium in the diet unless the patient consumes large quantities of green leafy vegetables like collard, turnip, and mustard greens. Other sources of calcium are in calcium-fortified soy or orange juice products.
	Try lactose-free, low-fat milk, soy milk, or lactase enzyme tablets with dairy products.
	Suggest that some patients are able to tolerate small amounts of up to less than one-half cup of milk per day. Some patients tolerate hard, aged cheeses like Parmesan and aged cheddar. Patients need vitamin D-rich foods (sardines, salmon, etc.) for adequate calcium absorption. Yogurt contains a good source of calcium and is usually well tolerated due to the fermentation from the live cultures.
	Don't:
	Don't allow dairy products.
	Don't allow foods that may cause distress, such as cold cuts and hot dogs that contain lactose filler.

Problem	*Do's and Don'ts*
Gas, Bloating, Cramping, and/or Diarrhea	Don't serve any mixes (cake, gravies, etc.) that contain lactose. Don't serve cheese products, particularly soft cheeses.

Source

Mahan, L. K., & Escott-Stump, S. (Eds.). "Medical Nutrition Therapy for Lower Gastrointestinal Tract Disorders." *Krause's Food, Nutrition & Diet Therapy* (11th ed.). Philadelphia, PA: W. B. Saunders. 2004. 719–720.

Inflammatory Bowel Disease (IBD)

(This disease refers to inflammation of the gastrointestinal tract of unknown etiology, including Crohn's disease and ulcerative colitis [UC].)

Author: Linda S. Cashman, MS, RD, CNSD

This list will assist the dietitian in answering food tolerance questions for patients with either Crohn's disease (most often affecting the small intestine) or ulcerative colitis (affecting only the large intestine). Some of the side effects of IBD may include diarrhea, nausea, recurrent abdominal pain, weight loss, and vitamin/mineral deficiencies. There is no specific diet for either Crohn's or ulcerative colitis, except to try to provide a well-balanced diet to assure adequate calories, vitamins, and minerals. Certain foods (listed as follows) may/may not have an impact on relieving the symptoms; however, individuals may have their own intolerances and would need to avoid/restrict those foods.

Problem	*Do's and Don'ts*
Diarrhea	**Do:** Severe diarrhea can cause malabsorption of nutrients, loss of electrolytes (especially sodium and potassium), minerals, and trace elements (especially zinc and magnesium). A trial with a clear liquid diet including fat-free broth, fruit ice, tea, and clear juices can usually be introduced. Oral glucose electrolyte solutions with added potassium can help to replace electrolytes and fluids. Physician management with intravenous hydration and electrolyte replacements may also be necessary depending on the severity of the diarrhea and the patient's ability to take in sufficient oral fluids. To control diarrhea and malabsorption of nutrients, a low-fat, low-fiber diet may be followed initially, such as white bread, cereals with fiber less than 3 gms, rice, potato, green beans, carrots, and canned peaches. Applesauce, which contains pectins, may also help the diarrhea. Low fiber helps to minimize the irritation to the inflamed bowel, slow the intestinal transit rate, and reduce stool frequency. Low fat may control the symptoms of steatorrhea (fat malabsorption). Gradually advance the diet as tolerated to also include protein foods, such as lean chicken, fish, pork, and beef.

Problem	*Do's and Don'ts*
Diarrhea	Total elimination of lactose products is not always necessary. Try lactase-treated milk or lactase pills if dairy causes GI upset. Require vitamin/mineral supplement given the severity of the diarrhea and/or vitamin and mineral losses. In Crohn's disease, resection of the distal small bowel can result in bile salt deficiency and subsequent fat malabsorption and fat-soluble vitamin (vitamins A, D, E, K) deficiency, therefore requiring vitamin repletion. If the ileum is resected, vitamin B_{12} deficiency can develop. Repletion with vitamin B_{12} injections is one option. **Don't:** Don't serve high-fiber foods, such as whole-grain breads, cereals, skins from fresh fruits and vegetables, nuts, and seeds. The amount of fiber tolerated varies between patients and usually can be increased when diarrhea subsides. Don't serve a prolonged low-fiber diet. Don't serve large amounts of sucrose found in table sugar, maple syrup, fruit, vegetables, honey, and in certain desserts and beverages. Don't consume large amounts of resistant (more difficult to digest) starches particularly found in legumes, cooked and cooled potatoes, rice and pasta, and under-ripe bananas. Don't ignore the effect of lactose in some patients. Some patients may require limiting lactose from dairy products. (In patients with Crohn's disease, lactose is absorbed in the small intestine.) However, oftentimes limiting lactose is based on individual tolerance level. Don't serve caffeinated and alcoholic beverages (particularly beer and wine) because they increase GI secretions and colonic motility. Don't forget to consult with the physician or dietitian before taking vitamin supplement except for a basic multivitamin/mineral. Certain fat-soluble vitamins can be toxic at high doses.
Nausea	**Do:** Depending on the severity of the nausea, provide a concomitant treatment with antiemetic therapy and a clear liquid diet (broth, fruit ice, black tea, gelatin), followed by

Problem	*Do's and Don'ts*
	toast (dry or with jelly) and crackers (saltines). If the patient continues to tolerate the diet, slowly resume low-fat, low-fiber diet.
	Have the patient drink fluids between meals rather than with meals.
	Don't:
	Don't serve high-fat, greasy meals.
	Don't forget to avoid food odors by eating cold food or food at room temperature.
	Don't allow the patient to eat 1 to 2 hours before lying down.
Abdominal Pain	**Do:**
	Continue with low-fat, low-fiber diet, but also incorporate small frequent feedings (eating approximately every 2–3 hours during the day).
	Don't:
	Don't serve large, high-fat meals.
Weight Loss	**Do:**
	Small frequent feedings with nutrient-dense foods should be included in diet. Snacks, such as peanut butter, cheddar cheese on crackers, low-fat yogurt, and puddings, as tolerated may be offered.
	Consider a high calorie/protein liquid oral supplement between meals. If the patient can tolerate ice cream, try adding it to the supplement for additional calories and protein.
	Don't:
	Don't consume large amounts of fruits, nonstarchy vegetables, and salads because these items are too low in calories.
	Don't consume large quantities of sugar-free/calorie-free beverages.

Sources

Morrison, G., & Hark, L. "Gastrointestinal Disease." Lichtenstein, G., & Burke, F. (Eds.). *Medical Nutrition & Disease* (2nd ed.). Malden, MA: Blackwell Science, Inc. 1999. 201–204.

Mahan, L. K., & Escott-Stump, S. (Eds.). "Medical Nutrition Therapy for Lower Gastrointestinal Tract Disorders." *Nutrition & Diet Therapy* (11th ed.). Philadelphia, PA: W. B. Saunders. 2004. 721–728.

Celiac Disease or Celiac Sprue (Gluten Sensitive Enteropathy)

Author: Linda S. Cashman, MS, RD, CNSD

This list will help the dietitian in providing nutrition guidelines to patients who have been diagnosed with celiac disease, which is the small intestinal malabsorption of gluten (gliadin is a fraction of gluten), a protein found in wheat, rye, barley, and possibly oats. The gluten damages the mucosal villi with the potential for malabsorption of all nutrients unless celiac disease is properly diagnosed and gluten is removed from the diet. When the gluten is removed from the diet, symptoms of abdominal pain, bloating, vomiting, and diarrhea are resolved. In undiagnosed children, growth failure can occur. Careful nutrition-label reading is key to eliminating gluten-containing products from the diet. Celiac sprue can develop for the first time at any age.

Problem	*Do's and Don'ts*
Diarrhea, Abnormal Stools, Vomiting, Abdominal Pain/Bloating	**Do:** Foods that are acceptable are corn, potato, rice, soybean (and flours derived from these products); also tapioca and arrowroot. It is important not to contaminate these products with gluten/gliadin-containing flour. Other acceptable foods are: all kinds of fresh meat, chicken, and fish. Limit milk and milk products initially, then reintroduce milk, aged cheeses such as cheddar, Parmesan, and Swiss, yogurt, and sour cream (however, check label for ingredients). Other acceptable foods are: all plain fruits and vegetables and white and sweet potatoes. Cereals that are allowed are cream of rice, puffed rice, Kellogg's Sugar Pops. Do provide a multivitamin/mineral supplement, particularly if the patient has been newly diagnosed with celiac disease because malabsorption of nutrients has more than likely been occurring. Common nutritional deficiencies are folate, iron, vitamin B_{12}, vitamin D, and calcium. **Don't:** Don't serve gliadin/gluten sources, such as wheat, rye, barley, bran, bulgar, graham, or oats. Recent studies have indicated that a small amount of oats are not harmful; however, oftentimes commercially available oats are contaminated with gluten.

Problem	*Do's and Don'ts*
	Don't serve egg noodles, spaghetti, etc.
	Don't serve prepared meats that contain wheat, barley, oats, or rye.
	Don't serve oat gum (added in certain cheeses).
	Don't serve certain creamed vegetables, some pie fillings, some commercial salad dressings, and candies.
	Don't serve most canned soups, bouillon, Ovaltine, beer, ale, distilled vodka, malted barley.
	Don't serve some catsup, mustard, chewing gum, distilled white vinegar, and some gravy extracts.
	Don't forget to read all nutrition labels and inquire about all food consumed at restaurants.

Sources

Mahan, L. K., & Escott-Stump, S. (Eds.). "Medical Nutrition Therapy for Lower Gastrointestinal Tract Disorders." *Krause's Food, Nutrition & Diet Therapy* (11th ed.). Philadelphia, PA: W. B. Saunders. 2004. 712–719.

American Dietetic Association. "Celiac Disease." *The Manual of Clinical Dietetics.* Chicago, IL: American Dietetic Association. 2000, 2005.

Cholecystitis (Inflammation of the Gallbladder) or Cholecystectomy (Gallbladder Removed)

Author: Linda S. Cashman, MS, RD, CNSD

This list will assist the dietitian in answering food tolerance questions pertaining to some of the symptoms of cholecystitis, such as abdominal pain, diarrhea, flatulence, and bloating.

Problem	*Do's and Don'ts*
Sharp Abdominal Pain, Burning Sensation in Abdomen	**Do:** In the acute phase, require the patient to keep NPO (nothing by mouth). When the acute phase has subsided, a trial of clear liquids, such as black tea, gelatin, clear juice, and broth without the fat can be initiated. If tolerated, then the patient may transition to a low-fat diet. Patients with either cholecystitis or who've had a cholecystectomy should transition to similar low-fat diets, such as fat-free or low-fat milk and cheese; lean meat, fish, and poultry; all plainly prepared fruits and vegetables. Choose plain bread, noodles, rice, and potato. Limit butter, margarine, or oils to 3 teaspoons per day (divided equally among three meals). Patients with gallbladders removed should also transition to a low-fat diet for at least the first few weeks after surgery. **Don't:** Don't serve moderate to high-fat foods because fat stimulates gallbladder contractions, which may result in pain. Don't forget to avoid: whole milk, cream, ice cream, and cream sauces; moderate to high amounts of butter, margarine, or oil; high-fat cheeses, fried or fatty meats; fried foods and high-fat desserts, such as donuts, muffins, pastries, and cakes.
Diarrhea	**Do:** Depending on the severity of the diarrhea, nutrient malabsorption, electrolyte losses, and dehydration may occur. Clear liquids with clear juices (apple or cranberry) and broth can be offered to replete the fluid and electrolyte losses. Advise the patient with copious stools to keep NPO until the diarrhea subsides. The PMD will likely prescribe fluid and electrolyte management.

Problem	*Do's and Don'ts*
	When the diarrhea is more manageable, advancing to a low-lactose, low-insoluble fiber, low-fat diet may be warranted. Soluble fibers in small amounts, such as unsweetened applesauce, canned peaches, bananas, and oatmeal, may help to solidify the stool.
	Lactose (found in all milk, cream, ice cream, and cheese) may or may not exacerbate the diarrhea; however, patients might want to try Lactaid low-fat milk and ice cream (or take lactase enzymes) and monitor for any change in frequency of diarrhea. Even though yogurt contains lactose, it's usually tolerated because of the fermentation; yogurt also may be beneficial in restoring some of the gut bacteria lost in frequent diarrhea.
	Don't:
	Don't serve moderate- to high-fat foods; fried and spicy foods should be kept to a minimum.
	Don't serve bran cereals or skins and seeds from fresh fruit and vegetables.
	Don't serve milk and lactose products.
Flatulence	**Do:**
	Have the patient eat slowly and chew with the mouth closed.
	Try to provide a low- to moderate-fiber diet (approximately less than 10 grams per day): cereals with fiber content of <2 grams per serving, canned fruits, fruit juices, cooked vegetables, such as green beans or carrots, lettuce in small amounts.
	Don't:
	Don't serve a high-fiber diet, such as whole-grain cereals, legumes (peas, kidney beans, lentils, etc), or cruciferous vegetables (broccoli, cauliflower, brussels sprouts, etc.).
	Don't serve chewing gum and don't talk while eating because an accumulation of gas is formed when swallowing.
Bloating	**Do:**
	Have the patient eat more slowly and chew food well. Provide a low-fat diet because fat takes longer to digest than carbohydrate or protein foods.
	Advise the patient that lactose (in dairy foods) may cause increased bloating.

Problem	*Do's and Don'ts*
Bloating	Low-lactose or Lactaid dairy products may be better tolerated.
	Don't:
	Don't serve moderate- to high-fat foods.
	Don't serve moderate- to high-fiber diets (approximately greater than 10 grams per day).

Source

Mahon, L. K., & Escott-Stump, S. (Eds.). "Medical Nutrition Therapy for Liver, Biliary System and Exocrine Pancreas Disorders." *Krause's Food, Nutrition & Diet Therapy* (11th ed.). Philadelphia, PA: W. B. Saunders. 2004. 757–760.

Colostomy/Ileostomy

Author: Linda S. Cashman, MS, RD, CNSD

This list will help guide dietitians in managing patients with either an ileostomy surgery (an opening into the ileum through a stoma in the abdominal wall) or colostomy (an opening into the colon) who may experience some of the following side effects: frequent loose stools, dehydration, electrolyte imbalance, bloating, cramping, and anorexia. These side effects occur more often in patients with ileostomies because of the area and amount of bowel that is usually resected, resulting in greater nutrient and fluid losses. However, many of these symptoms resolve or improve in 4 to 6 weeks after surgery. Loose stools, bloating, and ostomy odor may be an ongoing problem for some patients. Some other possible complications, particularly in ileostomy patients, would be ostomy blockages because of the smaller stoma (opening) size. Diet modification may help to alleviate some of these problems. However, there is no one recommendation for everyone; patients need to base their diets on their own individual symptoms.

Problem	*Do's and Don'ts*
Frequent Loose Stool/ Dehydration/ Electrolyte Imbalance	**Do:**
	Advise the patient that adult patients with large stool output (approximately greater than 700 cc per day) are at risk for dehydration and electrolyte imbalance. The PMD will manage the appropriate fluid, medications, and electrolyte replacement.
	Advise the patient that consistency of the stool, particularly after an ileostomy, is usually liquid, becoming less liquid in 7 to 10 days.
	Advise the patient that when he or she is able to take clear liquids, such as gelatin, cranberry juice, broth, and fruit ice, a clear liquid protein/carbohydrate supplement may be added to the diet for additional nutrients.
	Encourage water and other fluids (six to eight glasses per day) to maintain adequate hydration status. Increase fluid intake six to eight glasses per day, higher with excessive stool output, by taking additional broth to replenish the sodium.
	Advise the patient that potassium may need to be repleted by the PMD.
	As the diet advances, encourage foods such as unsweetened applesauce, bananas, breads, low-fiber cereals (less than 2 grams per serving), cheese, pasta, creamy peanut butter, and starchy foods to help thicken the stool.

Problem	*Do's and Don'ts*
Frequent Loose Stool/ Dehydration/ Electrolyte Imbalance	Suggest substituting milk with Lactaid milk; yogurt may help to restore the beneficial gut flora. Suggest that colostomy patients add extra fluids and slightly additional salt in the diet to maintain adequate fluids and electrolytes because there is less surface area for water and electrolyte absorption. Observe the effect of the stool consistency with foods consumed. Have the patient try new foods one at a time. **Don't:** Don't forget that in some cases, loose stools may be a result of eating certain foods. The following foods can cause loose stools: alcoholic beverages, grape juice, apple juice, prune juice, heavily spiced foods, broccoli, chocolate, baked beans. Don't serve large meals. Don't serve skins and seeds from fruits and vegetables.
Gas/Indigestion	**Do:** Have the patient consume at least three meals, preferably four to six smaller meals per day, particularly with a new ileostomy. It is important for the patient to chew food thoroughly. **Don't:** Don't allow the patient to lie down for about an hour after eating. Don't forget to use caution with foods that may cause gas, such as asparagus, beans, broccoli, cabbage, carbonated beverages, cauliflower, cucumber, pickles, fatty foods, melon, milk, and onions.
Constipation	**Do:** Counsel patients with a colostomy on the importance of fiber in the diet. Ask the patient to drink extra water and other fluids. Recommend more fruits, vegetables, and whole grains, such as oatmeal and whole-wheat bread; however, the patient should chew the food well. Encourage exercise that may help alleviate the constipation. However, obtain medical clearance before the patient begins to participate in any new exercise program.

Problem	*Do's and Don'ts*
	The PMD may also recommend the use of Metamucil or another oral fiber supplement. **Don't:** Don't consume large amounts of foods that tend to be constipating, such as cheese, rice, low-fiber grains (less than 2 grams per serving), etc.
Anorexia/ Weight Loss	**Do:** Suggest small frequent meals and nutrient-dense snacks (for example, creamy peanut butter on crackers, yogurt, avocados, cheese and crackers, high-calorie/protein supplement drink). **Don't:** Don't let the patient skip meals. Avoid serving liquids/water before mealtime.
Stoma Odor	**Do:** Advise the use of deodorants for the appliances, which are available and usually quite effective. Help the patient practice good hygiene. **Don't:** Don't allow odor-producing foods (for example, cauliflower, asparagus, baked beans, broccoli, onions, cabbage, highly spiced foods, and fish) if deodorants are not effective and the patient is concerned about offensive odors.
Prevent Stoma Blockages (undigested food blocking the stoma)	**Do:** Ask the patient to drink adequate fluids (approximately 2 quarts per day) to help maintain stoma patency. After approximately 4 to 6 weeks, reintroduce one new food and check the patient's tolerance. The patient should always chew food well. **Don't:** Don't eat large amounts of cabbage, celery, corn, coconut, dried fruit, mushrooms, seeds, popcorn, pineapple, peas, olives, nuts, popcorn, pickles, raw vegetables, and spinach, particularly in recent ileostomies (before 4 to 6 weeks). Don't serve tough, fibrous vegetables. Slowly add them back to the diet, one at a time.

Problem	*Do's and Don'ts*
Vitamin and Mineral Deficiency	**Do:**
	Counsel that oftentimes, patients with ileostomies avoid consuming or limit fruits and vegetables, resulting in low intake of vitamin A and C. A multivitamin and a vitamin C supplement may be required.
	If resected distal ileum, patients will require vitamin B_{12} supplementation, usually administered via intramuscular injection.
	Don't:
	Don't give high doses of vitamin/mineral supplementation unless advised to do so by PMD. High doses of fat-soluble vitamins (A, E, D, and K) can be toxic.

Sources

Mahon, L. K., & Escott-Stump, S. (Eds.). "Medical Nutrition Therapy for Lower Gastrointestinal Tract Disorders." *Krause's Food, Nutrition & Diet Therapy* (11th ed.). Philadelphia, PA: W. B. Saunders. 2004. 730–735.

Shield, J., & Mullen, M. *Patient Education Materials, Supplement to the Manual of Clinical Dietetics* (3rd ed.). Chicago, IL: American Dietetic Association. 1996.

Short-Bowel Syndrome

Author: Linda S. Cashman, MS, RD, CNSD

Short bowel syndrome (SBS) refers to the consequences with the loss of intestinal absorptive surface area that can result in diarrhea, dehydration, electrolyte imbalance, malabsorption, and progressive weight loss. In general, remaining small bowel of less than 200 cm (normal small bowel length is 300–500 cm) may lead to nutritional complications. Maintaining adequate hydration can be one of the biggest challenges. An adaptation phase (with villi or intestinal growth), in that the remaining bowel attempts to compensate for the loss of bowel, can occur up to a year. Different degrees of severity in SBS occur depending on factors such as length of small bowel remaining, loss of colon, loss of ileocecal valve, loss of ileum, etc. The following nutritional guidelines will assist the dietitian in managing patients with SBS.

Problem	*Do's and Don'ts*
Dehydration, Electrolyte Imbalance	**Do:** Use oral rehydration solutions (ORS) to help with fluid and electrolyte losses, preferably an isotonic (less than 300 mOsm/L) beverage such as Pedialyte, Enfalyte (both designed for children but can be used for adults), or Equalyte (for adults). Low osmolality will quickly leave the stomach and absorb easily into the intestines. Gatorade, although not as low in osmolality (349 mOsm/L) as above ORS, oftentimes is tolerated. Other lower osmolality beverages are diet cranberry juice, decaf tea, and diet soda. Water is encouraged to maintain hydration. **Don't:** Don't consume large quantities of high osmolality (hypertonic) beverages, such as apple juice, orange juice, and sodas. Don't consume large quantities of caffeine, which includes coffee, tea, and some soft drinks (no more than 1–2 cups per day).
Diarrhea, Abdominal Cramping/Pain	**Do:** With large stool outputs, a high-sodium diet may be appropriate to replete the sodium losses. The physician may prescribe medications to help slow down GI motility, GI secretions, and stool output. When the diet advances from clear liquids (tea, gelatin, low-fat broth, clear juice), small and frequent mini-meals are usually better tolerated. Food such as chicken, turkey (without the skin), fish, low-fat meat, low-fiber cereals (that is, Rice Krispies, Special K, cream of wheat) are usually tolerated.

Problem	*Do's and Don'ts*
Diarrhea, Abdominal Cramping/Pain	Also, canned fruits, bananas, and vegetables, such as green beans and butternut squash, are acceptable. Soluble fibers, such as applesauce, canned peaches, citrus fruits, rice bran, oatmeal, etc., are beneficial, particularly in patients who have the colon intact because soluble fibers metabolize into short chain fatty acids in the colon (preferred fuel for the colon), enhancing sodium and water absorption, thus counteracting the diarrhea. Also in these patients, dietary calcium, such as Lactaid milk and hard cheeses (aged cheddar, etc.), helps to decrease available oxalate, which in turn reduces the risk of kidney stones. Other suggestions for patients with an intact colon are a low-fat diet, which helps to decrease the diarrhea and also decreases the risk of cholesterol gallstones. However, patients without a colon have no benefit in a significant restriction of fat in the diet. A trial with a liquid oral nutritional supplement from a medical nutritional laboratory company (an elemental formula in predigested form) that contains medium-chain triglycerides (MCT) can be beneficial, particularly in fat malabsorption, because MCT does not require bile acids for absorption and may lessen the amount of diarrhea. Yogurt with live cultures helps restore the good bacteria (flora) in the gut. (Refer to ileostomy section for additional food tolerances/guidelines on page 253.) **Don't:** Don't forget that lactose (found in milk sugar, such as milk, cheese, ice cream) malabsorption is prevalent in SBS, so lactose restriction may lessen stool output. Don't serve large amounts of sweets. Don't serve high doses of vitamin C supplementation in patients with intact colon to decrease available oxalate, which can result in kidney stone formation. Patients without a colon are not at increased risk for oxalate formation. Don't serve high-sugar fluids (hypertonic), which can result in influx of water into intestines, resulting in greater fluid losses, particularly in patients without a colon. (Refer to ileostomy section for additional food intolerances on page 253.)

Problem	*Do's and Don'ts*
Vitamin/Mineral Deficiencies	**Do:** Depending on the specific parts of the bowel resected, significant vitamin and mineral deficiencies can occur. Loss of the distal ileum (site of vitamin B_{12} and bile acids) will require vitamin B_{12} supplementation (that is, intramuscular injections). Also with loss of ileum, calcium, zinc, and magnesium malabsorption may occur from the altered fatty acids. Fat-soluble vitamins (A, D, E, and K) may occur, which may require a multivitamin/mineral supplement to meet nutrition needs. **Don't:** Don't provide any individual vitamin and mineral supplement except a standard multivitamin/mineral unless advised by the physician. Certain vitamins (particularly fat-soluble vitamins) can be toxic at high levels and can also interfere with the absorption of other vitamins and minerals. Also, certain vitamins and minerals may be contraindicated depending on the area of small bowel or colon resected.
Weight Loss	**Do:** Small frequent meals are usually better tolerated. Encourage the patient to drink an oral high-calorie/protein supplement between meals. Consume nutrient-dense snacks, such as creamy peanut butter, custards, and puddings for extra calories. **Don't:** Don't allow large quantities of low-calorie fruits and vegetables. Don't forget to use caution with allowing water and low-calorie beverages with meals.

Sources

ASPEN. "Nutritional Considerations for Dealing with Intestinal Diseases in the Intensive Care Unit." Pipkin, W., & Gadacz, T. (Eds.). *Nutritional Considerations in the Intensive Care Unit, Science Rationale and Practice.* Dubuque, IA: Kendal Hunt Publishing. 2002. 281–282.

Mahon, L. K., & Escott-Stump, S. "Medical Nutrition Therapy for Lower Gastrointestinal Tract Disorders." *Krause's Food, Nutrition & Diet Therapy* (11th ed.). Philadelphia, PA: W. B. Saunders. 2004. 730–732.

Matarese, L., & Gottschlich, M. "Gastrointestinal and Pancreatic Disease." Wall-Alonso, E., Sullivan, M., & Byrne, T. (Eds.). *Contemporary Nutrition Support Practice, A Clinical Guide* (2nd ed.). Philadelphia, PA: Saunders. 2003. 428–429.

Liver Disease

Author: Elizabeth Winthrop, MS, RD, CNSD

The liver is the key organ in metabolism of carbohydrates, proteins, fats, alcohol, vitamins, and minerals. It produces bile for digestion, and most of the nutrients absorbed from the GI tract travel first to the liver for processing. The liver is also the largest organ, containing much of the body's blood supply. Disruption in fluid balances occur when blood cannot circulate normally through the liver and the liver fails to manufacture sufficient proteins to maintain serum oncotic pressure. With all the thousands of functions of the liver, it is not surprising that liver disease causes severe nutritional problems.

Problem	*Do's and Don'ts*
Fatty Liver or Nonalcoholic Steatohepatitis (NASH) Related to Overweight	**Do:** Counsel patients that fatty liver, due to overweight, can be resolved through achieving and maintaining a healthy body weight. See the section on weight management. Suggest the following Web sites for providing many tools for weight management: http://www.healthierus.gov/dietaryguidelines http://win.niddk.nih.gov/index.htm http://www.mypyramid.gov/ **Don't:** Don't allow consumption of low carbohydrate diets, which are high in fats and animal protein. Don't allow any very rapid weight loss regimen because it may increase risk of gallbladder disease and causes imbalances in fluids and electrolytes.
Fatty Liver Related to Diabetes	**Do:** Encourage careful control of diet, medications, self-monitoring, and exercise to achieve desirable blood glucose levels and to help resolve fatty liver due to diabetes. (See the section on the management of diabetes on page 92.) Discourage fasting due to the patient's lack of glycogen stores, which may result in hypoglycemia.
Fatty Liver Related to Alcohol	**Do:** Encourage abstinence from alcohol. The following Web site has a free guide for clinicians helping patients who drink too much: http://www.niaaa.nih.gov/publications/EducationTrainingMaterials/guide.htm.

Problem	*Do's and Don'ts*
	Don't: Don't give up on helping your patients to abstain from alcohol.
Fatty Liver Related to TPN	**Do:** Check baseline triglyceride levels and monitor triglycerides for any patients who are receiving lipid emulsion. A rapidly rising level or any triglyceride over 400 mg/dl should prompt discussion with the PMD for discontinuing IV lipid. Encourage careful control of blood sugars to also help prevent or resolve fatty liver in TPN patients. **Don't:** Don't forget to monitor blood sugars carefully. Make sure sliding scale insulin or an insulin drip is ordered by the PMD in addition to any insulin in the total parenteral nutrition (TPN) bag.
Self-Treatment with Herbal Supplements	**Do:** Research any herbal supplements carefully prior to the patient taking them. Liver disease patients should not take any supplements without discussion with their PMD. (Two supplements showing possible promise are SAMe, which may decrease pruritis in cholestasis, and milk thistle, recommended by the German Commission E as supportive therapy in chronic inflammatory liver conditions. The PMD must allow these supplements prior to use.) **Don't:** Don't use kava-containing dietary supplements that may be associated with severe liver injury. Don't use herbs with anticoagulant properties if coagulopathies are present, such as tree ear mushrooms (Auricularia polytricha used in Chinese cooking and garlic supplements). See herb table in the appendix on page 381.
Food Safety to Avoid Additional Liver Damage	**Do:** Pay careful attention to food safety rules for people with reduced immunity. See food safety and foodborne illness in the appendix on page 367. **Don't:** Don't use raw shellfish, particularly oysters, because it has been associated with outbreaks of vibrio. In people with liver disease, a vibrio infection may have up to a 50% risk of fatality.

Problem	*Do's and Don'ts*
Gallbladder Disease	**Do:** Maintain a healthy weight to reduce risk of gallbladder disease. Counsel obese patients that weight should be lost gradually and permanently using a diet with no more than 30% of calories from fat and including physical exercise. Encourage adequate intakes of calcium and dietary fiber that may also help to prevent gallstones. See the section on gallbladder disease on page 250. **Don't:** Don't allow crash dieting or yo-yo dieting if obese. Bariatric surgery also increases the risk for gallbladder disease. Don't serve high-fat meals because they may cause episodes of pain due to contraction of the gallbladder.
Hemochromatosis	**Do:** Hemochromatosis is a chronic and potentially fatal disorder in which excess iron builds up in the body. It is treated mainly by removing iron through phlebotomy. See http://www.cdc.gov/genomics/activities/ogdp/2003.htm for free patient education materials on this disorder. **Don't:** Don't allow raw fish or raw shellfish, and minimize alcohol intake. While iron-containing foods can be eaten, patients should avoid iron-containing supplements and limit supplemental vitamin C to 500 mg or less.
Wilson's Disease	**Do:** Advise patients that Wilson's Disease is a rare, inherited, and often fatal disorder in which excess copper builds up in the body, causing liver and neurological disease. Treat the disease with medications, which chelate copper and remove it from the body. Taking chelating agents (Trientine) within 2 hours of vitamin supplements containing iron or other minerals reduces the effectiveness of the medication. Use filtered or bottled water because tap water often flows through copper pipes. **Don't:** Don't serve high-copper foods (for example, mushrooms, nuts, liver, chocolate, molasses, broccoli, dried fruit, and shellfish). Don't use copper pots in cooking.

Problem	Do's and Don'ts
Gilbert's Syndrome	**Do:** Inform patients that the mild, chronic increase in bilirubin levels seen does not pose a nutritional risk. Caloric deprivation over a 24-hour period resulting in an increased bilirubin level is diagnostic for the disorder. **Don't:** Don't serve raw shellfish or excess doses of acetaminophen.
Portal Hypertension	**Do:** Inform patients that sodium restriction is important in portal hypertension as well as edema, ascites, and anasarca. The PMD may treat patients with portal hypertension with a "TIPS" procedure (transjugular intrahepatic portosystemic shunt). Because shunted blood bypasses the liver, ammonia and other toxins may reach the brain more easily, causing encephalopathy. Nutritional status generally improves after TIPS. **Don't:** Don't use salt or salty foods, such as canned soups, frozen dinners, salty nuts and snacks, cold cuts, pickles, packaged rice, noodle, gravy, or sauce mixes. The patient's status post-TIPS may need protein restriction (see recommendation in next section, but final decision should be up to the PMD).
Hepatic Encephalopathy (HE)	**Do:** Inform patients that an acute medical problem, hepatic encephalopathy (HE), which is often an emergency, is often precipitated in a patient with chronic liver disease. Characterized by changes in consciousness and behavior, as well as other neurological symptoms, treatment for HE involves removing the precipitating factor (infection, or blood in the GI tract). Limit or eliminate protein intake in the acute phase per the PMD's request. Give lactulose per the PMD's request to neutralize ammonia in the gut and to cause diarrhea to eliminate nitrogenous waste. Give neomycin per the PMD's request to reduce intestinal bacteria that produce ammonia. **Don't:** Don't jump directly to a branch-chain amino-acid containing formula for oral or tube feeding. It should be reserved for patients with intractable encephalopathy.

Problem	*Do's and Don'ts*
Hepatic Encephalopathy	Don't over-restrict protein, particularly after the patient is discharged; always check with the PMD for a desired level.
Hypoglycemia	**Do:** Inform patients to support blood sugar during nothing by mouth (NPO) periods glycogen stores are mobilized from the liver. Without adequate glycogen stores, liver patients must break down muscle tissue to glucose earlier, so that even brief fasts can cause muscle wasting. Advise liver patients to eat three meals and an evening snack daily. **Don't:** Don't allow patients to remain NPO without at least adding 5% dextrose to peripheral IV fluids. Plan for three meals and an evening snack for patients who are able to eat.
Steatorrhea	**Do:** Avoid high-fat foods. See the appendix for a low-fat diet on pages 356–357. Use MCT oil (medium chain triglyceride) to increase calories in the diet. (Note: MCT oil does not provide all the essential fatty acids.)
Vitamin K Deficiency Secondary to Fat Malabsorption	**Do:** Inform patients that vitamin K deficiency is likely in patients with primary biliary cirrhosis. Check prothrombin time. Provide foods high in vitamin K; include dark leafy green vegetables. Consider vitamin K supplements, with the PMD's approval. Inform patient about studies in probiotics for liver disease, which may increase the beneficial gut bacteria that produce vitamin K. **Don't:** Don't allow herbal preparations that affect coagulation. See the herb guide in the appendix.
Vitamin D Deficiency Secondary to Fat Malabsorption	**Do:** Inform patients that vitamin D deficiency is likely in patients with primary biliary cirrhosis. Fortified low-fat dairy products are a good dietary source of vitamin D, as well as protein and calcium.

Problem	*Do's and Don'ts*
	Supplement with vitamin D tablets if approved by the physician.
Vitamin A Deficiency Secondary to Fat Malabsorption	**Do:** Inform patients that vitamin A deficiency is likely in patients with primary biliary cirrhosis. **Don't:** Don't use vitamin A supplements without checking with the PMD because vitamin A overload can cause liver damage.
Nausea, Vomiting, and Anorexia	**Do:** Inform patients that liver disease itself may cause nausea, vomiting, and anorexia, or the upsets may be side effects of treatment for hepatitis C (interferon). Consume enough liquids to prevent dehydration, and work to increase calorie and protein intake. Choose small, frequent meals, calorie-dense foods, cold foods without strong odors, and ginger ale. **Don't:** Don't serve greasy fried foods. Patients with nausea may tend toward salty foods (for example, pretzels or crackers), which should be avoided in excess. Don't allow sports drinks (for example, Gatorade) because they contain appreciable sodium and should be avoided by patients on a low-sodium restriction. (See portal hypertension on page 263.)

Sources

http://www.healthierus.gov/dietaryguidelines.

http://win.niddk.nih.gov/index.htm.

http://www.mypyramid.gov/.

http://www.niaaa.nih.gov/publications/Practitioner/guide.pdf.

http://www.cfsan.fda.gov/~dms/aidseat.html.

Renal Calculi

Author: Sandra Allonen MEd, RD, LDN

This list will assist the dietitian in answering nutrition questions and serve as a guide to assist patients who have renal calculi. The most common side effect of renal calculi is pain in the pelvic region, ranging from mild to severe. This pain may be dependent on the size, shape, and/or location of the calculus. Secondary symptoms may include vomiting, fever and chills, and/or blood in the urine. There are four basic types of calculi described in this section.

Problem	*Do's and Don'ts*
Calcium-Based Calculi	**Do:**
	The most common type of calcium-based calculi is oxalate, which is a waste product of metabolism. Diet plays a role in stone formation.
	Have the patient drink at least 2.5–3 liters of water a day.
	Limit protein intake to 0.7–0.8 gm/kg of body weight.
	Keep vitamin C intake to RDA of 60 mg/day.
	Limit sodium to 1.5 gm/day.
	Have the patient consume adequate calcium of 1000 mg/day through foods, beverages, or supplements.
	Limit the diet intake to between 40–50 mg of oxalates per day.
	Don't:
	Don't restrict fluid intake. This will make urine more concentrated and increase the risk of stone formation.
	Don't allow consumption of a high-protein-style diet.
	Don't allow excessive amounts of vitamin C (1000 mg/day) through foods or supplements.
	Don't serve food and beverages that are high in sodium.
	Don't allow high-oxalate foods and beverages (for example, cocoa, tea, wheat bran, nuts, peanut butter, peanut oil, walnut oil, rhubarb, strawberries, beets, spinach, and Swiss chard).
	Don't restrict calcium intake.

Problem	Do's and Don'ts
Uric Acid—A Product of Purine Metabolism	Purines are found in all animal products and in many seeds and plants. **Do:** Advocate at least between 2.5–3 liters of water a day. Limit protein intake to 0.7–0.8 gm/kg of body weight. Limit sodium to 1.5 gm/day. Limit alcohol intake, especially beer and scotch. Alcohol increases purine production, leading to higher uric acid levels in the blood and urine. Limit high-fat foods because fat holds onto uric acid in the kidneys. Suggest adequate carbohydrates because carbohydrates help excrete extra uric acid in blood. Counsel overweight patients that weight loss should be done gradually because quick weight loss may increase uric acid levels. Recommend foods that are low in purines. See Table 4-1 on page 269. **Don't:** Don't restrict fluid intake. This will make urine more concentrated and increase risk of stone formation. Don't allow a high-animal-based protein diet; limit meat to 3 ounces per day. Don't provide food and beverages that are high in sodium. Don't serve foods and beverages that are high in purines (for example, high-fat breads, french fries, avocados, whole milk, cream, sour cream, high-fat cheeses, cheeses and cream sauces, large amounts of meats, organ meats, sardines, anchovies, herring, mackerel, scallops, and mussels). See Table 4-1 on page 269.
Cystine	**Do:** Certain persons have a rare genetic disorder that causes them to excrete too much of the amino acid, cystine, in the urine. The patient should drink at least 2–3 liters of fluids (especially water) to help keep urine as dilute as possible.

Problem	Do's and Don'ts
Struvite or Infected Stones	**Do:** Struvite or infected stones are generally found in paralyzed persons, persons with an abnormal urinary tract, and women with frequent urinary tract infections. The stones form in the presence of a long-standing infection with certain bacteria (for example, proteus, staphylococci) that converts urea into ammonia, alkalizing the urine and precipitating magnesium ammonium phosphate. Advise the patient that there are no dietary recommendations for persons with this type of stone.

Table 4-1 Foods Rich in Purine

Foods Highest in Purine		**Foods High in Purine**	
Sweetbreads	Salmon, canned	Bacon	Mutton
Anchovies	Gravies	Meat soups	Duck
Sardines, canned	Scallops	Beef	Shellfish
Liver	Herring	Perch	Goose
Kidneys	Smelts	Calf tongue	Trout
Heart	Roe	Pike	Halibut
Meat extracts, broths, bouillon	Yeast	Carp	Turkey
		Pork	Lentils
		Chicken soup	Veal
		Rabbit	Liver sausage
		Codfish	

Foods Moderately High in Purine		**Foods Containing Little Purine**
Asparagus	Shad	Beverages: Carbonated, fruit juices, Postum, chocolate, cocoa
Navy beans	Finnan haddie	Breads: White bread and crackers, cornbread
Bluefish	Spinach	Cereals and cereal products: Corn, macaroni, noodles, rice, tapioca, refined wheat
Oatmeal	Ham	Cheese of all kinds
Cauliflower	Tuna fish	Eggs
Oysters	Kidney beans	Fats (use only amounts allowed)
Chicken	White fish	Fruits of all kinds
Peas	Lima beans	Gelatin
Crab	Lobster	Milk in all forms
Salmon	Mushrooms	Nuts of all kinds
Eel		Pies except mincemeat
		Shad roe
		Sugar and sweets
		Vegetables of all kinds except those previously mentioned
		Vegetable and milk soups
		Vitamin concentrates

SECTION 5
Childhood Nutrition

Acute Nutrition Care Problems

Acute Diarrhea Illness and Symptoms in Infants and Young Children 272

Acute Diarrhea Illness and Symptoms in Infants and Young Children

Authors: Sharon Collier, MEd, RD, LDN; Amina Grunko, MS, RD, LDN; Colleen McLean, CNSD, RD

This section addresses the common nutrition-related causes of diarrhea, how to feed through it, and how to treat the consequences. All infants and young children with diarrhea should be under the care of their PMD.

Problem	*Do's and Don'ts*
Dehydration	**Do:** Initiate oral rehydration solution (ORS) therapy as per PMD diagnosis. If no dehydration, replace losses: • Greater than 10 kg: 60–120 mL/kg ORS for each diarrheal stool or vomiting episode • Less than 10 kg: 120–240 mL/kg ORS for each diarrheal stool or vomiting episode Some dehydration: • 50–100 mL/kg ORS over 4 hours and replacement of losses per above Severe dehydration: • 20 mL/kg IV hydration (lactated Ringer solution) • After pulse and state of consciousness return to normal, 100 mL/kg ORS over 4 hours and replacement of losses per no or some dehydration loss Continue to breast-feed and/or provide undiluted expressed human milk or formula ad lib to infants; encourage children to drink undiluted cow's milk. For infants treated for severe dehydration, wait until rehydration therapy has started before reinitiating usual beverages and monitor for signs and symptoms of lactose intolerance that may be more likely. **Don't:** Don't allow excessive intake of high-sugar-containing beverages (that is, fruit juice, fruit drink, soda). Don't avoid lactose-containing beverages unless lactose intolerance is documented by increased stool output.

Problem	*Do's and Don'ts*
Nutritional Intake	**Do:** Continue to breast-feed or provide undiluted formula ad lib to infants; encourage children to drink undiluted cow's milk; offer regular diet of complex carbohydrates, fruits, vegetables, and lean meats, as age appropriate; limit high-fat and sugary foods. See Dietary Reference Intake listings for age. **Don't:** Don't put on highly restrictive diets (that is, BRATT [banana, rice, applesauce, tea, and toast]—this is an unbalanced diet that is low in calories). Don't avoid lactose-containing beverages unless lactose intolerance is documented by increased stool output.
Excessive Simple Carbohydrate Intake	**Do:** Obtain diet history; assess diet for content of high-sugar-containing beverages (that is, fruit juice, fruit drink, soda) and foods/beverages containing sugar alcohol (that is, mannitol, sorbitol, xylitol, lactitol, isomalt, maltitol, and hydrogenated starch hydrolysates). **Don't:** Don't provide excessive amounts of simple carbohydrate foods or excessive juice and other high-sugar-containing beverages, defined as: Infants: > 4 ounces Toddlers and older children: > 8 ounces
Medication Induced	**Do:** Obtain history of medication use; consult your PMD or pharmacist as needed. **Don't:** Don't stop medications unless advised by your PMD.

Sources

Hendricks, K. M., & Duggan, C. (Eds.). *Manual of Pediatric Nutrition* (4th ed.). Lewiston, NY: BC Decker. 2005.

Kleinman, R. E. (Ed.). *Pediatric Nutrition Handbook* (5th ed.). Elk Grove Village, IL: American Academy of Pediatrics. 2004.

SECTION 6

Progressive Diets

Progressive Diets

Clear-Liquid Diet 276
Mechanical Soft Diet 277
Soft Diet 278

Table 6-1 Sample Menu for a Clear-Liquid Diet

Breakfast	Lunch	Dinner
Clear juice, 2/3 c	Clear juice, 2/3 c	Clear juice, 2/3 c
Coffee or tea	Broth (chicken, beef, or vegetable), 2/3 c	Broth (chicken, beef, or vegetable), 2/3 c
Sugar	Flavored gelatin, 1/2 c	Fruit ice or flavored gelatin, 1/2 c
	Coffee or tea	Coffee or tea
Snack	Sugar	Sugar
Juice, 2/3 c or broth, clear, 1/2 c	Snack Flavored ice, 1/2 c	Snack Carbonated beverage

Table 6-2 Foods Permitted in a Mechanical Soft Diet

Food Types	Foods Permitted
Milk	All forms
Cheeses	All forms
Eggs	Any cooked form
Breads	White, rye without seeds, refined whole wheat; cornbread; any cracker not made with whole grains; French toast made from permitted breads; spoonbread; pancakes, plain soft rolls
Cereals	All cooked, soft varieties; puffed flakes and noncoarse ready-to-eat varieties
Flour	All forms
Meats, fish, poultry	Small cubed and finely ground or minced forms; as ingredients in creamed dishes, soups, casseroles, and stews
Seafoods	Any variety of fish without bone (canned, fresh, or frozen; packaged prepared forms in cream sauces); minced, shredded, ground, and finely chopped shellfish
Legumes, nuts	Fine, smooth, creamy peanut butter; legumes (if tolerated) cooked tender, finely chopped, mashed, or minced
Potatoes	White potatoes: mashed, boiled, baked, creamed, scalloped, cakes, au gratin; sweet potatoes: boiled, baked, mashed
Soups	All varieties, preferably without hard solids, such as nuts and seeds
Fruits	Raw: avocado, banana; cooked and canned: fruit cocktail, cherries, apples, apricots, peaches, pears, sections of mandarin oranges, grapefruits, or oranges without membranes; all juices and nectars
Vegetables	All juices; all vegetables cooked tender, chopped, mashed, canned, or pureed; canned, pureed, or paste forms of tomato
Sweets	Marshmallow and chocolate sauces; preserves, marmalade, jelly, jam; candy: hard, chocolate, jelly beans, marshmallows, candy corn, butterscotch, gumdrops, plain fudge, lollipops, fondant mints; syrup: sorghum, maple, corn; sugar: granulated, brown, maple, confectioners'; honey, molasses
Desserts	All plain or certain flavored varieties (permitted flavorings include liquids, such as juice; finely chopped or pureed fruits without solid pieces of fruit, seeds, nuts, etc.); gelatins, puddings; ice cream, ice milk, sherbet; water ices; cakes, cookies, cake icing; cobblers
Fats	Butter, margarine, cream (or substitutes), oils and vegetable shortenings; salad dressings, tartar sauce, sour cream
Seasonings	Salt, pepper, soy sauce, vinegar, catsup; all other herbs, especially finely chopped or ground, that can be tolerated

Table 6-3 Sample Menu for a Soft Diet

Breakfast	Lunch	Dinner
Orange juice, 1/2 c	Tomato soup, 1/2 c	Soup, creamed, 1/2 c[a]
Farina, 1/2 c	Cod, broiled, 2–3 oz	Beef, stew meat, tender, 3–4 oz
Egg, soft-boiled, 1[a]	Potato, baked, no skin, medium, 1	White rice, 1/2 c
Bacon, crisp, 2 strips[a]	Toast, 1 slice	Asparagus, canned, 1/2 c
Toast, 1 slice	Butter or margarine, 1 tsp	Toast, 1 slice
Butter or margarine, 1 tsp	Pudding, plain, 1/2 c	Butter or margarine, 1 tsp
Jam, 1–3 tsp	Coffee or tea, 1–2 c	Gelatin, flavored, 1/2 c
Milk, 1 c	Sugar, 1–3 tsp	Coffee or tea, 1–2 c
Coffee or tea, 1–2 c	Cream, 1 Tbsp[a]	Cream, 1 Tbsp[a]
Sugar, 1–3 tsp	Salt, pepper	Sugar, 1–3 tsp
Cream, 1 Tbsp[a]		Salt, pepper
Salt, pepper		

[a]Egg, bacon, and cream may be omitted to lower the fat content of the diet.

SECTION 7

Appendices

A. Total Fat 281
B. Caffeine Values 282
C. Calculations and Conversions 284
D. Carbohydrates, Calories, and Glycemic Index of Commonly Consumed Foods 295
E. CPR 297
F. Dietary Guidelines for Americans 2005 298
G. Dietary Reference Intakes, 2000, and RDA, 1989 . . . 301
H. Diet and Drug Interactions 309
I. Ethnic, Cultural, and Religious Food Considerations 320
J. Energy Equations 326
K. Energy Expenditure of Activity 327
L. Exchange Lists for Meal Planning 328
M. Exchange List for Carbohydrate Counting 345
N. Fast Food Nutrients 346
O. Fat Sources 356
P. Food Labels 358
Q. Foodborne Illness 367
R. Glycemic Indexes for Foods 375
S. Growth Charts 376
T. Heimlich Maneuver 379
U. Herb Guide 381

V. Infant Formulas 385
W. Activity of Insulin Preparations 394
X. Micronutrients 396
Y. MyPyramid. 398
Z. Normal Nutritional Lab Values 401
AA. Nutrition Assessment Sheet 415
BB. Physical Indicators of Nutritional Status 418
CC. Enteral Formula Selection 430
DD. Vitamin and Mineral Food Sources 434
EE. Information Resources 435
FF. Food Sources of Selected Nutrients 446
GG. BMI Chart 458
HH. Super Recipes. 459
II. Sodium Content of Foods 461

Appendix A:
Total Fat

Table A-1 Amount of Total Fat That Provides 30 Percent of Calories and Saturated Fat That Provides 10 Percent

Total calories per day	Total fat (g) (no more than 30% of total calories)	Saturated fat (g) (no more than 10% of total calories)
1,600	53	18
2,000*	65	20
2,200	73	24
2,500*	80	25
2,800	93	31

* Percent Daily Values on Nutrition Facts Labels are based on a 2,000-calorie diet. Values for 2,000 and 2,500 calories are rounded to the nearest 5 g to be consistent with the label.

Source: U.S. Department of Agriculture and Department of Health and Human Services (2000).

Appendix B: Caffeine Values

Caffeine is a compound found mostly in coffee, tea, cola, cocoa, chocolate, and in foods containing these. Table B-1 lists the amounts of caffeine found in these beverages and foods.

Table B-1 Caffeine Values

Food	Serving size	Caffeine (mg)
Beverages		
Chocolate milk, includes malted milk	8 fl oz.	5–8
Chocolate shake	16 fl oz.	8
Cocoa, prepared from powder		
Regular	6 fl oz.	4–6
Sugar-free	6 fl oz.	15
Coffee, regular		
Brewed	6 fl oz.	103
Prepared from instant	6 fl oz.	57
Coffee, decaffeinated		
Brewed	6 fl oz.	2
Prepared from instant	6 fl oz.	2
Coffee liqueur	1.5 fl oz.	14
Cola or pepper-type, with caffeine	12 fl oz.	37
Diet cola, with caffeine	12 fl oz.	50
Tea, regular		
Brewed	6 fl oz.	36
Instant, prepared	8 fl oz.	26–36
Tea, chamomile	6 fl oz.	0
Tea, decaffeinated, brewed	6 fl oz.	2
Chocolate Foods		
Baking chocolate, unsweetened	1 square (1 oz.)	58
Brownies	1	1–3
Candies		
Dark chocolate	1.45-oz. bar	30
Milk chocolate bar	1.55-oz. bar	11
Semisweet chocolate chips	1/4 cup	26–28
Chocolate with other ingredients (nuts, crisped rice, etc.)	About 1.5 oz.	3–11
Cereal (containing cocoa)	1 oz.	1
Cocoa powder, unsweetened	1 Tbsp	12

Table B-1 Caffeine Values—*continued*

Food	Serving size	Caffeine (mg)
Cookies (chocolate chip, devil's food, chocolate sandwich)	1	1
Chocolate cupcake with chocolate frosting	1	1–2
Frosting	1/12 pkg (2 Tbsp)	1–2
Fudge	1 piece (about 3/4 oz.)	2–3
Ice cream/frozen yogurt	1/2 cup	2
Pudding		
Prepared from dry mix	1/2 cup	3
Ready-to-eat	4 oz.	6
Syrup		
Thin-type	1 Tbsp	3
Fudge-type	1 Tbsp	1

Source: U.S. Department of Agriculture, Agricultural Research Service (2000).

Appendix C: Calculations and Conversions

Energy from Food

grams carbohydrate × 4 kcal/g
grams protein × 4 kcal/g
grams fat × 9 kcal/g
grams alcohol × 7 kcal/g
total = energy from food

Example:			
	Carbohydrate	**275 g × 4 kcal/g =**	**1,100 kcal**
	Protein	**64 g × 4 kcal/g =**	**256 kcal**
	Fat	**60 g × 9 kcal/g =**	**540 kcal**
	Alcohol	**15 g × 7 kcal/g =**	**105 kcal**
	TOTAL ENERGY		**2,001 kcal**

Calculating the percentage of calories for each:

Carbohydrate	**(1,100 kcal ÷ 2,001 kcal) × 100 =**	**54.97%**	**(55%)**
Protein	**(256 kcal ÷ 2,001 kcal) × 100 =**	**12.79%**	**(13%)**
Fat	**(540 kcal ÷ 2,001 kcal) × 100 =**	**26.99%**	**(27%)**
Alcohol	**(105 kcal ÷ 2,001 kcal) × 100 =**	**5.25%**	**(5%)**

1 kilocalorie = 4.184 kilojoules
1 kilojoule = 0.239 kilocalories

Niacin Equivalents (NE)

Determining the amount of niacin from tryptophan:
NE = milligrams niacin
NE from tryptophan = grams excess protein ÷ 6
NE from tryptophan = (grams dietary protein − protein RDA) ÷ 6

Example: **Assume dietary protein = 86 g and protein RDA = 56 g**
NE from tryptophan = (86 g − 56 g) ÷ 6
NE from tryptophan = 5

Dietary Folate Equivalents (DFE)

Dietary folate equivalents account for differences in the absorption of food folate, synthetic folic acid in dietary supplements, and folic acid added to fortified foods. Food in the stomach also affects bioavailability. Folic acid taken as a supplement when fasting is two times more bioavailable than food folate. Folic acid taken with food and folic acid in fortified foods are 1.7 times more bioavailable than food folate.

1 μg DFE = 1 microgram of food folate
= 0.5 μg of folic acid supplement taken on an empty stomach
= 0.6 μg of folic acid supplement consumed with meals
= 0.6 μg of folic acid in fortified foods

1 μg folic acid as a fortificant = 1.7 μg DFE
1 μg folic acid as a supplement, fasting = 2.0 μg DFE

Example:

Food folate in cooked spinach	**100 μg = 100 μg DFE**
Ready-to-eat cereal fortified with folic acid	**100 μg = 170 μg DFE**
Supplemental folic acid taken without food	**100 μg = 200 μg DFE**

Estimating DFE from Daily Value:
DFE = %DV × DV × bioavailability factor

Example:
Assume that a serving of fortified breakfast cereal contains 10% of the Daily Value for folate
Daily Value = 400 μg folic acid

DFE = % DV × DV × bioavailability factor
DFE = 0.10 × 400 μg × 1.7
DFE = 68 μg, which can be rounded to 70 μg DFE

Retinal Activity Equivalents (RAE)

Retinol activity equivalents are a standardized measure of vitamin A activity that account for differences in the bioavailability of different sources of vitamin A. Of the provitamin A carotenoids, beta-carotene produces the most vitamin A.

1 μg RAE = 1 μg retinol
= 12 μg beta-carotene
= 24 μg of other vitamin A precursors

Although outdated, many vitamin supplements still report vitamin A content as International Units (IU).

1 μg RAE = 3.33 IU from retinol
= 10 IU from beta-carotene in supplements
= 20 IU from beta-carotene in foods

Vitamin D

Although outdated, many vitamin supplements still report vitamin D content as International Units (IU).

1 IU = 0.025 μg cholecalciferol
μg cholecalciferol = IU ÷ 40

Example:
A vitamin supplement contains 100 IU vitamin D
μg cholecalciferol = 100 ÷ 40 = 2.5

Vitamin E

Although outdated, many vitamin supplements still report vitamin E content as International Units (IU) rather than as milligrams of α-tocopherol. Two conversion factors are used to convert IU to milligrams of α-tocopherol. If the form of the supplement is "natural" or RRR-α-tocopherol (historically labeled as *d*-alpha-tocopherol), the conversion factor is 0.67 mg/IU. If the form of the supplement is *all rac*-α-tocopherol (historically labeled *dl*-α-tocopherol), the conversion factor is 0.45 mg/IU.

Examples:
A multivitamin supplement contains 30 IU of *d*-α-tocopherol
30 IU × 0.67 = 20 mg α-tocopherol
A multivitamin supplement contains 30 IU of *dl*-α-tocopherol
30 IU × 0.45 = 13.5 mg α-tocopherol

Estimating Energy Expenditure

The estimated energy requirement (EER) is defined as the dietary energy intake (in kilocalories per day) that is predicted to maintain energy balance in a healthy adult of a defined age, gender, weight, height, and level of physical activity consistent with good health.* The EER equations predict total energy expenditure (TEE).

Adult men (age 19 and older):

$$\mathbf{EER = 662 - 9.53 \times Age\ [yr] + PA \times (15.91 \times Weight\ [kg] + 539.6 \times Height\ [m])}$$

PA is the Physical Activity coefficient that represents physical activity level.

Sedentary	**PA = 1.0**
Low active	**PA = 1.11**
Active	**PA = 1.25**
Very active	**PA = 1.48**

Adult women (age 19 and older):

$$\mathbf{EER = 354 - 6.91 \times Age\ [yr] + PA \times (9.36 \times Weight\ [kg] + 726 \times Height\ [m])}$$

PA is the Physical Activity coefficient that represents physical activity level.

Sedentary	**PA = 1.0**
Low active	**PA = 1.12**
Active	**PA = 1.27**
Very active	**PA = 1.45**

Example: **A 21-year-old woman 5′4″ (1.6 m) tall, who weighs 120 pounds (54.5 kilograms) and is active.**

Example:
$$\begin{aligned} &= 354 - 6.91 \times 21\ \text{yr} + 1.27 \times (9.36 \times 54.5\ \text{kg} + 726 \times 1.6\ \text{m}) \\ &= 354 - 145.11 + 1.27 \times (510.12 + 1{,}161.6) \\ &= 354 - 145.11 + 1.27 \times 1{,}671.72 \\ &= 354 - 145.11 + 2{,}123.08 \\ &= 2{,}331.97 \\ &= 2{,}332\ \text{kcal/day} \end{aligned}$$

Total energy expenditure can also be estimated by first estimating resting energy expenditure (REE) and then adding additional energy to account for physical activity and the thermic effect of food.

*Source: Institute of Medicine, Food and Nutrition Board. *Dietary Reference Intakes for Energy, Carbohydrate, Fiber, Fat, Fatty Acids, Cholesterol, Protein, and Amino Acids.* Washington, DC: National Academy Press; 2002.

Resting Energy Expenditure (REE)

Harris-Benedict Equations

Adult men **REE = 66 + 13.7*W* + 5.0*H* − 6.8*A***

Adult women **REE = 655 + 9.6*W* + 1.8*H* − 4.7*A***

(*W* = weight in kilograms, *H* = height in centimeters, *A* = age)

Note: Harris-Benedict equations may overestimate resting energy expenditure (REE), especially for obese people.

Quick Estimate

Adult men **REE = weight (kg) × 1.0 kcal/kg × 24 hours**

REE = weight (kg) × 1.0 × 24

Adult women **REE = weight (kg) × 0.9 kcal/kg × 24 hours**

REE = weight (kg) × 0.9 × 24

Physical Activity (PA)

Physical activity can be estimated as a percentage of the resting energy expenditure (REE) based on the frequency and intensity of physical activity.

Percentage of REE	Activity Level	Description
20–39%	Sedentary	Mostly resting, with little or no activity
30–45%	Light	Occasional unplanned activity (for example, going for a stroll)
45–65%	Moderate	Daily planned activity, such as brisk walks
65–90%	Heavy	Daily workout routine requiring several hours of continuous exercise
90–120%	Exceptional	Daily vigorous workouts for extended hours; training for competition

Thermic Effect of Food (TEF)

The thermic effect of food can be estimated as 10% of the sum of REE + physical activity.

Total energy expenditure (TEE) = REE + PA + TEF

Example using quick estimate of REE:

A 175-pound (79.5 kg), 30-year-old man engages in moderate activity (60% of REE).

REE = 79.5 kg × 1.0 kcal/kg/hr × 24 hr/day
= 1,908 kcal/day

PA = 60% of REE
= 0.60 × 1,908 kcal/day
= 1,144.8 kcal/day

TEF = 10% of REE + PA
= 0.10 × (1,908 + 1,144.8 kcal/day)
= 0.10 × 3,052.8 kcal/day
= 305.3 kcal/day

TEE = REE + PA + TEF
= 1,908 + 1,144.8 + 305.3 kcal/day
= 3,358 kcal/day

Body Mass Index (BMI)

U.S. Formula

BMI = [weight in pounds ÷ (height in inches)^2] × 703

Example: **A 154-pound man is 5 ft 8 inches (68 inches) tall**
BMI = [154 ÷ (68 in × 68 in)] × 703
BMI = (154 ÷ 4,624) × 703
BMI = 23.41

Metric Formula

BMI = weight in kilograms ÷ [height in meters]^2
or
BMI = [weight in kilograms ÷ (height in cm)^2] × 10,000

Example: **A 70-kg man is 1.75 meters tall**
BMI = 70 kg ÷ (1.75 m × 1.75 m)
BMI = 70 ÷ 3.0625
BMI = 22.86

Metric Prefixes

giga-	G	1,000,000,000	deci-	d	0.1
mega-	M	1,000,000	centi-	c	0.01
kilo-	k	1,000	milli-	m	0.001
hecto-	h	100	micro-	μ	0.000001
deka-	da	10	nano-	n	0.000000001

Length: Metric and U.S. Equivalents

1 centimeter	0.3937 inch
1decimeter	3.937 inches
1 foot	0.3048 meter
1 inch	2.54 centimeters
1 meter	39.37 inches
	1.094 yards
1 micron	0.001 millimeter
	0.00003937 inch
1 millimeter	0.03937 inch
1 yard	0.9144 meter

Capacities or Volumes

1 cup, measuring	8 fluid ounces
	1/2 liquid pint
1 gallon (U.S.)	231 cubic inches
	3.785 liters
	0.833 British gallon
	128 U.S. fluid ounces
1 gallon (British Imperial)	277.42 cubic inches
	1.201 U.S. gallons
	4.546 liters
	160 British fluid ounces
1 liter	1.057 liquid quarts
	0.908 dry quart
	61.024 cubic inches
1 milliliter	0.0621 cubic inches
1 ounce, fluid or liquid (U.S.)	1.805 cubic inches
	29.574 milliliters
	1.041 British fluid ounces
1 pint, dry	33.600 cubic inches
	0.551 liter
1 pint, liquid	28.875 cubic inches
	0.473 liter
1 quart, dry (U.S.)	67.201 cubic inches
	1.101 liters
	0.969 British quart
1 quart, liquid (U.S.)	57.75 cubic inches
	0.946 liter
	0.833 British quart
1 quart (British)	69.354 cubic inches
	1.032 U.S. dry quarts
	1.201 U.S. liquid quarts
1 tablespoon, measuring	3 teaspoons
	1/2 fluid ounce
1 teaspoon, measuring	1/3 tablespoon
	1/6 fluid ounce
1 kilogram	2.205 pounds
1 microgram (μg)	0.000001 gram

Food Measurement Equivalents

16 tablespoons = 1 cup
12 tablespoons = $\frac{3}{4}$ cup
10 tablespoons + 2 teaspoons = $\frac{2}{3}$ cup
8 tablespoons = $\frac{1}{2}$ cup
6 tablespoons = $\frac{3}{8}$ cup
5 tablespoons + 1 teaspoon = $\frac{1}{3}$ cup
4 tablespoons = $\frac{1}{4}$ cup
2 tablespoons = $\frac{1}{8}$ cup
2 tablespoons + 2 teaspoons = $\frac{1}{6}$ cup
1 tablespoon = $\frac{1}{16}$ cup
2 cups = 1 pint
2 pints = 1 quart
3 teaspoons = 1 tablespoon
48 teaspoons = 1 cup

Food Measurement Conversions: Metric to U.S.

Capacity		**Weight**	
1 milliliter	$\frac{1}{5}$ teaspoon	1 gram	0.035 ounce
5 milliliters	1 teaspoon	100 grams	3.5 ounces
15 milliliters	1 tablespoon	500 grams	1.10 pounds
100 milliliters	3.4 fluid oz.	1 kilogram	2.205 pounds
240 milliliters	1 cup		35 ounces
1 liter	34 fluid oz.		
	4.2 cups		
	2.1 pints		
	1.06 quarts		
	0.26 gallon		

Food Measurement Conversions: U.S. to Metric

Capacity	
$\frac{1}{5}$ teaspoon	1 milliliter
1 teaspoon	5 milliliters
1 tablespoon	15 milliliters
1 fluid ounce	30 milliliters
$\frac{1}{5}$ cup	47 milliliters
1 cup	237 milliliters
2 cups (1 pint)	473 milliliters
4 cups (1 quart)	0.95 liter
4 quarts (1 gal.)	3.8 liters
Weight	
1 ounce	28 grams
1 pound	454 grams

Conversion Factors

To change	To	Multiply by
centimeters	inches	0.3937
centimeters	feet	0.03281
cubic feet	cubic meters	0.0283
cubic meters	cubic feet	35.3145
cubic meters	cubic yards	1.3079
cubic yards	cubic meters	0.7646
feet	meters	0.3048
gallons (U.S.)	liters	3.7853
grams	ounces avdp	0.0353
grams	pounds	0.002205
inches	millimeters	25.4000
inches	centimeters	2.5400
inches	meters	0.0254
kilograms	pounds	2.2046
liters	gallons (U.S.)	0.2642
liters	pints (dry)	1.8162
liters	pints (liquid)	2.1134
liters	quarts (dry)	0.9081
liters	quarts (liquid)	1.0567
meters	feet	3.2808
meters	yards	1.0936
millimeters	inches	0.0394
ounces avdp	grams	28.3495
ounces	pounds	0.0625
pints (dry)	liters	0.5506
pints (liquid)	liters	0.4732
pounds	kilograms	0.4536
pounds	ounces	16
quarts (dry)	liters	1.1012
quarts (liquid)	liters	0.9463

Fahrenheit and Celsius (Centigrade) Scales

°Celsius	°Fahrenheit	°Celsius	°Fahrenheit
−273.15	−459.67	30	86
−250	−418	35	95
−200	−328	40	104
−150	238	45	113
−100	148	50	122
−50	58	55	131
−40	40	60	140
−30	22	65	149
−20	−4	70	158
−10	−14	75	167
0	32	80	176
5	41	85	185
10	50	90	194
15	59	95	203
20	68	100	212
25	77		

Zero on the Fahrenheit scale represents the temperature produced by the mixing of equal weights of snow and common salt.

	°Fahrenheit	°Celsius
Boiling point of water	212°	100°
Freezing point of water	32°	0°
Normal body temperature	98.6°	37°
Comfortable room temperature	68–77°	20–25°
Absolute zero	459.6°	273.1°

Absolute zero is theoretically the lowest possible temperature, the point at which all molecular motion would cease.

To Convert Temperature Scales

To convert Fahrenheit to Celsius (Centigrade), subtract 32 and multiply by $^5/_9$.

$$°C = {}^5/_9(°F - 32)$$

To convert Celsius (Centigrade) to Fahrenheit, multiply by $^9/_5$ and add 32.

$$°F = ({}^9/_5 \times °C) + 32$$

Table C-1 Pound to Kilogram Conversion Chart

lb	kg	lb	kg	lb	kg	lb	kg	lg	kg
85.0	38.6	108.0	49.1	131.0	59.5	154.0	70.0	177.0	80.5
85.5	38.9	108.5	49.3	131.5	59.8	154.5	70.2	177.5	80.7
86.0	39.1	109.0	49.5	132.0	60.0	155.0	70.5	178.0	80.9
86.5	39.3	109.5	49.8	132.5	60.2	155.5	70.7	178.5	81.1
87.0	39.5	110.0	50.0	133.0	60.5	156.0	70.9	179.0	81.4
87.5	39.8	110.5	50.2	133.5	60.7	156.5	71.1	179.5	81.6
88.0	40.0	111.0	50.5	134.0	60.9	157.0	71.4	180.0	81.8
88.5	40.2	111.5	50.7	134.5	61.1	157.5	71.6	180.5	82.0
89.0	40.5	112.0	50.9	135.0	61.4	158.0	71.8	181.0	82.3
89.5	40.7	112.5	51.1	135.5	61.6	158.5	72.0	181.5	82.5
90.0	40.9	113.0	51.4	136.0	61.8	159.0	72.3	182.0	82.7
90.5	41.1	113.5	51.6	136.5	62.0	159.5	72.5	182.5	83.0
91.0	41.4	114.0	51.8	137.0	62.3	160.0	72.7	183.0	83.2
91.5	41.6	114.5	52.0	137.5	62.5	160.5	73.0	183.5	83.4
92.0	41.8	115.0	52.3	138.0	62.7	161.0	73.2	184.0	83.6
92.5	42.0	115.5	52.5	138.5	63.0	161.5	73.4	184.5	83.9
93.0	42.3	116.0	52.7	139.0	63.2	162.0	73.6	185.0	84.1
93.5	42.5	116.5	53.0	139.5	63.4	162.5	73.9	185.5	84.3
94.0	42.7	117.0	53.2	140.0	63.6	163.0	74.1	186.0	84.5
94.5	43.0	117.5	53.4	140.5	63.9	163.5	74.3	186.5	84.8
95.0	43.2	118.0	53.6	141.0	64.1	164.0	74.5	187.0	85.0
95.5	43.4	118.5	53.9	141.5	64.3	164.5	74.8	187.5	85.2
96.0	43.6	119.0	54.1	142.0	64.5	165.0	75.0	188.0	85.5
96.5	43.9	119.5	54.3	142.5	64.8	165.5	75.2	188.5	85.7
97.0	44.1	120.0	54.5	143.0	65.0	166.0	75.5	189.0	85.9
97.5	44.3	120.5	54.8	143.5	65.2	166.5	75.7	189.5	86.1
98.0	44.5	121.0	55.0	144.0	65.5	167.0	75.9	190.0	86.4
98.5	44.8	121.5	55.2	144.5	65.7	167.5	76.1	190.5	86.6
99.0	45.0	122.0	55.5	145.0	65.9	168.0	76.4	191.0	86.8
99.5	45.2	122.5	55.7	145.5	66.1	168.5	76.6	191.5	87.0
100.0	45.5	123.0	55.9	146.0	66.5	169.0	76.8	192.0	87.3
100.5	45.7	123.5	56.1	146.5	66.6	169.5	77.0	192.5	87.5
101.0	45.9	124.0	56.4	147.0	66.8	170.0	77.3	193.0	87.7
101.5	46.1	124.5	56.6	147.5	67.0	170.5	77.5	193.5	88.0
102.0	46.4	125.0	56.8	148.0	67.3	171.0	77.7	194.0	88.2
102.5	46.6	125.5	57.0	148.5	67.5	171.5	78.0	194.5	88.4
103.0	46.8	126.0	57.3	149.0	67.7	172.0	78.2	195.0	88.6
103.5	47.0	126.5	57.5	149.5	68.0	172.5	78.4	195.5	88.9
104.0	47.3	127.0	57.7	150.0	68.2	173.0	78.6	196.0	89.1
104.5	47.5	127.5	58.0	150.5	68.4	173.5	78.9	196.5	89.3
105.0	47.7	128.0	58.2	151.0	68.6	174.0	79.1	197.0	89.5
105.5	48.0	128.5	58.4	151.5	68.9	174.5	79.3	197.5	89.8
106.0	48.2	129.0	58.6	152.0	69.1	175.0	79.5	198.0	90.0
106.5	48.4	129.5	58.9	152.5	69.3	175.5	79.8	198.5	90.2
107.0	48.6	130.0	59.1	153.0	69.5	176.0	80.0	199.0	90.5
107.5	48.9	130.5	59.3	153.5	69.8	176.5	80.2	199.5	90.7

Appendix D: Carbohydrates, Calories, and Glycemic Index of Commonly Consumed Foods

Debra Wein, MS, RD, LDN, ACSM-HFI, NSCA-CPT

SECTION 7

Table D-1 High Carbohydrate Foods

	Carbohydrates (grams)	Total Calories	Glycemic Index (GI)
Cereals, cold and hot			
Grape-Nuts (1/2 cup)	46	200	Med–high
Shredded Wheat (1 cup)	37	180	Med–high
Raisin Bran (1 cup)	42	180	Med–high
All Bran (1 cup)	27	180	Med–high
Oatmeal (1 oz.)	30	140	Med–high
Cream of Wheat (1 oz.)	22	100	Med–high
Pancakes (2)	30	140	
Waffles , eggs (2)	34	240	Medium
Fruits			
Apple or orange	20	80	Medium
Banana	26	105	Medium
Raisins (1/2 cup)	60	240	Medium
Grapes (1 cup)	16	58	Medium
Applesauce (1/2 cup)	26	97	Medium
Dried apricots (8 halves)	30	120	Medium
Fruit yogurt (1 cup)	50	250	Low
Ice milk (1/2 cup)	22	120	Low
Spaghetti, macaroni, noodles (1 cup)	40	200	Medium
Rice (white/brown) (1 cup)	35	160	Medium
- parboiled rice			Low
Baked potato (1 large)	55	240	High
Stuffing (1 cup)	40	220	Medium
Starchy Vegetables			
Corn (1/2 cup)	18	80	High
Winter squash (1/2 cup)	15	65	High
Carrots (1, medium)	10	60	High
Peas (1/2 cup)	10	40	High
Tomato sauce (1/2 cup)	10	80	High

continues

Table D-1 High Carbohydrate Foods—*continued*

	Carbohydrates (grams)	Total Calories	Glycemic Index (GI)
Legumes			
Baked beans (1 cup)	50	330	Low
Lentils (1 cup)	40	215	Low
Kidney beans (1 cup)	33	204	Low
Lima beans (1 cup)	28	140	Low
Garbanzo beans (1 cup)	27	28	Low
Split-pea soup (11 oz.)	35	220	Low
Bread Products			
Whole grain (2 slices)	25	150	Med–high
Sub roll (8 inches)	60	280	Med–high
Bagel	30	210	Med–high
English muffin (1)	25	130	Med–high
Bran muffin (large)	45	320	Med–high
Corn bread (large slice)	29	198	Med–high
Graham crackers (2 squares)	11	60	Med–high

Appendix E: CPR

Table E-1 CPR

Procedure	Infants (younger than 1 year)	Children (1 year to onset of puberty)[1]	Adults
Airway	Head tilt-chin lift; jaw thrust if suspect spinal injury.	Head tilt-chin lift; jaw thrust if suspect spinal injury.	Head tilt-chin lift; jaw thrust if suspect spinal injury.
Breathing			
Initial Breaths	Two breaths with duration of 1 second each with enough volume to produce chest rise	Two breaths with duration of 1 second each with enough volume to produce chest rise	Two breaths with duration of 1 second each with enough volume to produce chest rise
Subsequent Breaths	One breath every 3 to 5 seconds (12–20 breaths per minute)	One breath every 3 to 5 seconds (12–20 breaths per minute)	One breath every 5 to 6 seconds (8–10 breaths per minute)
Circulation			
Pulse Check	Brachial artery	Carotid or femoral artery	Carotid or femoral artery
Compression Area	Just below nipple line	In the center of chest, between nipples	In the center of chest, between nipples
Compression Width	Two fingers or two-thumbs/hands-encircling technique	Heel of one hand or two hands	Two hands
Compression Depth	One-third to one-half depth of chest	One-third to one-half depth of chest	1½ inches to 2 inches
Compression Rate	100 per minute	100 per minute	100 per minute
Ratio of Compressions to Ventilations	30:2 (one rescuer); 15:2 (two rescuers)[2]	30:2 (one rescuer); 15:2 (two rescuers)[2]	30:2
Foreign Body Obstruction	Conscious: Back slaps and chest thrusts Unconscious: CPR	Conscious: Abdominal thrusts Unconscious: CPR	Conscious: Abdominal thrusts Unconscious: CPR

[1]Onset of puberty is approximately 12–14 years of age, as defined by secondary characteristics (for example, breast development in girls and armpit hair in boys).

[2]Pause the compressions to deliver ventilations.

Appendix F: Dietary Guidelines for Americans 2005

Adequate Nutrients Within Calorie Needs

Key Recommendations

- Consume a variety of nutrient-dense foods and beverages within and among the basic food groups while choosing foods that limit the intake of saturated and trans fats, cholesterol, added sugars, salt, and alcohol.
- Meet recommended intakes within energy needs by adopting a balanced eating pattern, such as the USDA Food Guide or the DASH Eating Plan.

Weight Management

Key Recommendations

- To maintain body weight in a healthy range, balance calories from foods and beverages with calories expended.
- To prevent gradual weight gain over time, make small decreases in food and beverage calories and increase physical activity.

Physical Activity

Key Recommendations

- Engage in regular physical activity and reduce sedentary activities to promote health, psychological well-being, and a healthy body weight.
- To reduce the risk of chronic disease in adulthood: Engage in at least 30 minutes of moderate-intensity physical activity, above usual activity, at work or home on most days of the week.
- For most people, greater health benefits can be obtained by engaging in physical activity of more vigorous intensity or longer duration.
- To help manage body weight and prevent gradual, unhealthy body weight gain in adulthood: Engage in approximately 60 minutes of moderate- to vigorous-intensity activity on most days of the week while not exceeding caloric intake requirements.
- To sustain weight loss in adulthood: Participate in at least 60 to 90 minutes of daily moderate-intensity physical activity while not exceeding caloric intake requirements. Some people may need to consult with a healthcare provider before participating in this level of activity.
- Achieve physical fitness by including cardiovascular conditioning, stretching exercises for flexibility, and resistance exercises or calisthenics for muscle strength and endurance.

Food Groups to Encourage

Key Recommendations

- Consume a sufficient amount of fruits and vegetables while staying within energy needs. Two cups of fruit and $2^1/_2$ cups of vegetables per day are recommended for a reference 2,000-calorie intake, with higher or lower amounts depending on the calorie level.
- Choose a variety of fruits and vegetables each day. In particular, select from all five vegetable subgroups (dark green, orange, legumes, starchy vegetables, and other vegetables) several times a week.
- Consume 3 or more ounce-equivalents of whole-grain products per day, with the rest of the recommended grains coming from enriched or whole-grain products. In general, at least half the grains should come from whole grains.
- Consume 3 cups per day of fat-free or low-fat milk or equivalent milk products.

Fats

Key Recommendations

- Consume less than 10 percent of calories from saturated fatty acids and less than 300 mg/day of cholesterol, and keep trans fatty acid consumption as low as possible.
- Keep total fat intake between 20 to 35 percent of calories, with most fats coming from sources of polyunsaturated and monounsaturated fatty acids, such as fish, nuts, and vegetable oils.
- When selecting and preparing meat, poultry, dry beans, and milk or milk products, make choices that are lean, low-fat, or fat-free.
- Limit intake of fats and oils high in saturated and/or trans fatty acids, and choose products low in such fats and oils.

Carbohydrates

Key Recommendations

- Choose fiber-rich fruits, vegetables, and whole grains often.
- Choose and prepare foods and beverages with minimal added sugars or caloric sweeteners, in keeping with amounts suggested by the USDA Food Guide and the DASH Eating Plan.
- Reduce the incidence of dental caries by practicing good oral hygiene and consuming sugar- and starch-containing foods and beverages less frequently.

Sodium and Potassium

Key Recommendations

- Consume less than 2,300 mg (approximately 1 tsp of salt) of sodium per day.
- Choose and prepare foods with little salt. At the same time, consume potassium-rich foods, such as fruits and vegetables.

Alcoholic Beverages

Key Recommendations

- Those who choose to drink alcoholic beverages should do so sensibly and in moderation—defined as the consumption of up to one drink per day for women and up to two drinks per day for men.
- Alcoholic beverages should not be consumed by some individuals, including those who cannot restrict their alcohol intake, women of childbearing age who may become pregnant, pregnant and lactating women, children and adolescents, individuals taking medications that can interact with alcohol, and those with specific medical conditions.
- Alcoholic beverages should be avoided by individuals engaging in activities that require attention, skill, or coordination, such as driving or operating machinery.

Food Safety

Key Recommendations

To avoid microbial food-borne illness:

- Clean hands, food contact surfaces, and fruits and vegetables. Meat and poultry should not be washed or rinsed.
- Separate raw, cooked, and ready-to-eat foods while shopping, preparing, or storing foods.
- Cook foods to a safe temperature to kill microorganisms.
- Chill (refrigerate) perishable food promptly and defrost foods properly.
- Avoid raw (unpasteurized) milk or any products made from unpasteurized milk, raw or partially cooked eggs or foods containing raw eggs, raw or undercooked meat and poultry, unpasteurized juices, and raw sprouts.

Appendix G:
Dietary Reference Intakes, 2000, and RDA, 1989

Table G-1 Dietary Reference Intakes: Recommended Intakes for Individuals. Food and Nutrition Board, the National Academies of Sciences

	Infants 0–6 mo	**Infants 7–12 mo**	**Children 1–2 y**	**Children 3–8 y**	**Males 9–13 y**	**Males 14–18 y**	**Females 9–13 y**	**Females 14–18 y**	**Pregnancy 14–18 y**	**Lactation 14–18 y**
Active PAL*EER (kcal/d)	Male **570** Female **520** (3 mo)	Male **743** Female **676** (9 mo)	Male **1,046** Female **932** (24 mo)	Male **1,742** Female **1,642** (6 y)	**2,279** (11 y)	**3,152** (16 y)	**2,071** (11 y)	**2,368** (16 y)	1st trimester **2,368** 2nd trimester **2,708** 3rd trimester **2,820**	1st 6 mo **2,698** 2nd 6 mo **2,768**
Carbohydrates			**130**	**130**	**130**	**130**	**130**	**130**	**175**	**210**
Total Fiber	ND[n]	ND	**19**	**25**	**31**	**48**	**26**	**26**	**28**	**29**
AI (g/d)[m] Fat	**31**	**30**	ND	ND	ND	ND	ND	ND	ND	ND
n-3 Polyunsaturated Fatty Acids (g/d) (α-Linoleic Acid)	**4.4**	**4.6**	**7**	**10**	**12**	**16**	**10**	**11**	**13**	**13**
Protein (g/kg/d)	**0.5**	**0.5**	**0.7**	**0.9**	**1.2**	**1.6**	**1.0**	**1.1**	**1.4**	**1.3**

continues

Table G-1 Dietary Reference Intakes: Recommended Intakes for Individuals—*continued*

	Infants 0–6 mo	Infants 7–12 mo	Children 1–2 y	Children 3–8 y	Males 9–13 y	Males 14–18 y	Females 9–13 y	Females 14–18 y	Pregnancy 14–18 y	Lactation 14–18 y
Vitamin A (μg/d)[a]	400*	500*	**300**	**400**	**600**	**900**	**600**	**700**	**750**	**1,200**
Vitamin C (mg/d)	40*	50*	**15**	**25**	**45**	**75**	**45**	**65**	**80**	**115**
Vitamin D (μg/d)[b,c]	5*	5*	5*	5*	5*	5*	5*	5*	5*	5*
Vitamin E (mg/d)[d]	4*	5*	**6**	**7**	**11**	**15**	**11**	**15**	**16**	**19**
Vitamin K (μg/d)	2.0*	2.5*	30*	55*	60*	75*	60*	75*	75*	75*
Thiamin (mg/d)	0.2*	0.3*	**0.5**	**0.6**	**0.9**	**1.2**	**0.9**	**1.0**	**1.4**	**1.4**
Riboflavin (mg/d)	0.3*	0.4*	**0.5**	**0.6**	**0.9**	**1.3**	**0.9**	**1.0**	**1.4**	**1.6**
Niacin (mg/d)[e]	2*	4*	**6**	**8**	**12**	**16**	**12**	**14**	**18**	**17**
Vitamin B_6 (mg/d)	0.1*	0.3*	**0.5**	**0.6**	**1.0**	**1.3**	**1.0**	**1.2**	**1.9**	**2.0**
Folate (μg/d)[f]	65*	60*	**150**	**200**	**300**	**400**	**300**	**400**[g]	**600**[h]	**500**
Vitamin B_{12} (mg/d)	0.4*	0.5*	**0.9**	**1.2**	**1.8**	**2.4**	**1.8**	**2.4**	**2.6**	**2.8**
Pantothenic Acid (mg/d)	1.7*	1.6*	2*	3*	4*	5*	4*	5*	6*	7*
Biotin (μg/d)	5*	6*	8*	12*	20*	25*	20*	25*	30*	35*
Choline (mg/d)	125*	125*	200*	250*	375*	550*	375*	400*	450*	550*
Calcium (mg/d)	210*	270*	500*	800*	1,300*	1,300*	1,300*	1,300*	1,300*	1,300*

Chromium (μg/d)	0.2*	5.5*	11*	15*	25*	35*	21*	24*	29*	**44**
Copper (μg/d)	200*	220*	**340**	**440**	**700**	**890**	**700**	**890**	**1,000**	**1,300**
Fluoride (mg/d)	0.01*	0.5*	0.7*	1*	2*	3*	2*	2*	3*	3*
Iodine (μg/d)	110*	130*	**90**	**90**	**120**	**150**	**120**	**150**	**220**	**290**
Iron (mg/d)	0.27*	**11**	**7**	**10**	**8**	**11**	**8**	**15**	**27**	**10**
Magnesium (mg/d)	30*	75*	**80**	**130**	**240**	**410**	**240**	**360**	**400**	**360**
Manganese (mg/d)	0.003*	0.6*	1.2*	1.5*	1.9*	2.2*	1.6*	1.6*	2.0*	2.6*
Molybdenum (μg/d)	2*	3*	**17**	**22**	**34**	**43**	**34**	**43**	**50**	**50**
Phosphorus (mg/d)	100*	275*	**460**	**500**	**1,250**	**1,250**	**1,250**	**1,250**	**1,250**	**1,250**
Selenium (μg/d)	15*	20*	**20**	**30**	**40**	**55**	**40**	**55**	**60**	**70**
Zinc (mg/d)	2*	**3**	**3**	**5**	**8**	**11**	**8**	**9**	**13**	**14**

Note: This table (taken from the DRI reports, see www.nap.edu) presents Recommended Dietary Allowances (RDAs) in **bold type** and Adequate Intakes (AIs) in ordinary type followed by an asterisk (*). RDAs and AIs may both be used as goals for individual intake. RDAs are set to meet the needs of almost all individuals in a group. For healthy breast-fed infants, the AI is the mean intake. The AI for other life stage and gender groups is believed to cover needs of all individuals in the group, but lack of data or uncertainty in the data prevent being able to specify with confidence the percentage of individuals covered by this intake.

[a] As retinol activity equivalents (RAEs). 1-RAE = 1 μg β-carotene, 24 μg α-carotene, or 24 μg β-cryptoxanthin in foods. To calculate RAEs from retinol equivalents (REs) of provitamin A carotenoids in foods, divide the REs by 2. For preformed vitamin A in foods or supplements and for provitamin A carotenoids in supplements, 1 RE = 1 RAE.

[b] Cholecalciferol, -1 μg cholecalciferol = 40 IU vitamin D.

[c] In the absence of adequate exposure to sunlight.

continues

Table G-1 Dietary Reference Intakes: Recommended Intakes for Individuals—*continued*

[d] As α-tocopherol, α-Tocopherol includes RRR-α-tocopherol, the only form of α-tocopherol that occurs naturally in foods, and the 2R-stereoisomeric forms of α-tocopherol (SRR-, SSR-, SRS-, and SSS-α-tocopherol), also found in fortified foods and supplements.

[e] As niacin equivalents (NE). 1 mg of niacin = 60 mg of tryptophan; 0-6 months = preformed niacin (not NE).

[f] As dietary folate equivalents (DFE). 1 DEF = 1 μg food folate = 0.6 μg of folic acid from fortified food or as a supplement consumed with food = 0.5 μg of a supplement taken on an empty stomach.

[g] In view of evidence linking folate intake with neural tube defects in the fetus, it is recommended that all women capable of becoming pregnant consume 400 μg from supplements or fortified foods in addition to intake of food folate from the diet.

[h] It is assumed that women will continue consuming 400 μg from supplements or fortified food until their pregnancy is confirmed and they enter prenatal care, which ordinarily occurs after the end of the preconceptional period—the critical time for formation of the neural tube.

[i] Although AIs have been set for choline, there are few data to assess whether a dietary supply of choline is needed at all stages of the life cycle, and it may be that the choline requirement can be met by endogenous synthesis at some of these stages.

[j] For healthy moderately active Americans and Canadians.

[k] PAL = physical activity letter, EER = estimated energy requirement, TEE = total energy expenditure. The intake that meets the average energy expenditure of individuals at the reference height, weight, and age.

[l] RDA = Recommended Dietary Allowance. The intake that meets the nutrient needs of almost all (97–98 percent) individuals in a group.

[m] AI – Adequate intake. The observed average or experimentally determined intake by a defined population or subgroup that appears to sustain a defined nutritional status, such as growth rate, normal circulating nutrient values, or other functional indicators of health. The AI is used if sufficient scientific evidence is not available to derive an Estimated Average Requirement (EAR). For healthy infants receiving human milk, the AI is the mean intake. The AI is not equivalent to an RDA. Based on 14 g/1000 kcal of required energy.

[n] ND = not determined. The observed average of experimentally determined intake by a defined population or subgroup that appears to sustain a defined nutritional status, such as growth rate, normal circulating nutrient values, or other functional indicators of health. The AI is used if sufficient scientific evidence is not available to derive an EAR. For healthy infants receiving human milk, the AI is the mean intake. The AI is not equivalent to an RDA.

No determined biological function in humans has been identified for the nutrients silicon and vanadium.

Table G-2 Dietary Reference Intakes (DRIs): Tolerable Upper Intake Levels (UL[a]), Food and Nutrition Board, the National Academies of Sciences

	Infants 0–6 mo	Infants 7–12 mo	Children 1–3 y	Children 4–8 y	Males/ Females 9–13 y	Males/ Females 14–18 y	Pregnancy ≤ 18	Lactation ≤ 18
Vitamin A (μg/d)[b]	600	600	600	900	1,700	2,800	2,800	2,800
Vitamin C (mg/d)	ND[f]	ND	400	650	1,200	1,600	1,800	1,800
Vitamin D (μg/d)	25	25	50	50	50	50	50	50
Vitamin E (μg/d)[c,d]	ND	ND	200	300	600	800	800	800
Vitamin K (μg/d)	ND	ND	ND	ND	ND	ND	ND	ND
Thiamin (mg/d)	ND	ND	ND	ND	ND	ND	ND	ND
Riboflavin (mg/d)	ND	ND	ND	ND	ND	ND	ND	ND
Niacin (mg/d)[d]	ND	ND	10	15	20	30	30	30
Vitamin B_6 (mg/d)	ND	ND	30	40	60	60	80	80
Folate (μg/d)[d]	ND	ND	300	400	600	BOO	800	800
Vitamin B_{12} (mg/d)	ND	ND	ND	ND	ND	ND	ND	ND
Pantothenic Acid (mg/d)	ND	ND	ND	ND	ND	ND	ND	ND
Biotin (μg/d)	ND	ND	ND	ND	ND	ND	ND	ND
Choline (mg/d)	ND	ND	1.0	1.0	2.0	3.0	3.0	3.0
Carotenoids[e]	ND	ND	ND	ND	ND	ND	ND	ND
Arsenic	ND	ND	ND	ND	ND	ND	ND	ND
Boron (mg/d)	ND	ND	3	6	11	17	17	17
Calcium (mg/d)	ND	ND	2.5	2.5	2.5	2.5	2.5	2.5
Chromium (μg/d)	ND	ND	ND	ND	ND	ND	ND	ND
Copper (μg/d)	ND	ND	1,000	3,000	5,000	8,000	8,000	8,000
Fluoride (mg/d)	.07	.09	1.3	2.2	10	10	10	10

continues

Table G-2 Dietary Reference Intakes (DRIs): Tolerable Upper Intake Levels (UL[a]), Food and Nutrition Board, the National Academies of Sciences—*continued*

	Infants 0–6 mo	Infants 7–12 mo	Children 1–3 y	Children 4–8 y	Males/ Females 9–13 y	Males/ Females 14–18 y	Pregnancy ≤ 18	Lactation ≤ 18
Iodine (μg/d)	ND	ND	200	300	600	900	900	900
Iron (mg/d)	40	40	40	40	40	45	45	45
Magnesium (mg/d)[c]	ND	ND	65	110	350	350	350	350
Manganese (mg/d)	ND	ND	2	3	6	9	9	9
Molybdenum (μg/d)	ND	ND	300	600	1,100	1,700	1,700	1,700
Nickel (mg/d)	ND	ND	0.2	0.3	0.6	1.0	1.0	1.0
Phosphorus (mg/d)	ND	ND	3	3	4	4	3.5	4
Selenium (μg/d)	45	60	90	150	280	400	400	400
Silicon[d]	ND	ND	ND	ND	ND	ND	ND	ND
Vanadium (mg/d)[e]	ND	ND	ND	ND	ND	ND	ND	ND
Zinc (mg/d)	4	5	7	12	23	34	34	34

[a]UL = The maximum level of daily nutrient intake that is likely to pose no risk of adverse effects. Unless otherwise specified, the UL represents total intake from food, water, and supplements. Due to lack of suitable data, ULs could not be established for vitamin K, thiamin, riboflavin, vitamin B_{12} pantothenic acid, biotin, or carotenoids. In the absences of ULs, extra caution may be warranted in consuming levels above recommended intakes.

[b]As preformed vitamin A only.

[c]As α-tocopherol; applies to any form of supplemental α-tocopherol.

[d]The ULs for vitamin E, niacin, and folate apply to synthetic forms obtained from supplements, fortified foods, or a combination of the two.

[e]β-Carotene supplements are advised only to serve as a provitamin A source for individuals at risk of vitamin A deficiency.

[f]ND = Not determinable due to lack of data of adverse effects in this age group and concern with regard to lack of ability to handle excess amounts.

Source: This table is taken from the DRI report: see www.nap.edu.

Table G-3 Dietary Reference Intakes (DRIs) During Pregnancy‡

	Females			Pregnancy		
Life Stage Group	**14–18 y**	**19–30 y**	**31–50 y**	**≤ 18y**	**19–30 y**	**31–50 y**
Calcium (mg/d)	1300*	1000*	1000*	1300*	1000*	1000*
Phosphorus (mg/d)	1250	700	700	1250	700	700
Magnesium (mg/d)	360	310	320	400	350	360
Vitamin A (μg/d)	700	700	700	750	770	770
Vitamin D (μg/d)[a,b]	5*	5*	5*	5*	5*	5*
Fluoride (mg/d)	3*	3*	3*	3*	3*	3*
Thiamin (mg/d)	1.0	1.1	1.1	1.4	1.4	1.4
Riboflavin (mg/d)	1.0	1.1	1.1	1.4	1.4	1.4
Niacin (mg/d)[c]	14	14	14	18	18	18
Vitamin B_6 (mg/d)	1.2	1.3	1.3	1.9	1.9	1.9
Folate (μg/d)[d]	400[g]	400[g]	400[g]	600[h]	600[h]	600[h]
Vitamin B_{12} (μg/d)	2.4	2.4	2.4	2.6	2.6	2.6
Pantothenic Acid (mg/d)	5*	5*	5*	6*	6*	6*
Biotin (μg/d)	25*	30*	30*	30*	30*	30*
Choline[e] (mg/d)	400*	425*	425*	450*	450*	450*
Vitamin C (mg/d)	65	75	75	80	85	85
Vitamin E[f] (mg/d)	15	15	15	15	15	15
Iron (mg/d)	15	18	18	27	27	27
Zinc (mg/d)	9	8	8	13	11	11
Copper (μg/d)	890	900	900	1000	1000	1000
Selenium (μg/d)	55	55	55	60	60	60
Iodine (μg/d)	150	150	150	220	220	220

‡ Institute of Medicine.

*Adequate Intakes (AI).

[a] As cholecalciferol. 1 μg cholecalciferol = 40 IU vitamin D.

[b] In the absence of adequate exposure to sunlight.

[c] As niacin equivalents (NE). 1 mg of niacin = 60 mg of tryptophan.

[d] As dietary folate equivalents (DFE). 1 DFE = 1 μg food folate = 0.6 μg folic acid from fortified food or as a supplement consumed with food = 0.5 μg of a supplement taken on an empty stomach.

[e] Although AIs have been set for choline, there is little data to assess whether a dietary supply of choline is needed at all stages of the life cycle, and it may be that the choline requirement can be met by endogenous synthesis at some of these stages.

[f] As α-tocopherol. α-tocopherol includes *RRR*-α-tocopherol, the only form of α-tocopherol that occurs naturally in foods, and the 2*R*-stereoisomeric forms of α-tocopherol (*SRR*-, *SSR*-, *SRS*-, and *SSS*-α-tocopherol), also found in fortified foods and supplements.

continues

SECTION 7

Table G-3 Dietary Reference Intakes (DRIs) During Pregnancy‡ —*continued*

[g] In view of evidence linking folate intake with neural tube defects in the fetus, it is recommended that all women capable of becoming pregnant consume 400 μg from supplements or fortified foods in addition to intake of food folate from a varied diet.

[h] It is assumed that women will continue consuming 400 μg from supplements or fortified food until their pregnancy is confirmed and they enter prenatal care, which ordinarily occurs after the end of the periconceptional period—the critical time for formation of the neural tube.

1a. Institute of Medicine. Vitamin A. In: *Dietary Intakes for Vitamin A, Vitamin K, Arsenic, Boron, Chromium, Copper, Iodine, Iron, Manganese, Molybdenum, Nickel, Silicon, Vanadium, and Zinc.* National Academy Press: 2001:65–126.

1b. Institute of Medicine FNB. Dietary Reference Intakes for Calcium, Phosphorus, Magnesium, Vitamin D, and Fluoride. Washington, DC: Institute of Medicine; 1997.

1c. Institute of Medicine FNB. Dietary Reference Intakes for Thiamin, Riboflavin, Niacin, Vitamin B_6, Folate, Vitamin B_{12}, Pantothenic Acid, Biotin, and Choline. Washington, DC: Institute of Medicine: 1998.

1d. Institute of Medicine FNB. Dietary Reference Intakes for Vitamin C, Vitamin E, Selenium, and Carotenoids. Washington, DC: Institute of Medicine: 2000.

Source: This table is taken from the DRI report: see www.nap.edu.

Appendix H: Diet and Drug Interactions

Allergies

Antihistamines are used to relieve or prevent the symptoms of colds, hay fever, and allergies. They limit or block histamine, which is released by the body when we are exposed to substances that cause allergic reactions. Antihistamines are available with and without a prescription (over-the-counter). These products vary in their ability to cause drowsiness and sleepiness.

Antihistamines

Some examples are:
Over-the-counter:
brompheniramine / DIMETANE, BROMPHEN
chlorpheniramine / CHLOR-TRIMETON
diphenhydramine / BENADRYL
clemastine / TAVIST

Prescription:
fexofenadine / ALLEGRA
loratadine / CLARITIN (now available over the counter)
cetirizine / ZYRTEC

Interaction
Food: It is best to take prescription antihistamines on an empty stomach to increase their effectiveness.
Alcohol: Some antihistamines may increase drowsiness and slow mental and motor performance. Use caution when operating machinery or driving.

Arthritis and Pain

Analgesic/Antipyretic

They treat mild to moderate pain and fever. An example is: acetaminophen / TYLENOL.

Interactions
Food: For rapid relief, take on an empty stomach because food may slow the body's absorption of acetaminophen.
Alcohol: Avoid or limit the use of alcohol because chronic alcohol use can increase your risk of liver damage or stomach bleeding. If you consume three or more alcoholic drinks per day talk to your doctor or pharmacist before taking these medications.

Non-Steroidal Anti-Inflammatory Drugs (NSAIDs)

NSAIDs reduce pain, fever, and inflammation.

Some examples are:
aspirin / BAYER, ECOTRIN
ibuprofen / MOTRIN, ADVIL
naproxen / ANAPROX, ALEVE, NAPROSYN
nabumetone / RELAF
celecoxis / CELEBREX

Interaction
Food: Because these medications can irritate the stomach, it is best to take them with food or milk.
Alcohol: Avoid or limit the use of alcohol because chronic alcohol use can increase your risk of liver damage or stomach bleeding. If you consume three or more alcoholic drinks per day, talk to your doctor or pharmacist before taking these medications. Buffered aspirin or enteric coated aspirin may be preferable to regular aspirin to decrease stomach bleeding.

Corticosteroids

They are used to provide relief to inflamed areas of the body. Corticosteroids reduce swelling and itching, and help relieve allergic, rheumatoid, and other conditions.

Some examples are:
methylprednisolone / MEDROL
prednisone / DELTASONE
prednisolone / PEDIAPRED, PRELONE
cortisone acetate / CORTEF

Interaction
Food: Take with food or milk to decrease stomach upset.

Narcotic Analgesics

Narcotic analgesics are available only with a prescription. They provide relief for moderate to severe pain. Codeine can also be used to suppress cough. Some of these medications can be found in combination with non-narcotic drugs such as acetaminophen, aspirin, or cough syrups. Use caution when taking these medications: take them only as directed by a doctor or pharmacist because they may be habit-forming and can cause serious side effects when used improperly.

Some examples are:
codeine combined with acetaminophen / TYLENOL #2, #3, and #4
morphine / ROXANOL, MS CONTIN
oxycodone combined with acetaminophen / PERCOCET, ROXICET
meperidine / DEMEROL
hydrocodone with acetaminophen / VICODIN, LORCET

Interaction
Alcohol: Avoid alcohol because it increases the sedative effects of the medications. Use caution when motor skills are required, including operating machinery and driving.

Asthma

Bronchodilators

Bronchodilators are used to treat the symptoms of bronchial asthma, chronic bronchitis, and emphysema. These medicines open air passages to the lungs to relieve wheezing, shortness of breath, and troubled breathing.

Some examples are:
theophylline / SLO-BID, THEO-DUR, THEO-DUR 24, UNIPHYL
albuterol / VENTOLIN, PROVENTIL, COMBIVENT
epinephrine / PRIMATENE MIST
montelukast / SINGULAIR
salmeterol xinefoate / SEREVENT

Interactions
Food: The effect of food on theophylline medications can vary widely. High-fat meals may increase the amount of theophylline in the body while high-protein, low-carb meals, and charcoal-broiled foods may decrease it. It is important to check with your pharmacist about which form you are taking because food can have different effects depending on the dose form (for example, regular release, sustained release, or sprinkles). For example, food has little effect on Theo-Dur and Slo-Bid, but food increases the absorption of Theo-24 and Uniphyl, which can result in side effects of nausea, vomiting, headache, and irritability. Food can also decrease absorption of products like Theo-Dur Sprinkles for children.
Caffeine: Avoid eating or drinking large amounts of foods and beverages that contain caffeine (for example, chocolate, colas, coffee, tea) because both oral bronchodilators and caffeine stimulate the central nervous system.
Alcohol: Avoid alcohol if you are taking theophylline medications because it can increase the risk of side effects such as nausea, vomiting, headache, and irritability.

Cardiovascular Disorders

There are numerous medications used to treat cardiovascular disorders such as high blood pressure, angina, irregular heartbeat, and high cholesterol. These drugs are often used in combination to enhance their effectiveness. Some classes of drugs can treat several conditions. For example, beta blockers can be used to treat high blood pressure, angina, and irregular heartbeats. Check with your doctor or pharmacist if you have questions on any of your medications. Some of the major cardiovascular drug classes are:

Diuretics

Sometimes called "water pills," diuretics help eliminate water, sodium, and chloride from the body. There are different types of diuretics.

Some examples are:
furosemide / LASIX
triamterene / hydrochlorothiazide / DYAZIDE, MAXZIDE
hydrochlorothiazide / HYDRODIURIL
triamterene / DYRENIUM
bumetamide / BUMEX
metolazone / ZAROXOLYN

Interaction
Food: Diuretics vary in their interactions with food and specific nutrients. Some diuretics cause loss of potassium, calcium, and magnesium. Triamterene, on the other hand, is known as a "potassium-sparing" diuretic. It blocks the kidneys' excretion of potassium, which can cause hyperkalemia (increased potassium). Excess potassium may result in irregular heartbeat and heart palpitations. When taking triamterene; avoid eating large amounts of potassium-rich foods such as bananas, oranges, and green leafy vegetables, or salt substitutes that contain potassium.

Beta Blockers

Beta blockers decrease the nerve impulses to the heart and blood vessels. This decreases the heart rate and the workload of the heart.

Some examples are:
atenolol / TENORMIN
metoprolol / LOPRESSOR
propranolol / INDERAL
nadolol / CORGARD

Interaction
Alcohol: Avoid drinking alcohol with propranolol / INDERAL because the combination lowers blood pressure too much.

Nitrates

Nitrates relax blood vessels and lower the demand for oxygen by the heart.

Some examples are:
isosorbide dinitrate / ISORDIL, SORBITRATE
nitroglycerin / NITRO, NITRO-DUR, TRANSDERM-NITRO, NITROSTAT, NITROLINGUAL SPRAY

Interaction
Alcohol: Avoid alcohol because it may add to the blood-vessel-relaxing effect of nitrates and result in dangerously low blood pressure.

Angiotensin Converting Enzyme (ACE) Inhibitors

ACE inhibitors relax blood vessels by preventing angiotensin II, a vasoconstrictor, from being formed.

Some examples are:
captopril / CAPOTEN
enalapril / VASOTEC
lisinopril / PRINIVIL, ZESTRIL
quinapril / ACCUPRIL
moexipril / UNIVASC

Interactions
Food: Food can decrease the absorption of captopril and moexipril. So take captopril and moexipril one hour before or two hours after meals. ACE inhibitors may increase the amount of potassium in your body. Too much potassium can be harmful. Make sure to tell your doctor if you are taking potassium supplements or diuretics (water pills) that may increase the amount of potassium in your body. Avoid eating large amounts of foods high in potassium such as bananas, green leafy vegetables, and oranges.

HMG-CoA Reductase Inhibitors/Statins

These medications are used to lower cholesterol. They work to reduce the rate of production of LDL (bad cholesterol). Some of these drugs also lower triglycerides. Recent studies have shown that pravastatin can reduce the risk of heart attack, stroke, or miniature stroke in certain patient populations.

Some examples are:
atorvastatin / LIPITOR
fluvastatin / LESCOL
lovastatin / MEVACOR
pravastatin / PRAVACHOL
simvastatin / ZOCOR

Interactions
Alcohol: Avoid drinking large amounts of alcohol because it may increase the risk of liver damage.
Food: Lovastatin (Mevacor) should be taken with the evening meal to enhance effectiveness.

Anticoagulants

Anticoagulants help to prevent the formation of blood clots.

An example is:
warfarin / COUMADIN

Interactions
Food: Vitamin K produces blood-clotting substances and may reduce the effectiveness of anticoagulants. So limit the amount of foods high in vitamin K (such as broccoli, spinach, kale, turnip greens, cauliflower, and brussels sprouts).
High doses of vitamin E (400 IU or more) may prolong clotting time and increase the risk of bleeding. Talk to your doctor before taking vitamin E supplements.

Infections

Antibiotics and Antifungals

Many different types of drugs are used to treat infections caused by bacteria and fungi. Some general advice to follow when taking any such product is:

- Tell your doctor about any skin rashes you may have had with antibiotics or that you get while taking this medication. A rash can be a symptom of an allergic reaction, and allergic reactions can be very serious.
- Tell your doctor if you experience diarrhea.
- If you are using birth control, consult with your healthcare provider because some methods may not work when taken with antibiotics.
- Be sure to finish all your medication even if you are feeling better.
- Take with plenty of water.

Antibiotics

Penicillin

Some examples are:
penicillin V / VEETIDS
amoxicillin / TRIMOX, AMOXIL
ampicillin / PRINCIPEN, OMNIPEN

Interaction
Food: Take on an empty stomach, but if it upsets your stomach, take it with food.

Quinolones

Some examples are:
ciprofloxacin / CIPRO
levofloxacin / LEVAQUIN
ofloxacin / FLOXIN

Interactions
Food: Take on an empty stomach one hour before or two hours after meals. If your stomach gets upset, take it with food. However, avoid calcium-containing products like milk, yogurt, vitamins or minerals containing iron, and antacids because they significantly decrease drug concentration.
Caffeine: Taking these medications with caffeine-containing products (for example, coffee, colas, tea, and chocolate) may increase caffeine levels, leading to excitability and nervousness.

Cephalosporins

Some examples are:
cefaclor / CECLOR, CECLOR CD
cefadroxil / DURICEF
cefixime / SUPRAX
cefprozil / CEFZIL
cephalexin / KEFLEX, KEFTAB

Interaction
Food: Take on an empty stomach one hour before or two hours after meals. If your stomach gets upset, take with food.

Macrolides

Some examples are:
azithromycin / ZITHROMAX
clarithromycin / BIAXIN
erythromycin / E-MYCIN, ERY-TAB, ERYC
erythromycin + sulfisoxazole / PEDIAZOLE

Interaction
Food: Take on an empty stomach one hour before or two hours after meals. If your stomach gets upset, take with food.

Sulfonamides

An example is:
sulfamethoxazole + trimethoprim / BACTRIM, SEPTRA

Interaction
Food: Take on an empty stomach one hour before or two hours after meals. If your stomach gets upset, take with food.

Tetracyclines

Some examples are:
tetracycline / ACHROMYCIN, SUMYCIN
doxycycline / VIBRAMYCIN
minocycline / MINOCIN

Interaction
Food: Take on an empty stomach one hour before or two hours after meals. If your stomach gets upset, take with food. However, it is important to avoid taking tetracycline / ACHROMYCIN, SUMYCIN with dairy products, antacids, and vitamins containing iron because these can interfere with the medication's effectiveness.

Nitroimidazole

An example is:
metronidazole / FLAGYL

Interaction
Alcohol: Avoid drinking alcohol or using medications that contain alcohol or eating foods prepared with alcohol while you are taking metronidazole and for at least three days after you finish the medication. Alcohol may cause nausea, abdominal cramps, vomiting, headaches, and flushing.

Antifungals

Some examples are:
fluconazole / DIFLUCAN
griseofulvin / GRIFULVIN
ketoconazole / NIZORAL
itraconazole / SPORANOX
terbinafine / LAMISIL

Interactions
Food: It is important to avoid taking these medications with dairy products (milk, cheeses, yogurt, ice cream) or antacids.
Alcohol: Avoid drinking alcohol, using medications that contain alcohol, or eating foods prepared with alcohol while you are taking ketoconazole/NIZORAL and for at least three days after you finish the medication. Alcohol may cause nausea, abdominal cramps, vomiting, headaches, and flushing.

Mood Disorders

Depression, Emotional, and Anxiety Disorders

Depression, panic disorder, and anxiety are a few examples of mood disorders—complex medical conditions with varying degrees of severity. When using medications to treat mood disorders it is important to follow your doctor's instructions. Remember to take your dose as directed even if you are feeling better, and do not stop unless you consult your doctor. In some cases it may take several weeks to see an improvement in symptoms.

Monoamine Oxidase (MAO) Inhibitors

Some examples are:
phenelzine / NARDIL
tranylcypromine / PARNATE

Interactions
MAO Inhibitors have many dietary restrictions, and people taking them need to follow the dietary guidelines and physician's instructions very carefully. A rapid, potentially fatal increase in blood pressure can occur if foods or alcoholic beverages containing tyramine are consumed while taking MAO Inhibitors.
Alcohol: Do not drink beer, red wine, other alcoholic beverages, non-alcoholic and reduced-alcohol beer, and red wine products.
Food: Foods high in tyramine that should be avoided include:

- American processed; cheddar, blue, brie, mozzarella, and Parmesan cheese; yogurt, sour cream.
- Beef or chicken liver; cured meats such as sausage and salami; game meat; caviar; dried fish.
- Avocados, bananas, yeast extracts, raisins, sauerkraut, soy sauce, miso soup.
- Broad (fava) beans, ginseng, caffeine-containing products (colas, chocolate, coffee, and tea).

Anti-Anxiety Drugs

Some examples are:
lorazepam / ATIVAN
diazepam / VALIUM
alprazolam / XANAX

Interactions
Alcohol: May impair mental and motor performance (e.g., driving, operating machinery).
Caffeine: May cause excitability, nervousness, and hyperactivity and lessen the anti-anxiety effects of the drugs.

Antidepressant Drugs

Some examples are:
paroxetine / PAXIL
sertraline / ZOLOFT
fluoxetine / PROZAC
citalopram / CELEXA

Interactions
Alcohol: Although alcohol may not significantly interact with these drugs to affect mental or motor skills, people who are depressed should not drink alcohol.
Food: These medications can be taken with or without food.

Stomach Conditions

Conditions like acid reflux, heartburn, acid indigestion, sour stomach, and gas are very common ailments. The goal of treatment is to relieve pain, promote healing, and prevent the irritation from returning. This is achieved by either reducing the acid the body creates or protecting the stomach from the acid. Lifestyle and dietary habits can play a large role in the symptoms of these conditions. For example, smoking cigarettes and consuming products that contain caffeine may make symptoms return.

Histamine Blockers

Some examples are:
cimetidine / TAGAMET or TAGAMET HB
famotidine / PEPCID or PEPCID AC
ranitidine / ZANTAC or ZANTAC 75
nizatadine / AXID or AXID AR

Interactions
Alcohol: Avoid alcohol while taking these products. Alcohol may irritate the stomach and make it more difficult for the stomach to heal.
Food: Can be taken with or without regard to meals.
Caffeine: Caffeine products (for example, cola, chocolate, tea, and coffee) may irritate the stomach.

Drug-to-Drug Interactions

Not only can drugs interact with food and alcohol, they can also interact with each other. Some drugs are given together on purpose for an added effect, like codeine and acetaminophen for pain relief. But other drug-to-drug interactions may be unintended and harmful. Prescription drugs can interact with each other or with over-the-counter (OTC) drugs, such as acetaminophen, aspirin, and cold medicine. Likewise, OTC drugs can interact with each other.

Sometimes the effect of one drug may be increased or decreased. For example, tricyclic antidepressants such as amitriptyline (ELAVIL), or nortriptyline (PAMELOR) can decrease the ability of clonidine (CATAPRES) to lower blood pressure. In other cases, the effects of a drug can increase the risk of serious side effects. For example, some antifungal medications such as itraconazole (SPORANOX) and ketoconazole (NIZORAL) can interfere with the way some cholesterol-lowering medications are broken down by the body. This can increase the risk of a serious side effect.

Doctors can often prescribe other medications to reduce the risk of drug-drug interactions. For example, two cholesterol-lowering drugs—pravastatin (PRAVACHOL) and fluvastatin (LESCOL)—are less likely to interact with antifungal medications. Be sure to tell your doctor about all medications—prescription and OTC—that you are taking.

Source: The National Consumers League 2004.

Appendix I: Ethnic, Cultural, and Religious Food Considerations

Author: Dianne Scheinberg, MS, RD, LD

Explanation: This section describes culture-specific foods. The foods with an asterisk (*) are foods that are high in saturated fat or total fat and should be de-emphasized or low-fat equivalents should be recommended.

Table I-1 Ethnic, Cultural, and Religious Food Considerations

Ethnic Group	Foods Commonly Eaten
Mexican	
Grain/starches	Corn, corn products, tortillas, rice, potatoes
Fruit	Lime, banana, avocado, pineapple, mango, papaya, coconut*, nopale, guava, orange, melon, cassava, kiwi
Vegetables	Tomatoes, squash, chili peppers, onions, beets, cabbage, pumpkins, sweet peppers, cacti
Protein	Beans: pinto beans, lentils, kidney beans, garbanzo beans, fava beans, fish, shellfish, meat, poultry, eggs
Dairy	Some cheese*
Fat	Soy*, corn*, olive oils*, pine nuts*, peanuts, seeds
Puerto Rican	
Grain/starches	Plantain, Puerto Rican bread, rice, viandas cornmeal, sweet potatoes, yams
Fruit	Guava, peaches, pears, pineapple, bananas, other tropical fruits
Vegetables	Onions, green peppers, tomatoes, beets, eggplant, carrots, green beans
Protein	Beans (red kidney beans, garbanzo beans), Eggs, pork, chicken, fish, dried salt cod *(Bacalao)*
Dairy	Aged cheese*, milk used in coffee—*café con leche* (lactose intolerance can be a problem)
Fat	Vegetable oils*
African American	
Grain/starches	Rice, potatoes, corn bread, biscuits, corn, grits, pasta, sweet potatoes, yams
Fruit	Melons, bananas, peaches
Vegetables	Kale, collard greens, mustard greens, okra, cabbage, tomatoes, summer squash
Protein	Beans, legumes, catfish, pork (chitterlings*, ham hocks*), chicken

Table I-1 Ethnic, Cultural, and Religious Food Considerations—*continued*

Ethnic Group	Foods Commonly Eaten
Dairy	Milk*, buttermilk*, cheese* (lactose intolerance is a problem for many)
Fat	Butter*, lard*, vegetable shortening*
Chinese	
Grain/Starches	Rice, noodles, taro, steamed buns, dumplings, wrappings, yams
Fruit	Melons, apples, oranges, Asian pears, lychee, all others
Vegetables	Mushrooms, sprouts, bok choy, broccoli, lima beans, string beans, baby corn, bamboo shoots, cabbage, eggplant, water chestnuts
Protein	Fish, pork, beef, poultry, shellfish, tofu, eel, duck*, eggs (chicken and duck), fresh and preserved
Dairy	Ice cream*, milk* (lactose intolerance is a problem for many), soy milk
Fat	Sesame oil*, peanut oil*
Japanese	
Grain/Starches	Rice, wheat noodles, yams,
Fruit	Pears, kiwi, persimmon, watermelon, oranges, plums, all others
Vegetables	Seaweed, bamboo shoots, water chestnuts, cabbage, cucumber, celery, pickled ginger, mushrooms, lotus root, watercress, all others
Protein	Shellfish, fish, beef, chicken, eggs, tofu, soybeans
Dairy	Soy milk (lactose intolerance is a problem for many)
Fats	Sesame oil*, peanut oil*
Korean	
Grain/Starches	Rice, barley, millet
Fruit	Apples, pears, oranges, melons, many others
Vegetables	Bean sprouts, greens, cabbage, radish
Protein	Beef, seafood, fish, chicken, soy beans, pine nuts*
Dairy	Generally not eaten
Fat	Vegetable oil*
Vietnamese	
Grain/Starches	Rice, noodles, French bread
Fruit	All
Vegetables	Onions, squash, broccoli, bitter melon, string beans, all others
Protein	Beef, fish, chicken, shellfish, legumes, soybeans, tofu
Dairy	Ice cream* (lactose intolerance may be a problem)
Fat	Vegetable oils*, peanut oil*

continues

Table I-1 Ethnic, Cultural, and Religious Food Considerations—*continued*

Ethnic Group	Foods Commonly Eaten
Thai	
Grain/Starches	Rice, noodles, tapioca
Fruit	Pineapple, papaya, mango, banana, lichee, oranges
Vegetables	Mushrooms, zucchini, turnips, radishes, corn, broccoli, celery, cucumber, bamboo, eggplant, peas
Protein	Shellfish, beef, tofu, chicken, duck*, nuts
Dairy	
Fat	Vegetable oil,* peanut sauce*
Native American	
Grain/Starches	Corn, wild oats, rice, bread
Fruit	Berries, cherries, apples, grapes, melon
Vegetables	Rhubarb, celery, wild mushrooms, squash, carrots, scallions, cacti
Protein	Game, seafood, acorns, hazelnuts, pine nuts*, beef, peanut butter*, rabbit
Dairy	(Lactose intolerance is a problem for many)
Fat	Lard*
Portuguese	
Grain/Starches	Rice, bread, farina, barley, cornmeal
Fruit	Figs, plums, peaches, grapes, cherries, bananas, oranges, apricot, pineapple, grapefruit, strawberries
Vegetables	Cabbage, kale, spinach, eggplant, cauliflower, green beans, leeks, onions, tomato, celery, greens, pumpkin
Protein	Fish, shellfish, beef, lamb, game, poultry, almonds*, beans
Dairy	Milk*, cheeses*
Fat	Vegetable oil*, peanut oil*, olive oil*, butter*
Italian	
Grain/Starches	Rice, pasta, focaccia, polenta, Italian bread
Fruit	Peaches, strawberries, oranges, apples, figs, grapes, pears
Vegetables	Celery, capers, onions, carrots, broccoli, peppers, zucchini, cauliflower, artichokes, tomatoes, eggplant, mushrooms, cabbage, asparagus
Protein	Lamb, chicken, pork, shellfish, fish, fava beans, beef, veal, sausage*, lentils, beans
Dairy	Cheeses*
Fat	Olive oil*

Table I-1 Ethnic, Cultural, and Religious Food Considerations—*continued*

Ethnic Group	Foods Commonly Eaten
Russian	
Grain/Starches	Oats, rice, wheat, farina, potatoes, buckwheat bread, rye bread
Fruit	Prunes, dried fruit, all others
Vegetables	Beets, carrots, cabbage, onions, artichokes, cucumbers, mushrooms, lima beans, green beans, Brussels sprouts
Protein	Ham, eggs, fish, chicken, Kielbasa*
Dairy	Curd cheese*, Swiss cheese*,
Fat	Sour cream*
Irish	
Grain/Starches	Potatoes, steel-cut oats, soda bread, barley
Fruit	Apples, strawberries
Vegetables	Carrots, cabbage, parsnips, onions, cauliflower, mushrooms, leeks, broccoli, turnips, peas, endive, asparagus
Protein	Beef (corned beef*), pork, mutton, lamb, ham
Dairy	Cheeses*, milk*, buttermilk*
Fat	Butter*
Mediterranean	
Grain/Starches	Couscous, polenta, potatoes, pasta, rice
Fruit	Avocado, apples, oranges, grapes, strawberries
Vegetables	Tomatoes, eggplant, lettuce, mushrooms, onion, garlic, legumes, beans
Protein	Fish, poultry, eggs
Dairy	Cheese*, yogurt*
Fat	Olive oil*
Middle Eastern	
Grain/Starches	Pita bread, rice, couscous, bulgur, wheat
Fruit	Figs, peaches, dates
Vegetables	Grape leaves, tomatoes, peppers, onions, squash, fennel, okra, peas, eggplant/baba ghanouj, parsley, artichoke, spinach
Protein	Lamb, chicken
Dairy	Feta cheese*, yogurt*
Fat	Olive oil*
Arabic	
Grain/Starches	Couscous, millet, pita, rice, bulgur
Fruit	Figs, apples, apricots, plums, grapes, bananas, cantaloupe, watermelon, tangerines

continues

Table I-1 Ethnic, Cultural, and Religious Food Considerations—*continued*

Ethnic Group	Foods Commonly Eaten
Vegetables	Onion, cauliflower, spinach, cucumber, okra, artichokes, potato, eggplant, cabbage, squash
Protein	Garbanzo beans/hummus, beef, chicken, lamb, lentils, pine nuts*, almonds*, pistachios
Dairy	Yogurt*, buttermilk*, goat milk*
Fat	Olive oil*, tahini/sesame paste*
Indian	
Grain/Starches	Rice, roti, basmati rice, chapati, millet, bulgur, potato
Fruit	Papaya, mango, grapes, figs, chutney, banana, melon, dates
Vegetables	Onions, tomatoes, turnips, carrots, plantains, eggplant, broccoli, cucumber, cabbage, squash
Protein	Almonds, cashews, chicken, chickpeas, beef, lamb, shrimp, lentils
Dairy	Yogurt*
Fat	Coconut oil*, peanut oil*, butter* (ghee)
Religion	**Food Restrictions and Practices**
Jewish	Ⓤ or **K** on food products denote that they are Kosher Do not eat meat and dairy together at the same meal. Do not eat pork, fish without scales and fins, and shellfish.
Hindu	Do not consume alcohol, beef, pork products.
Mormon (LDS)	Abstain from alcohol, coffee, and tea. Limit meat.
Muslim	Do not consume pork, carnivorous animals, birds of prey, and alcohol. Slaughter meat in a prescribed manner. Permitted foods are called *halal.*

Table I-1 Ethnic, Cultural, and Religious Food Considerations—*continued*

Religion	Food Restrictions and Practices
Seventh Day Adventist	Prohibit pork, shellfish, caffeine, and alcohol. Some Seventh Day Adventists are lacto-ovo vegetarians. Avoid condiments such as black pepper.

Sources:

Eating Healthy with Ethnic Food. Department of Health and Human Services. www.nhlbi.nih.go/health/public/heart/obesity/lose_wt/eth_dine/htm.

Eating in America: A look at Culturally Diverse Populations. Kraft Foods. www.kraftfoods.com/kf/HealthyLiving/NutritionUpdate/ArticleforProfessionals.

Ethnic Dining the Heart Healthy Way. Colorado State University. www.ext.colostate.edu/pubs/columnnn/nn990922.html.

Ethnic and Cultural Diversity. Medic Direct. www.medicdirect.com.uk/diet/default.ihtml?step=4&pid=1313.

Ireland: What to Eat. Global Gourmet. www.globalgourmet.com/destinations/ireland/irelandwhat.html.

Latin American Diet Pyramid. Oldways. www.oldwayspt.org/pyramids/latin/p_latin.html.

Lutz, C., & Przytulski, K. *NutriNotes*. Philadelphia, PA: F.A. Davis Company. 2004.

Mediterranean Diet Pyramid. Oldways. www.oldwayspt.org/images/pyra-med.jpg.

Mexico. Sally's Place. www.sallys-place.com/food/ethnic_cusine/mexico.htm.

Middle East. Global Gourmet. www.globalgourmet.com/destinations/mideast/mestwhat.html.

Native American Food Pyramid. United States Department of Agriculture. www.nal.usda.go/fnic/Fpyr/NAmFGP.html.

Food Pyramids: Indian, Arabic, Russian, Italian, Portuguese, Thai, Japanese, Mexican, Chinese. Southeastern Michigan Dietetic Association. www.semda.org/info/pyramid.asp?ID=1.

Traditional Healthy Asian Diet Pyramid. Oldways. www.oldwayspt.org/images/pyra-asian.jpg.

Vietnam. Sally's Place. www.sallys-place.com/food/ethnic_cusine/vietnam.htm.

Appendix J: Energy Equations

Table J-1 Equations for Predicting Energy Requirements

Origin	Energy Determination	Gender	Age	Equation
Harris-Benedict	BMR	Male	Unspecified	66.47 + 13.75 W + 5.0 H − 6.76 A
		Female		655.1 + 9.56 W + 1.85 H − 4.68 A
World Health Organization (WHO)	REE	Male	0–3 y	60.9 W − 54
			3–10 y	22.7 W + 495
		Female	0–3 y	61 W − 51
			3–10 y	22.5 W + 499
Schofield	REE	Male	<3 y	0.17 W + 1.517 H − 617.6
			3–10 y	19.6 W + .1303 H + 414.9
			10–18 y	16.3 W + .1372 H + 515.5
		Female	<3 y	16.25 W + 1.0232 H − 413.5
			3–10 y	16.97 W + 161.8 H + 371.2
			10–18 y	8.365 W + 4.65 H + 200.0
Altman and Dittmer	REE	Male	3–16 y	19.56 W + 506.16
		Female		18.67 W + 578.64
Maffeis et al.	REE	Male	6–10 y	1287 + 28.6 W + 23.6 H − 69.1 A
		Female		1552 + 35.8 W + 15.6 H − 36.3 A
Piero et al. (for surgical infants)	REE	Unspecified	Infants	Cal/min = −74.436 + 34.661 W + 4.96 × HR + (0.78 × age in days)

W = weight in kilograms; A = age in years; H = height in centimeters; HR = heart rate in beats per minute

Source: See data from individual endnote references.

Appendix K: Energy Expenditure of Activity

Table K-1 Approximate Energy Expenditure for Various Activities in Relation to Resting Needs for Males and Females of Average Size*

Activity Category‡	Representative Value for Activity Factor per Unit Time of Activity
Resting Sleeping, reclining	REE × 1.0
Very light Seated and standing activities, painting trades, driving, laboratory work, typing, sewing, ironing, cooking, playing cards, playing a musical instrument	REE × 1.5
Light Walking on a level surface at 2.5 to 3 mph, garage work, electrical trades, carpentry, restaurant trades, house-cleaning, child care, golf, sailing, table tennis	REE × 2.5
Moderate Walking 3.5–4 mph, weeding and hoeing, carrying a load, cycling, skiing, tennis, dancing	REE × 5.0
Heavy Walking with load uphill, tree felling, heavy manual digging, basketball, climbing, football, soccer	REE × 7.0

*Data from references 26 and 34.

‡When reported as multiples of basal needs, the expenditures of males and females are similar.

Source: Reprinted with permission from *Recommended Dietary Allowances,* 10th ed., © 1989 by the National Academy of Sciences. Published by National Academy Press.

Appendix L: Exchange Lists for Meal Planning

Starch List

Cereals, grains, pasta, crackers, snacks, starchy vegetables, and cooked beans, peas, and lentils are starches. In general one starch is:

- 1/2 cup of cooked cereal, grain, or starchy vegetable
- 1/3 cup of cooked rice or pasta
- 1 ounce of a bread product, such as 1 slice of bread
- 3/4 to 1 ounce of most snack foods (some snack foods may also have added fat)

One starch exchange equals
15 grams carbohydrate,
3 grams protein,
0–1 gram fat,
and 80 calories.

Bread

Bagel	1/4 (1 oz.)
Bread, reduced-calorie	2 slices (1 1/2 oz.)
Bread, white, whole-wheat, pumpernickel, rye	1 slice (1 oz.)
Bread sticks, crisp, 4 in. long × 1/2 in.	4 (2/3 oz.)
English muffin	1/2
Hot dog or hamburger bun	1/2 (1 oz.)
Naan, 8 × 2 in.	1/4
Pancake, 4 in. across, 1/4 in. thick	1
Pita, 6 in. across	1/2
Roll, plain, small	1 (1 oz.)
Raisin bread, unfrosted	1 slice (1 oz.)
Tortilla, corn, 6 in. across	1
Tortilla, flour, 6 in. across	1
Tortilla, flour, 10 in. across	1/3
Waffle, 4 in. square, reduced-fat	1

Cereals and Grains

Bran cereals	1/2 cup
Bulgur	1/2 cup
Cereals, cooked	1/2 cup
Cereals, unsweetened, ready-to-eat	3/4 cup
Cornmeal (dry)	3 Tbsp
Couscous	1/3 cup
Flour (dry)	3 Tbsp
Granola, low-fat	1/4 cup
Grape-Nuts	1/4 cup

Grits	1/2 cup
Kasha	1/2 cup
Millet	1/3 cup
Muesli	1/4 cup
Oats	1/2 cup
Pasta	1/3 cup
Puffed cereal	1 1/2 cups
Rice, white or brown	1/3 cup
Shredded Wheat	1/2 cup
Sugar-frosted cereal	1/2 cup
Wheat germ	3 Tbsp

Starchy Vegetables

Baked beans	1/3 cup
Corn	1/2 cup
Corn on cob, large	1/2 cob (5 oz)
Mixed vegetables with corn, peas, or pasta	1 cup
Peas, green	1/2 cup
Plantain	1/2 cup
Potato, baked with skin	1/4 large (3 oz.)
Potato, boiled	1/2 cup or 1/2 medium (3 oz.)
Potato, mashed	1/2 cup
Squash, winter (acorn, butternut, pumpkin)	1 cup
Yam, sweet potato, plain	1/2 cup

Crackers and Snacks

Animal crackers	8
Graham crackers, 2 1/2 in. square	3
Matzoh	3/4 oz.
Melba toast	4 slices
Oyster crackers	24
Popcorn (popped, no fat added, or low-fat microwave)	3 cups
Pretzels	3/4 oz.
Rice cakes, 4 in. across	2
Saltine-type crackers	6
Snack chips, fat-free or baked (tortilla, potato)	15–20 (3/4 oz.)
Whole-wheat crackers, no fat added	2–5 (3/4 oz.)

Beans, Peas, and Lentils
(Count as 1 starch exchange, plus 1 very lean meat exchange.)

Beans and peas (garbanzo, pinto, kidney, white, split, black-eyed)	1/2 cup
Lima beans	2/3 cup
Lentils	1/2 cup
Miso	3 Tbsp

= 400 mg or more of sodium per serving.

Starchy Foods Prepared with Fat
(Count as 1 starch exchange, plus 1 fat exchange.)

Biscuit, 2½ in. across 1
Chow mein noodles .... ½ cup
Corn bread, 2 in. cube .... 1 (2 oz.)
Crackers, round butter type 6
Croutons .... 1 cup
French-fried potatoes (oven-baked) .... 1 cup (2 oz.)
Granola .... ¼ cup
Hummus .... ⅓ cup
Muffin, 5 oz. .... ⅕ (1 oz.)
Popcorn, microwave .... 3 cups
Sandwich crackers, cheese or peanut butter filling 3
Snack chips (potato, tortilla) .... 9–13 (¾ oz.)
Stuffing, bread (prepared) .... ⅓ cup
Taco shell, 6 in. across 2
Waffle, 4 in. square or across 1
Whole-wheat crackers, fat added .... 4–6 (1 oz.)

Fruit List

Fresh, frozen, canned, and dried fruits and fruit juices are on this list. In general, one fruit exchange is:

- 1 small fresh fruit (4 oz.)
- ½ cup of canned or fresh fruit or unsweetened fruit juice
- ¼ cup of dried fruit

One fruit exchange equals
15 grams carbohydrate and
60 calories.
The weight includes skin, core, seeds, and rind.

Fruit

Apple, unpeeled, small .... 1 (4 oz.)
Applesauce, unsweetened .... ½ cup
Apples, dried .... 4 rings
Apricots, fresh .... 4 whole (5½ oz.)
Apricots, dried .... 8 halves
Apricots, dried .... ½ cup
Banana, small .... 1 (4 oz.)
Blackberries .... ¾ cup
Blueberries .... ¾ cup
Cantaloupe, small .... ⅓ melon (11 oz.) or 1 cup cubes

Cherries, sweet, fresh	12 (3 oz.)
Cherries, sweet, canned	$\frac{1}{2}$ cup
Dates	3
Figs, fresh	$1\frac{1}{2}$ large or 2 medium ($3\frac{1}{2}$ oz.)
Figs, dried	$1\frac{1}{2}$
Fruit cocktail	$\frac{1}{2}$ cup
Grapefruit, large	$\frac{1}{2}$ (11 oz.)
Grapefruit sections, canned	$\frac{3}{4}$ cup
Grapes, small	17 (3 oz.)
Honeydew melon	1 slice (10 oz.) or 1 cup cubes
Kiwi	1 ($3\frac{1}{2}$ oz.)
Mandarin oranges, canned	$\frac{3}{4}$ cup
Mango, small	$\frac{1}{2}$ fruit ($5\frac{1}{2}$ oz.) or $\frac{1}{2}$ cup
Nectarine, small	1 (5 oz.)
Orange, small	1 ($6\frac{1}{2}$ oz.)
Papaya	$\frac{1}{2}$ fruit (8 oz.) or 1 cup cubes
Peach, medium, fresh	1 (4 oz.)
Peaches, canned	$\frac{1}{2}$ cup
Pear, large, fresh	$\frac{1}{2}$ (4 oz.)
Pears, canned	$\frac{1}{2}$ cup
Pineapple, fresh	$\frac{3}{4}$ cup
Pineapple, canned	$\frac{1}{2}$ cup
Plums, small	2 (5 oz.)
Plums, canned	$\frac{1}{2}$ cup
Plums, dried (prunes)	3
Raisins	2 Tbsp
Raspberries	1 cup
Strawberries	$1\frac{1}{4}$ cup whole berries
Tangerines, small	2 (8 oz.)
Watermelon	1 slice ($13\frac{1}{2}$ oz.) or $1\frac{1}{4}$ cup cubes

Fruit Juice

Apple juice/cider	$\frac{1}{2}$ cup
Cranberry juice cocktail	$\frac{1}{3}$ cup
Cranberry juice cocktail, reduced-calorie	1 cup
Fruit juice blends, 100% juice	$\frac{1}{3}$ cup
Grape juice	$\frac{1}{3}$ cup
Grapefruit juice	$\frac{1}{2}$ cup
Orange juice	$\frac{1}{2}$ cup
Pineapple juice	$\frac{1}{2}$ cup
Prune juice	$\frac{1}{2}$ cup

Milk List

Different types of milk and milk products are on this list. Cheeses are on the Meat and Meat Substitutes list, and cream and other dairy fats are on the Fat list. Based on the amount of fat they contain, milks are divided into fat-free/low-fat milk, reduced-fat milk, and whole milk. One choice of these includes the following.

	Carbohydrate (grams)	Protein (grams)	Fat (grams)	Calories
Fat-free/low-fat (½% or 1%)	12	8	0–3	90
Reduced-fat (2%)	12	8	5	120
Whole	12	8	8	150

One milk exchange equals 12 grams carbohydrate and 8 grams protein.

Fat-Free and Low-Fat Milk
(0–3 grams fat per serving)

½% milk .... 1 cup
1% milk .... 1 cup
Buttermilk, fat-free or low-fat .... 1 cup
Evaporated fat-free milk .... ½ cup
Fat-free dry milk .... ⅓ cup dry
Fat-free milk .... 1 cup
Nonfat flavored yogurt sweetened with non-nutritive sweetener and fructose .... ⅔ cup (6 oz.)
Plain nonfat yogurt .... ⅔ cup (6 oz.)
Soy milk, low-fat or fat-free .... 1 cup

Reduced-Fat
(5 grams fat per serving)

2% milk .... 1 cup
Plain low-fat yogurt .... ¾ cup
Soy milk .... 1 cup
Sweet acidophilus milk .... 1 cup

Whole Milk
(8 grams fat per serving)

Evaporated whole milk .... ½ cup
Goat milk .... 1 cup
Kefir .... 1 cup
Whole milk .... 1 cup
Yogurt, plain (made from whole milk) .... ¾ cup

Other Carbohydrates List

Substitute food choices from this list for a starch, fruit, or milk choice on your meal plan. Some choices will also count as one or more fat choices.

One exchange equals
15 grams carbohydrate
or 1 starch,
or 1 fruit,
or 1 milk.

Food	Serving Size	Exchanges per Serving
Angel food cake, unfrosted	1/12th cake (about 2 oz.)	2 carbohydrates
Brownie, small, unfrosted	2 in. square (about 1 oz.)	1 carbohydrate, 1 fat
Cake, unfrosted	2 in. square (about 1 oz.)	1 carbohydrate, 1 fat
Cake, frosted	2 in. square (about 2 oz.)	2 carbohydrates, 1 fat
Cookie or sandwich cookie with creme filling	2 small (about 2/3 oz.)	1 carbohydrate, 1 fat
Cookie, sugar-free	3 small or 1 large (3/4–1 oz.)	1 carbohydrate, 1–2 fats
Cranberry sauce, jellied	1/4 cup	1 1/2 carbohydrates
Cupcake, frosted	1 small (about 2 oz.)	2 carbohydrates, 1 fat
Doughnut, plain cake	1 medium (1 1/2 oz.)	1 1/2 carbohydrates, 2 fats
Doughnut, glazed	3 3/4 in. across (2 oz.)	2 carbohydrates, 2 fats
Energy, sport, or breakfast bar	1 bar (1 1/3 oz.)	1 1/2 carbohydrates, 0–1 fat
Energy, sport, or breakfast bar	1 bar (2 oz.)	2 carbohydrates, 1 fat
Fruit cobbler	1/2 cup (3 1/2 oz.)	3 carbohydrates, 1 fat
Fruit juice bars, frozen, 100% juice	1 bar (3 oz.)	1 carbohydrate
Fruit snacks, chewy (pureed fruit concentrate)	1 roll (3/4 oz.)	1 carbohydrate
Fruit spreads, 100% fruit	1 1/2 Tbsp	1 carbohydrate
Gelatin, regular	1/2 cup	1 carbohydrate
Gingersnaps	3	1 carbohydrate
Granola or snack bar, regular or low fat	1 bar (1 oz.)	1 1/2 carbohydrates
Honey	1 Tbsp	1 carbohydrate
Ice cream	1/2 cup	1 carbohydrate, 1 fat

Ice cream, low-fat	1/2 cup	1 carbohydrate
Ice cream, fat-free, no sugar added	1/2 cup	1 carbohydrate
Jam or jelly, regular	1 Tbsp	1 carbohydrate
Milk, chocolate, whole	1 cup	2 carbohydrates, 1 fat
Pie, fruit, 2 crusts	1/6 pie of 8 in. commercially prepared pie	3 carbohydrates, 2 fats
Pie, pumpkin or custard	1/8 pie of 8 in. commercially prepared pie	2 carbohydrates, 2 fats
Pudding, regular (made with reduced-fat milk)	1/2 cup	2 carbohydrates
Pudding, sugar-free or sugar-free and fat-free (made with fat-free milk)	1/2 cup	1 carbohydrate
Reduced-calorie meal replacement (shake)	1 can (10–11 oz.)	1 1/2 carbohydrates, 0–1 fat
Rice milk, low-fat or fat-free, plain	1 cup	1 carbohydrate
Rice milk, low-fat, flavored	1 cup	1 1/2 carbohydrates
Salad dressing, fat-free	1/4 cup	1 carbohydrate
Sherbet, sorbet	1/2 cup	2 carbohydrates
Spaghetti or pasta sauce, canned	1/2 cup	1 carbohydrate, 1 fat
Sports drinks	8 oz. (1 cup)	1 carbohydrate
Sugar	1 Tbsp	1 carbohydrate
Sweet roll or Danish	1 (2 1/2 oz.)	2 1/2 carbohydrates, 2 fats
Syrup, light	2 Tbsp	1 carbohydrate
Syrup, regular	1 Tbsp	1 carbohydrate
Syrup, regular	1/4 cup	4 carbohydrates
Vanilla wafers	5	1 carbohydrate, 1 fat
Yogurt, frozen	1/2 cup	1 carbohydrate, 0–1 fat
Yogurt, frozen fat-free	1/3 cup	1 carbohydrate
Yogurt, low-fat with fruit	1 cup	3 carbohydrates, 0–1 fat

Vegetable List

Vegetables that contain small amounts of carbohydrates and calories are on this list. In general, one vegetable exchange is:

- 1/2 cup of cooked vegetables or vegetable juice
- 1 cup of raw vegetables

If you eat 3 cups or more of raw vegetables or 1 1/2 cups of cooked vegetables at one meal, count them as 1 carbohydrate choice.

One vegetable exchange equals
5 grams carbohydrate,
2 grams protein,
0 grams fat, and
25 calories.

Artichoke
Artichoke hearts
Asparagus
Beans (green, wax, Italian)
Bean sprouts
Beets
Broccoli
Brussels sprouts
Cabbage
Carrots
Cauliflower
Celery
Cucumber
Eggplant
Green onions or scallions
Greens (collard, kale, mustard, turnip)
Kohlrabi
Leeks
Mixed vegetables (without corn, peas, or pasta)
Mushrooms
Okra
Onions
Pea pods
Peppers (all varieties)
Radishes
Salad greens (endive, escarole, lettuce, romaine, spinach)
Sauerkraut
Spinach
Summer squash
Tomato
Tomatoes, canned
Tomato sauce
Tomato/vegetable juice
Turnips
Water chestnuts
Watercress
Zucchini

= 400 mg or more of sodium per serving.

Meat and Meat Substitutes List

Meat and meat substitutes that contain both protein and fat are on this list. In general, one meat exchange is:

- 1 oz. meat, fish, poultry, or cheese
- 1/2 cup beans, peas, or lentils

Based on the amount of fat they contain, meats are divided into very lean, lean, medium-fat, and high-fat lists. One ounce (one exchange) of each of these includes the following.

	Carbohydrate (grams)	Protein (grams)	Fat (grams)	Calories
Very lean	0	7	0–1	35
Lean	0	7	3	55
Medium-fat	0	7	5	75
High-fat	0	7	8	100

Very Lean Meat and Substitutes List

One exchange equals
0 grams carbohydrate,
7 grams protein,
0–1 gram fat,
and 35 calories.

One very lean meat exchange is equal to any one of the following items.

Poultry: Chicken or turkey (white meat, no skin), Cornish hen (no skin) .... 1 oz.
Fish: Fresh or frozen cod, flounder, haddock, halibut, lox (smoked salmon), trout, tuna (fresh or canned in water) .... 1 oz.
Shellfish: Clams, crab, lobster, scallops, shrimp, imitation shellfish .... 1 oz.
Game: Duck or pheasant (no skin), venison, buffalo, ostrich .... 1 oz.
Cheese with 1 gram or less fat per ounce:
Fat-free or low-fat cottage cheese .... 1/4 cup
Fat-free cheese .... 1 oz.
Other: Processed sandwich meats with 1 gram or less fat per ounce, such as deli thin, shaved meats, chipped beef .... 1 oz.
Turkey ham .... 1 oz.
Egg whites 2
Egg substitutes, plain .... 1/4 cup
Hot dogs with 1 gram or less fat per ounce .... 1 oz.

= 400 mg or more of sodium per serving.

Kidney (high in cholesterol)	1 oz.
Sausage with 1 gram or less fat per ounce	1 oz.
Count as one very lean meat and one starch exchange:	
Beans, peas, lentils (cooked)	1/2 cup

Lean Meat and Substitutes List

One exchange equals
0 grams carbohydrate,
7 grams protein,
3 grams fat,
and 55 calories.

One lean meat exchange is equal to any one of the following items.

Beef: USDA Select or Choice grades of lean beef trimmed of fat, such as round, sirloin, and flank steak; tenderloin; roast (rib, chuck, rump); steak (T-bone, porterhouse, cubed); ground round	1 oz.
Pork: Lean pork, such as fresh ham; canned, cured, or boiled ham; Canadian bacon; tenderloin, center loin chop	1 oz.
Lamb: Roast, chop, leg	1 oz.
Veal: Lean chop, roast	1 oz.
Poultry: Chicken, turkey (dark meat, no skin), chicken (white meat with skin), domestic duck or goose (well-drained of fat, no skin)	1 oz.
Fish:	
Herring (uncreamed or smoked)	1 oz.
Oysters	6 medium
Salmon (fresh or canned), catfish	1 oz.
Sardines (canned)	2 medium
Tuna (canned in oil, drained)	1 oz.
Game: Goose (no skin), rabbit	1 oz.
Cheese:	
4.5%-fat cottage cheese	1/4 cup
Grated Parmesan	2 Tbsp
Cheeses with 3 grams or less fat per ounce	1 oz.
Other:	
Hot dogs with 3 grams or less fat per ounce	1 1/2 oz.
Processed sandwich meat with 3 grams or less fat per ounce, such as turkey pastrami or kielbasa	1 oz.
Liver, heart (high in cholesterol)	1 oz.

SECTION 7

= 400 mg or more of sodium per serving.

Medium-Fat Meat and Substitutes List

One exception equals
0 grams carbohydrate,
7 grams protein,
5 grams fat,
and 75 calories.
One medium-fat meat exchange is equal to any one of the following items.

Beef: Most beef products fall into this category (ground beef, meatloaf, corned beef, short ribs, prime grades of meat trimmed of fat, such as prime rib) .... 1 oz.
Pork: Top loin, chop, Boston butt, cutlet .... 1 oz.
Lamb: Rib roast, ground .... 1 oz.
Veal: Cutlet (ground or cubed, unbreaded) .... 1 oz.
Poultry: Chicken dark meat (with skin), ground turkey or ground chicken, fried chicken (with skin) .... 1 oz.
Fish: Any fried fish product .... 1 oz.
Cheese: With 5 grams or less fat per ounce .... 1 oz.
Feta .... 1 oz.
Mozzarella .... 1 oz.
Ricotta .... 1/4 cup (2 oz.)
Other:
Egg (high in cholesterol, limit to 3 per week) 1
Sausage with 5 grams or less fat per ounce .... 1 oz.
Tempeh .... 1/4 cup
Tofu .... 4 oz. or 1/2 cup

High-Fat Meat and Substitutes List

One exchange equals
0 grams carbohydrate,
7 grams protein,
8 grams fat,
and 100 calories.
One high-fat meat exchange is equal to any one of the following items.

Pork: Spareribs, ground pork, pork sausage .... 1 oz.
Cheese: All regular cheeses, such as American, cheddar, Monterey Jack, Swiss .... 1 oz.

= 400 mg or more of sodium per serving.

Other: Processed sandwich meats with 8 grams or less fat per ounce,
such as bologna, pimento loaf, salami .... 1 oz.
Sausage, such as bratwurst, Italian, knockwurst, Polish, smoked .... 1 oz.
Hot dog (turkey or chicken) ✎ 1 (10/lb)
Bacon .... 3 slices (20 slices/lb)
Count as one high-fat meat plus one fat exchange:
Hot dog (beef, pork, or combination) ✎ 1 (10/lb)

Fat List

Fats are divided into three groups, based on the main type of fat they contain: monounsaturated, polyunsaturated, and saturated. Monounsaturated and polyunsaturated fats in the foods we eat are linked with good health benefits. Saturated fats and fats called trans fatty acids or trans unsaturated fatty acids are linked with heart disease. In general, one fat exchange is:

- 1 teaspoon of regular margarine or vegetable oil
- 1 tablespoon of regular salad dressing

Monounsaturated Fats List

One fat exchange equals
5 grams fat and
45 calories.

Avocado, medium .... 2 Tbsp (1 oz.)
Oil (canola, olive, peanut) .... 1 tsp
Olives
  ripe (black) .... 8 large
  green, stuffed .... 10 large
Nuts
  almonds, cashews .... 6 nuts
  mixed (50% peanuts) .... 6 nuts
  peanuts .... 10 nuts
  pecans .... 4 halves
Peanut butter, smooth or crunchy .... ½ Tbsp
Sesame seeds .... 1 Tbsp
Tahini or sesame paste .... 2 tsp

✎ = 400 mg or more of sodium per serving.

Polyunsaturated Fats List

One fat exchange equals
5 grams fat and
45 calories.

Margarine	
stick, tub, or squeeze	1 tsp
lower-fat spread (30% to 50% vegetable oil)	1 Tbsp
Mayonnaise	
regular	1 tsp
reduced-fat	1 Tbsp
Nuts, walnuts, English	4 halves
Oil (corn, safflower, soybean)	1 tsp
Salad dressing	
regular	1 Tbsp
reduced-fat	2 Tbsp
Miracle Whip Salad Dressing	
regular	2 tsp
reduced-fat	1 Tbsp
Seeds (pumpkin, sunflower)	1 Tbsp

Saturated Fats List

One fat exchange equals
5 grams of fat and
45 calories.

Bacon, cooked	1 slice (20 slices/lb)
Bacon, grease	1 tsp
Butter	
stick	1 tsp
whipped	2 tsp
reduced-fat	1 Tbsp
Chitterlings, boiled	2 Tbsp (1/2 oz.)
Coconut, sweetened, shredded	2 Tbsp
Coconut milk	1 Tbsp
Cream, half and half	2 Tbsp
Cream cheese	
regular	1 Tbsp (1/2 oz.)
reduced-fat	1 1/2 Tbsp (3/4 oz.)
Fatback or salt pork, see below‡	
Shortening or lard	1 tsp
Sour cream	
regular	2 Tbsp
reduced-fat	3 Tbsp

‡Use a piece 1 in. × 1 in. × 1/4 in. if you plan to eat the fatback cooked with vegetables. Use a piece 2 in. × 2 in. × 1/2 in. when eating only the vegetables with the fatback removed.

= 400 mg or more of sodium per serving.

Free Foods List

A *free food* is any food or drink that contains less than 20 calories or less than 5 grams of carbohydrate per serving. Foods with a serving size listed should be limited to three servings per day. Foods listed without a serving size can be eaten as often as you like.

Fat-Free or Reduced-Fat Foods

Cream cheese, fat-free.......1 Tsp ($^1/_2$ oz.)
Creamers, nondairy, liquid.......1 Tbsp
Creamers, nondairy, powdered.......2 tsp
Mayonnaise, fat-free.......1 Tbsp
Mayonnaise, reduced-fat.......1 tsp
Margarine spread, fat-free.......4 Tbsp
Margarine spread, reduced-fat.......1 tsp
Miracle Whip, fat-free.......1 Tbsp
Miracle Whip, reduced-fat.......1 tsp
Nonstick cooking spray
Salad dressing, fat-free or low-fat.......1 Tbsp
Salad dressing, fat-free, Italian.......2 Tbsp
Sour cream, fat-free, reduced-fat.......1 Tbsp
Whipped topping, regular.......1 Tbsp
Whipped topping, light or fat-free.......2 Tbsp

Sugar-Free Foods

Candy, hard, sugar-free.......1 candy
Gelatin dessert, sugar-free
Gelatin, unflavored
Gum, sugar-free
Jam or jelly, light.......2 tsp
Sugar substitutes‡
Syrup, sugar-free.......2 Tbsp

‡Sugar substitutes, alternatives, or replacements that are approved by the Food and Drug Administration (FDA) are safe to use. Common brand names include:
Equal (aspartame)
Splenda (sucralose)
Sprinkle Sweet (saccharin)
Sweet One (acesulfame K)
Sweet-10 (saccharin)
Sugar Twin (saccharin)
Sweet 'n Low (saccharin)

Drinks

Bouillon, broth, consommé
Bouillon or broth, low-sodium
Carbonated or mineral water
Club soda
Cocoa powder, unsweetened .... 1 Tbsp
Coffee
Diet soft drinks, sugar-free
Drink mixes, sugar-free
Tea
Tonic water, sugar-free

Condiments

Ketchup .... 1 Tbsp
Horseradish
Lemon juice
Lime juice
Mustard
Pickle relish .... 1 Tbsp
Pickles, dill .... 1½ medium
Pickles, sweet (bread and butter) .... 2 slices
Pickles, sweet (gherkin) .... ¾ oz.
Salsa .... ¼ cup
Soy sauce, regular or light .... 1 Tbsp
Taco sauce .... 1 Tbsp
Vinegar
Yogurt .... 2 Tbsp

Seasonings

Be careful with seasonings that contain sodium or are salts, such as garlic or celery salt, and lemon pepper.

Flavoring extracts
Garlic
Herbs, fresh or dried
Pimento
Spices
Tabasco or hot pepper sauce
Wine, used in cooking
Worcestershire sauce

= 400 mg or more of sodium per serving.

Combination Foods List

Many of the foods we eat are mixed together in various combinations. These combination foods do not fit into any one exchange list. This is a list of exchanges for some typical combination foods.

Entrees	Serving Size	Exchanges per Serving
Tuna noodle casserole, lasagna, spaghetti with meatballs, chili with beans, macaroni and cheese	1 cup (8 oz.)	2 carbohydrates, 2 medium-fat meats
Chow mein (without noodles or rice)	2 cups (16 oz.)	1 carbohydrate, 2 lean meats
Tuna or chicken salad	½ cup (3½ oz.)	½ carbohydrate, 2 lean meats, 1 fat
Frozen Entrees and Meals		
Dinner-type meal 🧂	generally 14–17 oz.	3 carbohydrates, 3 medium-fat meats, 3 fats
Meatless burger, soy based	3 oz.	½ carbohydrate, 2 lean meats
Meatless burger, vegetable and starch based	3 oz.	1 carbohydrate, 1 lean meat,
Pizza, cheese, thin crust 🧂	¼ of 12 in. (6 oz.)	2 carbohydrates 2 medium-fat meats, 1 fat,
Pizza, meat topping, thin crust 🧂	¼ of 12 in. (6 oz.)	2 carbohydrates 2 medium-fat meats, 2 fats
Pot pie 🧂	1 (7 oz.)	2½ carbohydrates, 1 medium-fat meat, 3 fats
Entree or meal with less than 340 calories 🧂	about 8–11 oz.	2–3 carbohydrates, 1–2 lean meats
Soups		
Bean 🧂	1 cup	1 carbohydrate, 1 very lean meat
Cream (made with water) 🧂	1 cup (8 oz.)	1 carbohydrate, 1 fat
Instant 🧂	6 oz. prepared	1 carbohydrate
Instant with beans/lentils 🧂	8 oz. prepared	2½ carbohydrates, 1 very lean meat
Split pea (made with water) 🧂	½ cup (4 oz.)	1 carbohydrate
Tomato (made with water) 🧂	1 cup (8 oz.)	1 carbohydrate
Vegetable beef, chicken noodle, or other broth-type 🧂	1 cup (8 oz.)	1 carbohydrate

🧂 = 400 mg or more of sodium per serving.

Fast Foods List*

Food	Serving Size	Exchanges per Serving
Burritos with beef	1 (5–7 oz.)	3 carbohydrates, 1 medium-fat meat, 1 fat
Chicken nuggets	6	1 carbohydrate, 2 medium-fat meats, 1 fat
Chicken breast and wing, breaded and fried	1 each	1 carbohydrate, 4 medium-fat meats, 2 fats
Chicken sandwich, grilled	1	2 carbohydrates, 3 very lean meats
Chicken wings, hot	6 (5 oz.)	1 carbohydrate, 3 medium-fat meats, 4 fats
Fish sandwich/tartar sauce	1	3 carbohydrates, 1 medium-fat meat, 3 fats
French fries	1 medium serving (5 oz.)	4 carbohydrates, 4 fats
Hamburger, regular	1	2 carbohydrates, 2 medium-fat meats
Hamburger, large	1	2 carbohydrates, 3 medium-fat meats, 1 fat
Hot dog with bun	1	1 carbohydrate, 1 high-fat meat, 1 fat
Individual pan pizza	1	5 carbohydrates, 3 medium-fat meats, 3 fats,
Pizza, cheese, thin		2½ carbohydrates
crust	¼ of 12 in. (about 6 oz.)	2 medium-fat meats,
Pizza, meat, thin		2½ carbohydrates
crust	¼ of 12 in. (about 6 oz.)	2 medium-fat meats, 1 fat
Soft-serve cone	1 small (5 oz.)	2½ carbohydrates, 1 fat
Submarine sandwich	1 sub (6 in.)	3 carbohydrates, 1 vegetable, 2 medium-fat meats, 1 fat
Submarine sandwich (less than 6 grams fat)	1 sub (6 in.)	2½ carbohydrates, 2 lean meats,
Taco, hard or soft		1 carbohydrate
shell	1 (3–3½ oz.)	1 medium-fat meat, 1 fat

*Ask at your fast-food restaurant for nutrition information about your favorite fast foods or check Web sites.

Source: *Exchange Lists for Meal Planning*. The American Diabetes Association, Alexandria, VA, and The American Dietetic Association, Chicago, IL. 1995.

= 400 mg or more of sodium per serving.

Appendix M: Exchange List for Carbohydrate Counting

Table M-1 Nutrient Content of Exchanges

Groups/List	Carbohydrates (grams)	Protein (grams)	Fat (grams)	Calories
Carbohydrate Group				
Starch	15	3	0–1	80
Fruit	15	—	—	60
Milk				
Fat-free, low-fat	12	8	0–3	90
Reduced-fat	12	8	5	120
Whole	12	8	8	150
Other carbohydrates	15	Varies	Varies	Varies
Nonstarchy vegetables	5	2	—	25
Meat and Meat Substitutes Group				
Very lean	—	7	0–1	35
Lean	—	7	3	55
Medium fat	—	7	5	75
High fat	—	7	8	100
Fat Group	—	—	5	45

Source: Reprinted by permission from the American Dietetic Association. *Exchange Lists for Meal Planning,* © 2003. American Diabetes Association, Inc.

Appendix N: Fast Food Nutrients

ERA, EatRight Analysis CD-ROM; **AMT,** amount; **WT,** weight; **CAL,** calories; **PROT,** protein; **CARB,** carbohydrate; **FIBR,** fiber; **FAT,** fat; **SATF,** saturated fat; **MONO,** monounsaturated fat; **POLY,** polyunsaturated fat; **CHOL,** cholesterol

ERA CODE	FOOD DESCRIPTION	AMT	UNIT	WT (g)	CAL (kcal)	PROT (g)	CARB (g)	FIBR (g)	FAT (g)	SATF (g)	MONO (g)	POLY (g)	CHOL (mg)
Fast Foods/Restaurants													
Arby's													
6432	Arby's Curly Fries	1	ea	99.222	310	4	39	3	15	3.5	9.6	1.9	0
69045	Arby's Q Sandwich	1	ea	186	360	16	40	2	14	4	6.5	3.5	70
53256	Arby's Sauce	1	ea	14	15	0	4	0	0	0	0	0	0
69056	Beef 'n' Cheddar Sandwich	1	ea	198	460	23	43	2	23	9	8.9	5.1	50
57015	Cheddar Fries, Serving	1	ea	170	460	6	54	4	24	6	15.4	2.6	5
69046	Grill Chicken Deluxe Sandwich	1	ea	252	450	29	37	2	22	4			110
69048	Italian Sub Sandwich	1	ea	312	780	29	49	3	53	15	24.6	13.4	120
69055	Philly Beef 'n' Swiss Sandwich	1	ea	311	670	36	46	4	40	16	16.3	7.7	75
56336	Roast Beef Sandwich, Reg	1	ea	157	330	21	35	2	14	7			45
56337	Roast Beef Sandwich, Jr	1	ea	129	290	16	34	2	12	5	4.7	2.3	40
69049	Roast Beef Sub Sandwich	1	ea	334	730	35	48	3	46	16	19.7	10.3	75
69042	Roast Chicken Club Sandwich	1	ea	278	520	29	38	2	28	7	10.2	10.8	115
69052	Roast Chicken Sandwich, Lt, Deluxe	1	ea	194	276	23	33	3	5	1	2.1	1.9	40
69044	Turkey Sub Sandwich	1	ea	306	630	26	51	2	37	9	12.9	15.1	100
Boston Market													
52103	Chicken Salad, Chunky	0.75	cup	158	370	28	3	1	27	4.5			120
28257	Red Beans+Rice, Low Fat	1	cup	227	260	8	45	4	5	0			5
50300	Tomato Bisque	1	cup	230	280	4	16	2	23	10			50
Burger King													
57002	BK Broiler Chicken Sandwich	1	ea	258	550	30	52	3	25	5			105
56360	Chicken Sandwich	1	ea	224	660	25	53	3	39	8			70
57001	Double Cheeseburger	1	ea	197	570	35	32	2	34	17			110
56362	Ocean Catch Fish Filet	1	ea	263	710	24	67	4	38	14			50
56363	Onion Rings, Serving	1	ea	91	320	4	40	3	16	4	8	4	0
56999	Whopper Jr Sandwich	1	ea	167	410	18	32	2	23	7			50
57000	Whopper Jr Sandwich+ Cheese	1	ea	180	460	21	33	2	27	10			60
56354	Whopper Sandwich	1	ea	278	680	29	53	4	39	12			80
56355	Whopper Sandwich+ Cheese	1	ea	303	780	34	55	4	47	17			105

WTR, water; **V,** vitamin; **THI,** thiamin; **RIB,** riboflavin; **NIA,** niacin; **FOL,** folate; **CALC,** calcium; **PHOS,** phosphorus; **SOD,** sodium; **POT,** potassium; **MAG,** magnesium

WTR (g)	V-A (RE)	THI (mg)	RIB (mg)	NIA (mg)	V-B6 (mg)	FOL (g)	V-B12 (g)	V-C (mg)	V-E (mg)	CALC (mg)	PHOS (mg)	SOD (mg)	POT (mg)	MAG (mg)	IRON (mg)	ZINC (mg)
	0	0.1	0.1	2			0	12		0		770	724		1.4	0.6
		0.3	0.4	9				5		80		1,530	456		3.6	
								1		0		180	28		0	
		0.4	0.6	10				1		100		1,170	328		3.6	3
		0.1	0.2	2.4			0	15		60		1,290	888		1.8	1.1
	88	0.3	0.3	14.9				1		60		1,050	722		2.7	
	105	1	0.5	8.6				2		250		2,440	594		2.7	
		0.4	0.7	13.9				9		300		1,850	646		2.7	5.9
	0	0.3	0.5	11.1	0.2	14		0		60	122	890	427	16	3.6	3.8
		0.3	0.4	9.6	0.1	10				60	87	700	291	12	2.7	2.2
	110	0.6	0.8	11.1				2		300		2,140	775		4.5	
		0.6	0.8	12.4				2		150		1,440	624		2.7	2.6
	40	0.4	0.7	9.4				2		100		1,010	390		2.7	
	22	14.6	0.6	20.8				2		200		2,170	552		0.4	
	20							4		20		800			0.7	
	40							12		60		1,050			2.7	
	150							21		60		1,280			3.6	
	60							6		60		1,110			3.6	
	20							0		80		1,330			2.7	
	100							0		250		1,020			4.5	
	20							0		80		1,200			3.6	
	0						0	0		100		460			0	
	40							5		80		520			3.6	
	80							5		150		740			3.6	
	100							9		100		940			5.4	
	150							9		250		1,390			5.4	

ERA, EatRight Analysis CD-ROM; **AMT,** amount; **WT,** weight; **CAL,** calories; **PROT,** protein; **CARB,** carbohydrate; **FIBR,** fiber; **FAT,** fat; **SATF,** saturated fat; **MONO,** monounsaturated fat; **POLY,** polyunsaturated fat; **CHOL,** cholesterol

ERA CODE	FOOD DESCRIPTION	AMT	UNIT	WT (g)	CAL (kcal)	PROT (g)	CARB (g)	FIBR (g)	FAT (g)	SATF (g)	MONO (g)	POLY (g)	CHOL (mg)
Fast Foods/Restaurants (continued)													
Carl's Junior													
91408	Chicken Sandwich, Charbroiled Club	1	ea	239	460	32	33	2	22	7			90
91410	Chicken Sandwich, Crispy Ranch	1	ea	266	730	29	76	4	34	7.1			59
91413	Fish Sandwich, Carl's Catch	1	ea	201	510	18	50	1	27	7			80
Dairy Queen													
2131	Banana Split	1	ea	369	510	8	96	3	12	8			30
2132	Blizzard, Heath Flavor	1	ea	404	820	14	119	1	33	20			60
2227	Blizzard, Strawberry, Regular	1	ea	383	570	12	95	1	16	11			50
2133	Buster Bar	1	ea	149	450	10	41	2	28	12			15
2222	Cone, Chocolate, Reg	1	ea	198	340	8	53	0	11	7			30
2135	Dilly Bar	1	ea	85	210	3	21	0	13	7			10
2136	Dipped Cone, Regular	1	ea	220	490	8	59	1	24	13			30
69027	Double Bacon Cheeseburger	1	ea	269	670	40	29	2	43	19			135
13236	Hot Dog, Super, 1/4-lb	1	ea	198	580	20	39	2	37	13			75
56374	Hot Dog	1	ea	99	240	9	19	1	14	5			25
56375	Hot Dog+Cheese	1	ea	11	290	12	20	1	18	8	8	2	40
2145	Malt, Regular, Vanilla	1	ea	418	610	13	106	<1	14	8	2	2	45
2151	Peanut Buster Parfait	1	ea	305	730	16	99	2	31	17			35
2224	Shake, Chocolate, Reg	1	ea	539	770	17	130	0	20	13			70
56371	Single Cheeseburger	1	ea	152	340	20	29	2	17	8			55
56368	Single Hamburger	1	ea	138	290	17	29	2	12	5			45
2154	Sundae, Chocolate, Regular	1	ea	234	400	8	71	0	10	6			30
Generic Fast Food													
56606	Croissant + Egg & Cheese	1	ea	127	368	13	24		25	14.1	7.5	1.4	216
42064	English Muffin+Butter	1	ea	63	189	5	30	2	6	2.4	1.5	1.3	13
5463	Hashbrown Potatoes, Svg	0.5	cup	72	151	2	16		9	4.3	3.9	0.5	9
15177	Hot Wings, Pieces	6	pce	135	471	27	18	2	33	8			150
56667	Hot Dog + Chili	1	ea	114	296	14	31		13	4.9	6.6	1.2	51
66004	Hot Dog/Frankfurter & Bun	1	ea	98	242	10	18		15	5.1	6.9	1.7	44
56639	Nachos, Chips + Cheese	7	pce	113	346	9	36		19	7.8	8	2.2	18
6176	Onion Rings, Serving	8.5	pce	83	276	4	31		16	7	6.7	0.7	14
2022	Strawberry Milkshake	1	cup	283	320	10	53	1	8	4.9	2.2	0.3	31
2033	Strawberry Sundae	1	ea	153	268	6	45	0	8	3.7	2.7	1	21
Hardees													
56411	Biscuit 'n' Gravy	1	ea	221	530	10	56		30	9			15
2247	Cool Twist Cone, Vanilla/ Chocolate	1	ea	118	180	4	34		2	1			10

WTR, water; **V,** vitamin; **THI,** thiamin; **RIB,** riboflavin; **NIA,** niacin; **FOL,** folate; **CALC,** calcium; **PHOS,** phosphorus; **SOD,** sodium; **POT,** potassium; **MAG,** magnesium

WTR (g)	V-A (RE)	THI (mg)	RIB (mg)	NIA (mg)	V-B6 (mg)	FOL (g)	V-B12 (g)	V-C (mg)	V-E (mg)	CALC (mg)	PHOS (mg)	SOD (mg)	POT (mg)	MAG (mg)	IRON (mg)	ZINC (mg)
	80							6		200		1,110			2.7	
	71							6		176		1,435			4.2	
	60							2		150		1,030			1.8	
	200							15		250		180			1.8	
	300	0.2	0.8					1		450	450	580	730		1.8	
	300	0.2	0.7					9		450	350	260	700		1.8	
	80							0		150		280			1.1	
	150							1		250		160			1.8	
	60							0		100		75			0.4	
	150							2		250		190			1.8	
	150							9		250		1,210			4.5	
	0							0		250		1,710			4.5	
	20							4		60		730			1.8	
	60	0.2	0.2	2				4		150	150	950	180		1.8	
	80	0.1	0.6	0.8	0.2			<1		400	350	230	570		1.4	
	150							1		300		400			1.8	
	400							2		600		420			2.7	
	100							4		150		850			3.6	
	40							4		60		630			2.7	
	150							0		250		210			1.4	
58	282	0.2	0.4	1.5	0.1	47	0.8	<1		244	348	551	174	22	2.2	1.8
21	33	0.3	0.3	2.6	<0.1	57	<0.1	1	0.1	103	85	386	69	13	1.6	0.4
43	3	0.1	<0.1	1.1	0.2	8	<0.1	5	0.1	7	69	290	267	16	0.5	0.2
	20							1		40		1,230			1.4	
54	7	0.2	0.4	3.7	<0.1	73	0.3	3		19	192	480	166	10	3.3	0.8
53	0	0.2	0.3	3.6	<0.1	48	0.5	<1	0.3	24	97	670	143	13	2.3	2
46	154	0.2	0.4	1.5	0.2	10	0.8	1		272	276	816	172	55	1.3	1.8
31	2	0.1	0.1	0.9	0.1	55	0.1	1	0.3	73	86	430	129	16	0.8	0.3
210	74	0.1	0.6	0.5	0.1	8	0.9	2	0.4	320	283	235	515	37	0.3	1
93	60	0.1	0.3	0.9	0.1	18	0.6	2	0.8	161	154	92	271	24	0.3	0.7
												1,550				
												120				

ERA, EatRight Analysis CD-ROM; **AMT,** amount; **WT,** weight; **CAL,** calories; **PROT,** protein; **CARB,** carbohydrate; **FIBR,** fiber; **FAT,** fat; **SATF,** saturated fat; **MONO,** monounsaturated fat; **POLY,** polyunsaturated fat; **CHOL,** cholesterol

ERA CODE	FOOD DESCRIPTION	AMT	UNIT	WT (g)	CAL (kcal)	PROT (g)	CARB (g)	FIBR (g)	FAT (g)	SATF (g)	MONO (g)	POLY (g)	CHOL (mg)
Fast Foods/Restaurants (continued)													
Hardees (continued)													
69061	Frisco Hamburger	1	ea	219	717	33	37	2	49	13.9			100
56420	Hot Ham 'n' Cheese Sandwich	1	ea	201	421	23	43	3	17	9.6			78
56418	Roast Beef Sandwich, Regular	1	ea	123	310	17	26	2	16	6			43
Jack in the Box													
69032	Bacon Cheeseburger	1	ea	274	760	39	39	2	50	17	21.2	11.8	135
56430	Breakfast Jack Sandwich	1	ea	126	280	17	28	1	12	5	4.7	2.3	190
56441	Chicken Fajita Pita	1	ea	230	320	24	34	3	10	4.5	4	1.5	55
69035	Chicken Sandwich	1	ea	164	400	15	38	3	21	3			40
69033	Grilled Sourdough Burger	1	ea	233	690	34	37	2	45	15	20.8	9.2	105
56436	Jumbo Jack Burger	1	ea	271	550	27	43	2	30	10	12.4	7.6	75
56437	Jumbo Jack Burger+ Cheese	1	ea	296	640	31	44	2	38	15	14.4	8.6	105
69040	Sourdough Breakfast Sandwich	1	ea	162	450	21	36	2	24	8			205
Kentucky Fried Chicken													
15169	Chicken Breast, Extra Crispy	1	ea	168	470	39	17	1	28	8	16.7	3.3	160
15163	Chicken Breast, Original	1	ea	153	400	29	16	1	24	6	14.4	3.6	135
15170	Chicken Leg, Extra Crispy	1	ea	67	195	15	7	1	12	3	7.4	1.6	77
15165	Chicken Leg, Original	1	ea	61	140	13	4	0	9	2	5.3	1.7	75
15184	Hot & Spicy Chicken Drumstick	1	ea	64	175	13	9	1	10	3			77
15187	Hot & Spicy Chicken Wing	1	ea	55	210	10	9	1	15	4			55
Long John Silver's													
69030	Fish Sandwich Batter Dip	1	ea	174.3	430	16	46		20	5			35
57003	Fish+LemCrumb Dinner, 3 piece	1	ea	470.6	730	31	89		29	6			60
56461	Fish, Batter Fried, Serving	1	pce	92.14	230	12	16		13	4			30
27110	Malt Vinegar, Serving	1	ea	7.94	0	0	0	0	0	0	0	0	
McDonald's													
69010	Big Mac Sandwich	1	ea	216	590	24	47	3	34	11			85
42332	Biscuit+Biscuit Spread	1	ea	69	240	4	30	1	11	2.5			0
56675	Breakfast Burrito	1	ea	113	290	13	24	2	16	6			170
69009	Cheeseburger	1	ea	121	330	15	36	2	14	6			45
15174	Chicken McNuggets	1	ea	72	190	10	13	1	11	2.5			35
42335	Danish, Apple	1	ea	105	340	5	47	2	15	3			20
69005	Egg McMuffin	1	ea	136	290	17	27	1	12	4.5			235
69013	Filet-O-Fish Sandwich	1	ea	156	470	15	45	1	26	5			50
5462	French Fries, Medium	1	ea	147	450	6	57	5	22	4			0

WTR, water; **V,** vitamin; **THI,** thiamin; **RIB,** riboflavin; **NIA,** niacin; **FOL,** folate; **CALC,** calcium; **PHOS,** phosphorus; **SOD,** sodium; **POT,** potassium; **MAG,** magnesium

WTR (g)	V-A (RE)	THI (mg)	RIB (mg)	NIA (mg)	V-B6 (mg)	FOL (g)	V-B12 (g)	V-C (mg)	V-E (mg)	CALC (mg)	PHOS (mg)	SOD (mg)	POT (mg)	MAG (mg)	IRON (mg)	ZINC (mg)
101												1,079				
												1,831				
												804				
	150	0.3	0.5	10	0.4			9		250		1,570	530		4.5	
	80	0.5	0.4	3.1				10		150		750	120		3.6	
	200	0.9	0.2	7.3				15		200		850	410		2.7	
	40							5		100		770	200		2.7	
	150	0.7	0.5	8.4	0.3			9		200		1,180	480		4.5	
	100	0.4	0.3	2.1				9		150		880	490		4.5	
	150	0.4	0.5	2				9		250		1,340	530		4.5	
	100							4		200		1,040	220		2.7	
	20							1		20		874			1.1	
	20							1		40		1,116			1.1	
	20							1		20		375			0.7	
	20							1		20		422			0.7	
	20							1		20		360			0.7	
	20							1		20		350			0.7	
												1,150				
												1,720				
												700				
												15				
	60	0.5	0.4	6.1	0.3	49	2.3	4	1	300	267	1,090	455	46	4.5	4.8
	2	0.3	0.2	2	<0.1	4		0	0.7	40	321	640	95	8	1.8	0.3
	100							12		150		680			2.7	
	60	0.3	0.3	3.8	0.1	24	1.2	2	0.5	250	176	830	279	27	2.7	2.6
	0	0.1	0.1	4.9	0.2		0.2	0	0.9	9	191	360	202	16	0.7	0.7
	100	0.3	0.2	2				15		60	0	340	113		1.4	
	100	0.5	0.4	3.3	0.1	33	0.7	1	0.8	200	268	790	197	23	2.7	1.5
	40	0.3	0.2	2.8	0.1	32	0.6	0	1.6	200	197	890	286	34	1.8	0.8
	0	0.117	0	4.19	0.526	55.27	0	18	1.793	20	189.6	290	1,013	57.18	1.08	0.692

ERA, EatRight Analysis CD-ROM; **AMT,** amount; **WT,** weight; **CAL,** calories; **PROT,** protein; **CARB,** carbohydrate; **FIBR,** fiber; **FAT,** fat; **SATF,** saturated fat; **MONO,** monounsaturated fat; **POLY,** polyunsaturated fat; **CHOL,** cholesterol

ERA CODE	FOOD DESCRIPTION	AMT	UNIT	WT (g)	CAL (kcal)	PROT (g)	CARB (g)	FIBR (g)	FAT (g)	SATF (g)	MONO (g)	POLY (g)	CHOL (mg)
Fast Foods/Restaurants (continued)													
McDonald's (continued)													
2166	Frozen Yogurt Cone, Vanilla	1	ea	90	150	4	23	0	4	3			20
4732	Grill Chicken Deluxe Sand w/o Mayo	1	ea	215	340	26	45	2	7	1.5			50
69008	Hamburger	1	ea	107	280	12	35	2	10	4			30
6155	Hashbrown Potatoes	1	ea	53	130	1	14	1	8	1.5			0
45069	Hotcakes+Marg+Syrup	1	ea	228	600	9	104	0	17	3			20
47147	McDonaldland Cookies	1	ea	57	230	3	38	1	8	2			0
69011	Quarter Pounder	1	ea	172	430	23	37	2	21	8			70
69012	Quarter Pounder+Cheese	1	ea	200	530	28	38	2	30	13			95
69006	Sausage McMuffin	1	ea	112	360	13	26	1	23	8			45
19579	Scrambled Eggs, 1 svg	1	ea	102	160	13	1	0	11	3.5			425
2167	Shake, Low-Fat, Chocolate	1	ea	294.6	360	11	60	1	9	6			40
2168	Shake, Low-Fat, Strawberry	1	ea	294	360	11	60	0	9	6			40
2169	Shake, Low-Fat, Vanilla	1	ea	293.4	360	11	59	0	9	6			40
Pizza Hut													
56481	Cheese Pizza, Pan Style	1	pce	110	290	12	28	2	14	6			10
56490	Pepperoni Pizza, Hand Tossed	1	pce	116	280	13	28	2	13	6			20
56482	Pepperoni Pizza, Pan Style	1	pce	106	280	11	28	2	14	5			15
56493	Pepperoni Pizza, Personal Pan	1	ea	257	620	26	70	5	28	11			30
56486	Pepperoni Pizza, Thin/Crispy	1	pce	81	190	9	21	2	9	4			15
56483	Supreme Pizza, Pan Style	1	pce	133	320	13	29	3	17	6			20
56487	Supreme Pizza, Thin/Crispy	1	pce	117	250	12	23	2	13	6			20
Subway													
52127	Chicken Taco Salad	1	ea	370	250	18	15	2	14	5			52
69117	Club Sandwich (6-inch)	1	ea	255	320	24	46	4	6	2			35
52120	Cold Cut Salad	1	ea	316	230	14	11	3	15	6			55
69129	Meatball Sandwich (6-inch)	1	ea	287	530	24	53	6	26	10			55
52121	Pizza Salad	1	ea	335	277	12	13	2	20	8			50
52116	Seafood/Crab Salad	1	ea	314	200	9	17	4	11	3.5			25
52118	Tuna Salad	1	ea	314	240	13	10	3	16	4			40
69107	Tuna Sandwich (6-inch)	1	ea	168	330	13	36	3	16	4.5			25
69109	Veggie Sandwich (6-inch)	1	ea	166	230	9	44	4	3	1			0
Taco Bell													
56691	7 Layer Burrito	1	ea	283	530	16	66	13	23	7			25
56690	Big Beef Burrito Supreme	1	ea	298	520	24	54	11	23	10			55
56688	Chicken Burrito	1	ea	171	345	17	41		13	5			57

WTR, water; **V,** vitamin; **THI,** thiamin; **RIB,** riboflavin; **NIA,** niacin; **FOL,** folate; **CALC,** calcium; **PHOS,** phosphorus; **SOD,** sodium; **POT,** potassium; **MAG,** magnesium

WTR (g)	V-A (RE)	THI (mg)	RIB (mg)	NIA (mg)	V-B6 (mg)	FOL (g)	V-B12 (g)	V-C (mg)	V-E (mg)	CALC (mg)	PHOS (mg)	SOD (mg)	POT (mg)	MAG (mg)	IRON (mg)	ZINC (mg)
	60							1		100		75			0.4	
	40							6		200		890			2.7	
	22	0.3	0.3	3.8	0.1	21	1	2	0.2	200	111	590	258	24	2.7	2.2
	0	0.1	<0.1	0.9	0.1	8	0	2	0.6	7	51	330	212	11	0.4	0.2
	80	0.2	0.3	1.9	0.1	<1	0.3	<1	1.2	100	516	770	292	28	4.5	0.5
	0	0.2	0.2	2	<0.1			0	1	20	71	250	63	11	1.8	0.4
	20	0.4	0.3	6.8	0.2	28	2.6	2	0.4	200	208	840	408	34	4.5	4.7
	100	0.4	0.4	6.8	0.3	33	2.9	2	0.8	350		1,310			4.5	
	40	0.6	0.3	3.8	0.1	16	0.5	0	0.7	200	156	740	191	22	1.8	1.5
	150	0.1	0.5	0.1	0.1	44	1.1	0	0.9	40	172	170	126	10	1.1	1.1
	60	0.1	0.5	0.4	0.1			1		350	354	250	542		0.7	
	60	0.1	0.5	0.4	0.1			6		350	329	180	542		0.7	
	60	0.1	0.5	0.3				1		350	327	250	534		0.4	
	150							2		200		590			1.8	
	150							24		200		790			1.8	
	100							2		100		610			1.8	
	250							6		300		1,430			4.5	
	100							2.4		100		610			1.44	
	100							6		150		670			1.8	
	100							9		150		710			1.8	
	361							35		115		990			3	
	60							21		60		1,300			5.4	
	200							30		150		1,370			1.8	
	150							27		150		1,360			5.4	
	390							33		100		1,336			2	
	200							30		100		970			1.1	
	200							30		100		880			1.1	
	80							12		150		830			3.6	
	60							21		60		510			3.6	
	300							6		200		1,280			3.6	
	600							5		150		1,520			2.7	
	440							1		140		854			2.5	

SECTION 7

ERA, EatRight Analysis CD-ROM; **AMT,** amount; **WT,** weight; **CAL,** calories; **PROT,** protein; **CARB,** carbohydrate; **FIBR,** fiber; **FAT,** fat; **SATF,** saturated fat; **MONO,** monounsaturated fat; **POLY,** polyunsaturated fat; **CHOL,** cholesterol

ERA CODE	FOOD DESCRIPTION	AMT	UNIT	WT (g)	CAL (kcal)	PROT (g)	CARB (g)	FIBR (g)	FAT (g)	SATF (g)	MONO (g)	POLY (g)	CHOL (mg)
Fast Foods/Restaurants (continued)													
Taco Bell (continued)													
56689	Chicken Soft Taco	1	ea	121	200	14	21	2	7	2.5			35
45585	Cinnamon Twists, 1 svg	1	ea	28	140	1	19	0	6	0			0
56531	Mexican Pizza	1	ea	220	570	21	42	8	35	10			45
56534	Nachos Bellgrande, 1 svg	1	ea	312	770	21	84	17	39	11			35
56684	Nachos Supreme, 1 svg	1	ea	198	450	14	45	9	24	.8			30
56536	Pintos+Cheese+Red Sauce	1	ea	120	190	9	18	10	9	4			15
56526	Soft Taco Supreme	1	ea	142	260	12	23	3	14	7			35
56693	Steak Soft Taco	1	ea	128	230	15	20	2	10	2.5			25
56524	Taco	1	ea	78	180	9	12	3	10	4			25
56692	Taco Supreme	1	ea	113	220	10	14	3	14	7			35
Taco Time													
56540	Crispy Bean Burrito	1	ea	164.2	427	15	53	9	18	5			12
56541	Crispy Meat Burrito	1	ea	162.8	552	34	39	7	30	10			58
56553	Mexi, Fries, Serving	1	ea	114.2	266	3	27		17				0
56546	Natural Super Taco	1	ea	312.4	609	40	58	14	26	12.6			80
56544	Soft Combo Burrito	1	ea	272	617	39	66	18	23	10			63
Wendy's													
56571	Bacon Cheeseburger	1	ea	165	380	20	34	2	18	7			55
56574	Big Classic Burger+Cheese	1	ea	282	570	34	46	3	29	12			100
2177	Frosty Dairy Dessert, Medium	1	ea	298	440	11	73	0	11	7			50
69059	Grilled Chicken Sandwich	1	ea	188	300	24	36	2	7	1.5			55
69058	Junior Cheeseburger Deluxe	1	ea	179	350	17	37	2	16	6			45
69057	Junior Hamburger	1	ea	117	270	14	34	2	9	3			30
56566	Single Burger, Deluxe	1	ea	218	410	24	37	2	19	7			70

WTR, water; **V,** vitamin; **THI,** thiamin; **RIB,** riboflavin; **NIA,** niacin; **FOL,** folate; **CALC,** calcium; **PHOS,** phosphorus; **SOD,** sodium; **POT,** potassium; **MAG,** magnesium

WTR (g)	V-A (RE)	THI (mg)	RIB (mg)	NIA (mg)	V-B6 (mg)	FOL (g)	V-B12 (g)	V-C (mg)	V-E (mg)	CALC (mg)	PHOS (mg)	SOD (mg)	POT (mg)	MAG (mg)	IRON (mg)	ZINC (mg)
	60							1		80		540			0.7	
	40	0.1	<0.1	0.6	<0.1			0		0		190	22		0.4	
	400	0.3	0.3	2.9	1.1	59		5		250		1,040	403	79	3.6	5.3
	150	0.1	0.4	2.4				4		200		1,310	733		3.6	
	100-							4		150		810			2.7	
	500	0.1	0.1	0.4	0.2	64	0	0		150		650	360	103	1.8	2
	150							4		100		590			1.8	
	40							0		80		1,020			1.4	
	100	0.1	0.1	1.2	0.1			0		8		350	159		1.1	
	150							0		100		350			1.1	
	26	0.4	0.2	2.2	0.4	14				158	238	453	383		4.4	2.2
	60	0.3	0.4	5.5	0.4	74		2		197	276	1,000	506		4.4	4.4
	0	0.1	<0.1	0.9			0	4		11	40	799	277		0.9	
186	166	0.5	0.5	5.5	0.6	82		6		331	457	889	827		7.7	5.5
	116	0.5	0.5	5.3	0.6	75		5		292	418	1,343	760		7.5	5.3
	80							9		150		890	320		3.6	
	150							15		200		1,460	580		5.4	
	200							0		400		260	770		1.4	
	40							9		80		740	430		2.7	
	100							9		150		890	320		3.6	
	20							4		100		600	220		3.6	
	60							9		100		890	440		5.4	

Appendix O: Fat Sources

Table O-1 Saturated Fat, Total Fat, Cholesterol, and Omega-3 Content of Meat, Fish, and Poultry in 3-Ounce Portions Cooked Without Added Fat

Source	Saturated Fat g/3 oz.	Total Fat g/3 oz.	Cholesterol mg/3 oz.	Omega-3 g/3 oz.
Lean Red Meats				
Beef (rump roast, shank, bottom round, sirloin)	1.4	4.2	71	
Lamb (shank roast, sirloin roast, shoulder roast, loin chops, sirloin chops, center leg chop)	2.8	7.8	78	
Pork (sirloin cutlet, loin roast, sirloin roast, center roast, butterfly chops, loin chops)	3.0	8.6	71	
Veal (blade roast, sirloin chops, shoulder roast, loin chops, rump roast, shank)	2.0	4.9	93	
Organ Meats				
Liver				
Beef	1.6	4.2	331	
Calf	2.2	5.9	477	
Chicken	1.6	4.6	537	
Sweetbread	7.3	21.3	250	
Kidney	0.9	2.9	329	
Brains	2.5	10.7	1,747	
Heart	1.4	4.8	164	

Table O-1 Saturated Fat, Total Fat, Cholesterol, and Omega-3 Content of Meat, Fish, and Poultry in 3-Ounce Portions Cooked Without Added Fat—*continued*

Source	Saturated Fat g/3 oz.	Total Fat g/3 oz.	Cholesterol mg/3 oz.	Omega-3 g/3 oz.
Poultry				
Chicken (without skin)				
Light (roasted)	1.1	3.8	72	
Dark (roasted)	2.3	8.3	71	
Turkey (without skin)				
Light (roasted)	0.9	2.7	59	
Dark (roasted)	2.0	6.1	72	
Fish				
Haddock	0.1	0.8	63	0.22
Flounder	0.3	1.3	58	0.47
Salmon	1.7	7.0	54	1.88
Tuna, light, canned in water	0.2	0.7	25	0.24
Shellfish				
Crustaceans				
Lobster	0.1	0.5	61	0.07
Crab meat				
Alaskan King Crab	0.1	1.3	45	0.38
Blue Crab	0.2	1.5	85	0.45
Shrimp	0.2	0.9	166	0.28
Mollusks				
Abalone	0.3	1.3	144	0.15
Clams	0.2	1.7	57	0.33
Mussels	0.7	3.8	48	0.70
Oysters	1.3	4.2	93	1.06
Scallops	0.1	1.2	56	0.36
Squid	0.6	2.4	400	0.84

Source: Dietary Guidelines for Americans. 2000. Washington, DC: USDA.

Appendix P: Food Labels

Prepared by Karlyn Grimes, MS, RD

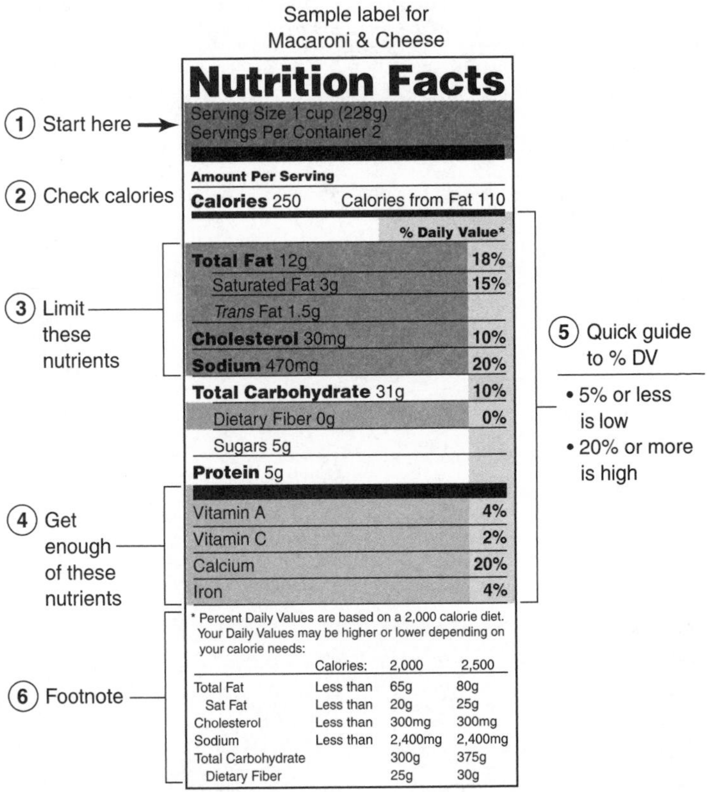

Figure P-1 Sample label for Macaroni & Cheese. *Source:* U.S. Food and Drug Administration. http://www.cfsan.fda.gov/~dms/foodlab.html.

① **Table P-1** Serving Size and Servings per Container

Description	Comments
✓ ***Serving Sizes*** are presented in both common household units—cups, tablespoons, 1 piece—followed by metric units (grams or milliliters). A ***Serving Size*** represents the amounts that individuals typically eat, allowing for comparison of foods within a food category. ✓ ***Servings Per Container*** indicate the number of servings per package, box, can, or other unit.	✓ Instruct individuals to pay close attention to how many servings are contained in a package so they can compare it to how much they typically eat. ✓ ***For Example:*** If an individual eats 2 cups of macaroni and cheese, they must multiply all of the nutrients listed between total fat and protein by two, and do the same for the percentages listed next to the four vitamins and minerals represented on the label—vitamin A, vitamin C, calcium, and iron.

② **Table P-2** Calories and Calories from Fat

Description	Comments
✓ ***Calories*** represent the total food energy provided per serving. ✓ ***Calories from Fat*** indicate the number of total calories that come exclusively from fat.	✓ Educate individuals to monitor their calorie intake to ensure they meet, but do not exceed, their daily energy requirements. Link excess calories to overweight and obesity. ✓ ***General Guide to Calories (based on a 2,000 calorie diet):*** • 40 calories is low • 100 calories is moderate • 400 calories is high

③ **Table P-3** Limit These Nutrients

Description	Comments
✓ ***Total Fat, Saturated Fat, Trans Fat, Cholesterol,*** and ***Sodium*** are the nutrients that Americans tend to receive in adequate or excessive quantities. Eating too much of these nutrients is linked to various chronic diseases such as heart disease, diabetes, and certain cancers.	✓ Reputable health authorities recommend that individuals keep their intake of saturated fat, trans fat, and cholesterol as low as possible to promote an optimal health profile. ✓ ***Daily Values (DV) for Food Labels (based on a 2,000 calorie diet):*** • *Total Fat*: 65 grams (30% of total calories) • *Saturated Fat*: 20 grams (10% of total calories) • *Trans Fat*: Not established, but was required on all food labels starting in January, 2006. • *Cholesterol*: 300 mg • *Sodium*: 2,400 mg

④ **Table P-4** Get Enough of These

Description	Comments
✓ Studies show that Americans generally receive inadequate amounts of ***Dietary Fiber, Vitamin A, Vitamin C, Calcium,*** and ***Iron*** in their diets, prompting the FDA to include this data up front and center on the Nutrition Facts Food Label.	✓ Encourage individuals to get at least 100% of the DV for each of these nutrients on a daily basis, preferably from foods rather than supplements. ✓ ***Daily Values for Food Labels:*** • *Fiber*: 25 grams or 11.5 grams per 1,000 calories consumed • *Vitamin A*: 5,000 IU (regardless of calorie intake) • *Vitamin C*: 60 mg (regardless of calorie intake) • *Calcium*: 1,000 mg (regardless of calorie intake) • *Iron*: 18 mg (regardless of calorie intake)

⑤ Table P-5 The Percent Daily Value (% DV)

Description	Comments
✓ The ***Percent Daily Value (%DV)*** is based on a 2,000 calorie diet and indicates whether a given food provides significant or insignificant amounts of a given nutrient. ✓ For an individual following a 2,000 calorie diet, the %DV for the foods and beverages consumed should add up to 100%. Some individuals require fewer than 2,000 calories a day so they should aim for less than or equal to 80% of the DV while others need more calories and should strive for 120% plus of the DV. ✓ In general, ***5%DV or less is low*** and ***20%DV or more is high*** for all the nutrients listed on the Nutrition Facts panel.	✓ There is no DV for trans fats, sugars, and protein. • ***Trans Fats:*** Fats linked with raising LDL ("**L**ethal") blood cholesterol levels, which increase your risk of coronary heart disease. Information about trans fats is insufficient to establish a DV. • ***Sugars:*** Sugars listed on the food label include naturally occurring (like those in fruits and milk) *and* added sugars. The primary recommendation established for sugars is to limit *added* sugars to 25% or less of total daily calories, but no DV is currently listed on the Nutrition Facts panel. • ***Protein:*** A %DV is only required when a claim is made with regard to a food's protein content or the food is marketed for infants and children under 4 years old. Approximately 50 grams or 10% of total daily calories is recommended for a 2,000 calorie diet.

SECTION 7

⑥ **Table P-6** Footnotes	
Description	**Comments**
✓ The asterisk (*) that follows the *% Daily Value* below the *Calories from Fat* statement refers to the footnote in the lower part of the nutrition label indicating that the %DV used on the label is based on a 2,000 calorie diet. ✓ The ***footnote*** provides specific guidelines for six key nutrients based on a 2,000 and 2,500 calorie diet.	✓ The full footnote is not required on small labels, but when it appears, it always contains the same information. ✓ Note how the cholesterol and sodium recommendations remain the same regardless of energy intake (calories) whereas total fat, saturated fat, total carbohydrate, and dietary fiber vary with total calorie intake. ✓ Generally below the footnotes, you will find the ingredients listed in descending order of predominance by weight.

Table P-7 Dissecting the Nutrition Facts Food Label	
Energy Terms	
Descriptive Term	**Legal Definition**
Calorie-free	✓ Less than 5 calories per reference amount and per labeled serving
Low-calorie	✓ 40 calories or less per reference amount ✓ *Meals and Main Dishes*: 120 calories or less per 100 gram serving
Reduced/Less calorie(s)	✓ At least 25% fewer calories per reference amount than an appropriate reference food

Table P-7 Dissecting the Nutrition Facts Food Label—*continued*

Fat Terms All Food Products, Excluding Meats, Poultry, Seafood, and Game Meats	
Descriptive Term	**Legal Definition**
Fat-free	✓ Less than 0.5 grams of fat per reference amount and per labeled serving ✓ *Meals and Main Dishes*: less than 0.5 grams of fat per labeled serving
Low-fat	✓ 3 grams of fat or less per reference amount ✓ *Meals and Main Dishes*: 3 grams of fat or less per 100 gram serving and not more than 30% of calories from fat
Reduced/Less fat	✓ At least 25% less fat per reference amount than an appropriate reference food
Percent fat-free	✓ Must satisfy the legal definition for low-fat
Saturated fat-free	✓ Less than 0.5 grams saturated fat and less than 0.5 grams trans fatty acids per reference amount and per labeled serving ✓ *Meals and Main Dishes*: less than 0.5 grams saturated fat and less than 0.5 grams trans fatty acids per labeled serving
Low-saturated fat	✓ 1 gram or less of saturated fat per reference amount and 15% or less of calories from saturated fat ✓ *Meals and Main Dishes*: 1 gram or less of saturated fat per 100 gram serving and less than 10% of calories from saturated fat
Reduced/Less saturated fat	✓ At least 25% less saturated fat per reference amount than an appropriate reference food
Trans-fat free	✓ Less than 0.5 grams of trans fat and less than 0.5 grams of saturated fat per serving
Fat Terms Meat, Poultry, Seafood, and Game Meats	
Descriptive Term	**Legal Definition**
Extra Lean	✓ On meat, poultry, seafood, and game meats that contain less than 5 g total fat, less than 2 g saturated fat, and less than 95 mg cholesterol per reference amount and per 100 g serving ✓ *Meals and Main Dishes*: meets criteria per 100 g and per labeled serving

continues

Table P-7 Dissecting the Nutrition Facts Food Label—*continued*

Descriptive Term	Legal Definition
Lean	✓ On meat, poultry, seafood, and game meats that contain less than 10 g total fat, 4.5 g or less saturated fat, and less than 95 mg cholesterol per reference amount and per 100 g ✓ *Meals and Main Dishes*: meets criteria per 100 g serving and per labeled serving
	Cholesterol Terms
Descriptive Term	**Legal Definition**
Cholesterol-free	✓ Less than 2 mg of cholesterol per reference amount and per labeled serving ✓ *Meals and Main Dishes*: less than 2 mg of cholesterol per labeled serving
Low-cholesterol	✓ 20 mg or less of cholesterol per reference amount ✓ *Meals and Main Dishes*: 20 mg of cholesterol or less per 100 g serving
Reduced or less cholesterol	✓ At least 25% less cholesterol per reference amount than an appropriate reference food
	Fiber Terms
Descriptive Term	**Legal Definition**
High-fiber	✓ 5 g of fiber or more per serving
Good source of fiber	✓ 2.5 g to 4.9 g of fiber per serving
More or added fiber	✓ At least 2.5 g more fiber per serving than an appropriate reference food
	Sodium Terms
Descriptive Term	**Legal Definition**
Sodium-free	✓ Less than 5 mg of sodium per reference amount and per labeled serving ✓ *Meals and Main Dishes*: less than 5 mg per labeled serving
Very-low-sodium	✓ 35 mg or less per reference amount ✓ *Meals and Main Dishes*: 35 mg or less per 100 g serving
Low-sodium	✓ 140 mg of sodium or less per reference amount ✓ *Meals and Main Dishes*: 140 mg or less per 100 g serving

Table P-7 Dissecting the Nutrition Facts Food Label—*continued*

Descriptive Term	Legal Definition
Reduced sodium	✓ At least 25% less sodium per reference amount than an appropriate reference food
Other Terms	
Descriptive Term	**Legal Definition**
Fresh	✓ A raw food that has not been frozen, heat processed, or otherwise preserved
Good source	✓ 10–19% of the Daily Value per serving
Healthy	✓ Low in fat, saturated fat, trans fat, cholesterol, and sodium, and containing at least 10% of the Daily Value for vitamin A, vitamin C, iron, calcium, protein, or fiber
High in	✓ 20% or more of the Daily Value for a given nutrient per serving
Light	✓ One-third fewer calories or 50% less fat ✓ *Meals and Main Dishes*: contains at least 50% less fat (low-fat) or one-third fewer calories (low-calorie) than a reference 100 gram serving and per labeled serving
More, extra	✓ At least 10% more of the Daily Value than a reference food

Source: U.S. Food and Drug Administration Center for Food Safety and Applied Nutrition http://www.cfsan.fda.gov/~dms/flg-6a.html.

Table P-8 Health Claims

Food and beverage manufacturers can make claims on food labels linking nutrients with disease states. The FDA maintains a ranking system, which assigns the letters **A** through **D** to health claims allowed on food labels. Health claims that receive an **A** possess a high level of confidence based on scientific evidence. At the other extreme, those health claims ranked as a **D** have very little scientific evidence to support the claim. A statement indicating the degree of scientific evidence supporting the claim must accompany **B, C,** and **D** claims, but not **A** claims because they have better scientific backing.

A Guide to Grade A Health Claims

- ✓ Adequate calcium intake and a reduced risk of osteoporosis
- ✓ A diet low in sodium and a reduced risk of hypertension
- ✓ A diet low in saturated fat and cholesterol and reduced risk of coronary heart disease
- ✓ A diet low in dietary fat intake and reduced risk of cancer
- ✓ A diet high in fiber-containing grain products, fruits, and vegetables and a reduced risk of cancer
- ✓ A diet high in fruits, vegetables, and grain products that contain fiber, particularly soluble fiber, and reduced risk of coronary heart disease
- ✓ Low-fat diets rich in fruits and vegetables, and a reduced risk of cancer
- ✓ Healthful diets with adequate folate and a reduced risk of neural tube defects
- ✓ A diet focusing on sugar alcohols versus regular sugars and starches and a reduced risk of dental caries
- ✓ Soluble fiber from oat bran, rolled oats (or oatmeal), whole oat flour, or psyllium seed husk and a reduced risk of coronary heart disease
- ✓ Soy protein as part of a diet low in saturated fat and cholesterol and a reduced risk of heart disease
- ✓ Plant sterol–stanol esters and a reduced risk of coronary heart disease
- ✓ A diet rich in whole-grain foods and a reduced risk of heart disease and certain cancers
- ✓ Diets high in potassium and low in sodium and a reduced risk of high blood pressure and stroke

Appendix Q: Foodborne Illness

Author: Elizabeth Scott, PhD

This list will assist the dietitian in understanding the common causes and symptoms of foodborne illness and offer information on how to prevent the acquisition and transmission of illness. Those most vulnerable to foodborne illness include children under five, seniors over 65, pregnant women, and other immuno-compromised/suppressed individuals. The illnesses listed are those commonly seen in the United States.

Preventing cross-contamination in the kitchen is a universal precaution for reducing the risk of foodborne illness. Prevention methods include keeping raw meat and poultry separate from other foods, sanitizing work surfaces after contact with raw meat, and thorough hand washing after handling all raw foods. Avoid hand-to-mouth contact while handling raw foods and do not taste raw foods of animal origin—poultry, meats, and eggs. Cook all foods of animal origin (meat, fish, and eggs) to a minimum internal temperature of 160°F for 15 seconds. Cook poultry to a minimum internal temperature of 165°F for 15 seconds. This can be best measured with an instant-read thermometer or by the following observations: cook fish until the flesh flakes with a fork; cook eggs and egg dishes until the yolks and whites are firm; cook all meats until the juices run clear and the meat is not pink or raw when cut open.

Additional advice is listed under the **Prevention** column.

Table Q-1 Common Foodborne Illnesses

Disease Agent (and Name of Disease)	Symptoms	Length of Illness	Complications	Common Sources of the Pathogen	Prevention
BACTERIA					
Campylobacter jejuni (campylobacteriosis)	•Mild to severe diarrhea, stomach pains, fever, and nausea, usually 1–10 days after exposure •Blood may be seen in feces •Vomiting less common •Can mimic appendicitis	•Usually lasts from 2–5 days and rarely more than 10 days •May be more severe and last longer in adults	•Complications include arthritis, Guillain-Barré syndrome, and meningitis	•Raw or undercooked poultry, beef, pork, shellfish, untreated milk, and water •Contact with infected cats, dogs, birds, human, and animal feces	•Prevent cross-contamination. •Ensure thorough cooking. •Do not put hands to mouth while handling meat. •Keep pets off kitchen counters and wash hands after contact with animals.
E.coli O157:H7 (Hamburger disease)	•Mild to severe bloody diarrhea, usually 2–5 days after exposure	•Usually up to 8 days	•Neurological symptoms, stroke, and hemolytic uremic syndrome (HUS), which can cause kidney failure and death, especially in young children	•Undercooked ground beef products, untreated milk, juices and any food or water contaminated with cow feces •Person-to-person spread can occur	•Thoroughly cook beef products, especially hamburgers. •Prevent cross-contamination. •Wash hands after handling ground beef. •Do not put hands to mouth.
Salmonella (salmonellosis)	•Mild to severe diarrhea, vomiting, and fever, for usually	•Usually lasts from 1–7 days	•Septicemia, meningitis, and joint infections	•Raw or undercooked poultry and other meats, eggs,	•Prevent cross-contamination. •Thorough cooking.

	6–72 hours after exposure	•May be more severe in the young, elderly, and immunocompromised •Some individuals may excrete the pathogen for many weeks after symptoms have stopped and can act as a source of the disease.		and untreated milk •Also foods as diverse as chocolate and bean sprouts •Contact with infected pets: reptiles, dogs, and cats •Person-to-person spread can occur as well as transmission by contact with contaminated environmental surfaces.	•Cool and refrigerate foods within 2 hours of cooking. •Handle raw eggs carefully and avoid foods containing raw egg. •Keep pets out of kitchen and wash hands after handling pets. •Do not clean out animal tanks at kitchen sink. •Keep young children away from dogs and cats suffering from diarrhea. •Decontaminate environmental surfaces such as floors when sick pets are present.
Listeria monocytogenes (listeriosis)	•Can range from mild flu-like illness to meningitis, from 2–30 days after consumption	•Varies according to the severity of the symptoms	•Damage to heart muscle, internal abscesses, septicemia, meningitis, fetal damage, and abortion	•Untreated milk, soft cheeses, pate, seafood products, frozen cooked crabmeat, cooked shrimp, and packaged salad vegetables	•Prevent cross-contamination. •Thoroughly wash fresh vegetables, salads, and prepackaged salads.

continues

Table Q-1 Common Foodborne Illnesses—*continued*

Disease Agent (and Name of Disease)	Symptoms	Length of Illness	Complications	Common Sources of the Pathogen	Prevention
			•Pregnant women and their fetuses and those with depressed immunity are at most risk of serious illness		•Vulnerable individuals should avoid high-risk foods.
Shigella (shigellosis or bacillary dysentery)	•Diarrhea, fever, nausea, vomiting, and stomach cramps, 1–7 days after consumption •Blood and mucus may be seen in stools.	•Varies with age, nutritional status, and species of Shigella •Most feel better within 4–7days, if no complications	•Convulsions in young children and possibility of kidney failure	•Food or drink contaminated with human feces •Contact with contaminated environmental surfaces •Contact with infected individuals	•High standards of personal hygiene, special attention to hand washing. •Infected individuals should not prepare food. •Decontaminate environmental surfaces in the bathroom when sick individuals are present.
Staphylococcus aureus (staphylococcal food poisoning) A toxin produced in the food causes illness.	•Diarrhea, vomiting, nausea, stomach pain, and cramps, within 30 minutes to 8 hours	•Symptoms usually last for 1-2 days. •Symptoms can be very intense and result in admission to hospital.	•Rare	Nose, throat, and skin of healthy carriers •Septic spots and wounds	•Minimize hand contact with foods and ensure that all skin wounds and sores are covered

				•Foods that require a lot of handling in their preparation such as sandwiches, cream-filled pastries, cold cuts, pasta, tuna-potato salads, and other foods left out of the refrigerator	with a waterproof dressing. •Do not allow foods to stay at room temperature for more than 2 hours (either keep food hot or cool and refrigerate). •Cooking may not destroy the toxin.
Clostridium botulinum (botulism) Illness is caused by a toxin produced in the food.	•Symptoms of nerve dysfunction, such as blurred or double vision, difficulty in swallowing, and also vomiting, diarrhea, or constipation usually occur within 18–36 hours. •Can occur from within 4 hours to 10 days. •Later symptoms include paralysis.	•Symptoms are severe. •Death occurs in 5–10% of cases. •Most common in communities that preserve foods at home.	•Recovery can take many months.	•Improperly canned and bottled foods, such as canned vegetables, tuna, soups, and liver pate •Also, smoked and salted meats and fish, sausage, and garlic in oil •Improperly handled baked potatoes wrapped in foil •Especially home-preserved foods	•Careful home canning and bottling procedures following instructions •Discard any cans or bottles (commercial or home-produced) that show signs of damage, dents, or distortion.
VIRUSES					
Hepatitis A	•Onset of first symptoms usually 4–6 weeks after exposure	•Weeks to months depending on severity of illness	•Rarely, liver damage and death in severe cases •Severity increases with age.	•Raw shellfish from sewage-polluted water •Contaminated raw fruit and vegetables	•Attention to personal hygiene and sanitation of kitchen surfaces

continues

Table Q-1 Common Foodborne Illnesses—*continued*

Disease Agent (and Name of Disease)	Symptoms	Length of Illness	Complications	Common Sources of the Pathogen	Prevention
	•Early symptoms include malaise, fever, nausea, vomiting, and lack of appetite. •Followed 3–10 days later by jaundice and darkened urine			•Any food handled by an infected handler •Fecal-oral transmission from person to person	•Infected individuals should avoid food handling. •Shellfish should be steamed at 194°F.
Calcivirus or Norovirus	•Acute onset of diarrhea, nausea, vomiting, stomach pains, headache, and mild fever occur within 1 to 3 days.	•Usually 24–48 hours	•Rare	•Raw shellfish from sewage-polluted water •Ready-to-eat foods such as sandwiches and salads that have been handled by an infected person •Also, possible airborne transmission as a result of projectile vomiting and via contact with contaminated environmental surfaces	•Attention to personal hygiene and sanitation of surfaces, especially when individuals with diarrhea and vomiting are present •Shellfish should be steamed for a minimum of 4 minutes at 194°F.

PROTOZOA *Cyclospora cayetanensis*	•Watery stools, nausea, stomach pain, fatigue, and weight loss	•Several days to many weeks	•Diarrhea can last for months in immuno-depressed individuals.	•Contaminated drinking or swimming water •Foods that have been in contact with contaminated water such as fruit, especially berries and vegetables	-Attention to personal hygiene for infected individuals -Infected individuals should avoid handling foods that will not be cooked before eating. -Avoid untreated drinking water, especially in undeveloped regions.
Cryptosporidium (cryptosporidiosis)	•Profuse watery stools, stomach pain, loss of appetite, nausea, and vomiting occur within 1 to 14 days of infection.	•Usually up to 21 days	•Illness can be mild to very severe and death can occur in immuno-depressed individuals.	•Fecal-oral route, including person-to-person, waterborne, and foodborne	-Attention to personal hygiene for infected individuals -Infected individuals should avoid handling foods that will not be cooked before eating. -Boil contaminated drinking water for at least 1 minute.
Giardia lamblia (giardiasis)	•Diarrhea, stomach cramp, bloating, fatigue, or weight loss within 5 days to 3 weeks of infection	•Weeks to months	•Severe infection, damage to digestive tract, arthritis	•Fecal-oral route, including person-to-person, and waterborne	-Attention to personal hygiene -Boil contaminated drinking water.

continues

Table Q-1 Common Foodborne Illnesses—*continued*

Disease Agent (and Name of Disease)	Symptoms	Length of Illness	Complications	Common Sources of the Pathogen	Prevention
Toxoplasma gondii (toxoplasmosis)	•Flu-like symptoms, rash, diarrhea within 10–13 days	•Weeks to months	•Miscarriage, stillbirth, severe birth defects including epilepsy, mental retardation, retinitis •Immuno-deficient individuals: confusion, weakness, paralysis, seizures, coma	•Raw or undercooked meats and unwashed fruit and vegetables •Contact with cat feces	•Thorough cooking of meat products, wash raw fruit and vegetables •Pregnant women should avoid handling contaminated cat litter.

Sources:
Foodborne Diseases. NIAID Fact Sheet. www.niaid.nih.gov/factsheets/foodbornedis.htm.
Insel, P.M., Turner, R.E., Ross, D. *Discovering Nutrition*. Sudbury, MA: Jones and Bartlett Publishers. 2003.
Nester, E.W., Anderson, D.G., Roberts, C.E., Pearsall, N.N., Nester, M.T. *Microbiology: A Human Perspective* (4th ed) New York, NY: McGraw-Hill. 2004.
Scott, E., Sockett, P. *How to Prevent Food Poisoning. A Practical Guide to Safe Cooking, Eating, and Food Handling*. New York, NY: John Wiley & Sons. 1998.

Other Sources:
Call the **U.S. Food and Drug Administration Food Information Line** at: 1-888-SAFE FOOD for more information regarding food safety.

Appendix R: Glycemic Indexes for Foods

The table below shows values of the Glycemic Index (GI) and Glycemic Load (GL) for a few common foods. GIs of 55 or below are considered low, and 70 or above are considered high. GLs of 10 or below are considered low, and 20 or above are considered high.

Table R-1 GI and GL for Common Foods

Food	GI	Serving Size	Net Carbs	GL
Peanuts	14	4 oz. (113 g)	15	2
Bean sprouts	25	1 cup (104 g)	4	1
Grapefruit	25	½ large (166 g)	11	3
Pizza	30	2 slices (260 g)	42	13
Low-fat yogurt	33	1 cup (245 g)	47	16
Apples	38	1 medium (138 g)	16	6
Spaghetti	42	1 cup (140 g)	38	16
Carrots	47	1 large (72 g)	5	2
Oranges	48	1 medium (131 g)	12	6
Bananas	52	1 large (136 g)	27	14
Potato chips	54	4 oz. (114 g)	55	30
Snickers bar	55	1 bar (113 g)	64	35
Brown rice	55	1 cup (195 g)	42	23
Honey	55	1 Tbsp (21 g)	17	9
Oatmeal	58	1 cup (234 g)	21	12
Ice cream	61	1 cup (72 g)	16	10
Macaroni and cheese	64	1 serving (166 g)	47	30
Raisins	64	1 small box (43 g)	32	20
White rice	64	1 cup (186 g)	52	33
Sugar (sucrose)	68	1 Tbsp (12 g)	12	8
White bread	70	1 slice (30 g)	14	10
Watermelon	72	1 cup (154 g)	11	8
Popcorn	72	2 cups (16 g)	10	7
Baked potato	85	1 medium (173 g)	33	28
Glucose	100	(50 g)	50	50

Data courtesy of: nutritiondata.com

Appendix S: Growth Charts

NAME ______________________

Weight-for-stature percentiles: Boys

RECORD # ____________

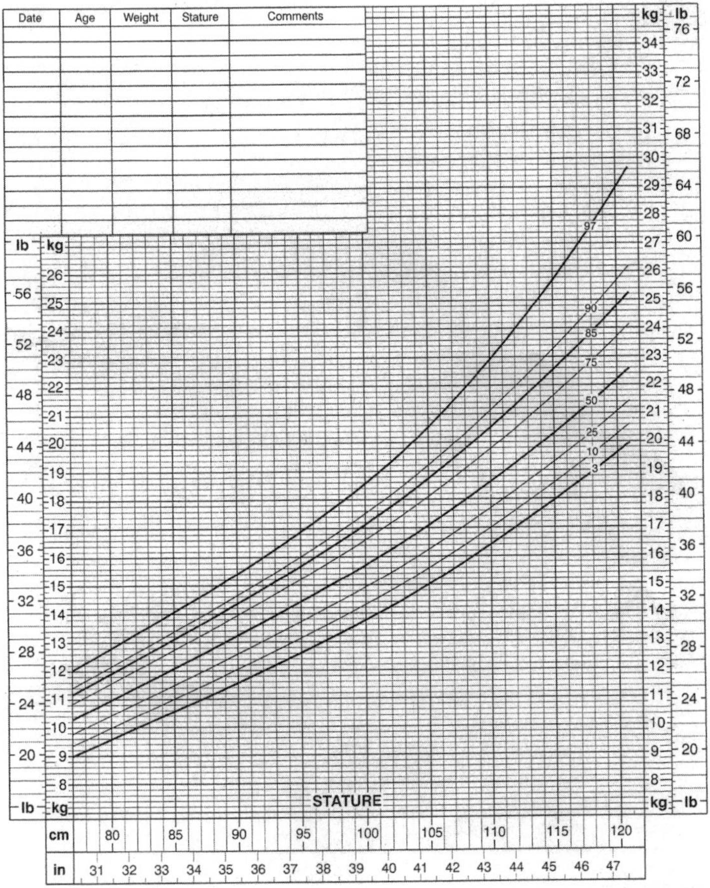

Published May 30, 2000 (modified 10/16/00).
SOURCE: Developed by the National Center for Health Statistics in collaboration with the National Center for Chronic Disease Prevention and Health Promotion (2000).
http://www.cdc.gov/growthcharts

SAFER · HEALTHIER · PEOPLE

NAME ______________________

Weight-for-stature percentiles: Girls

RECORD # ____________

Date	Age	Weight	Stature	Comments

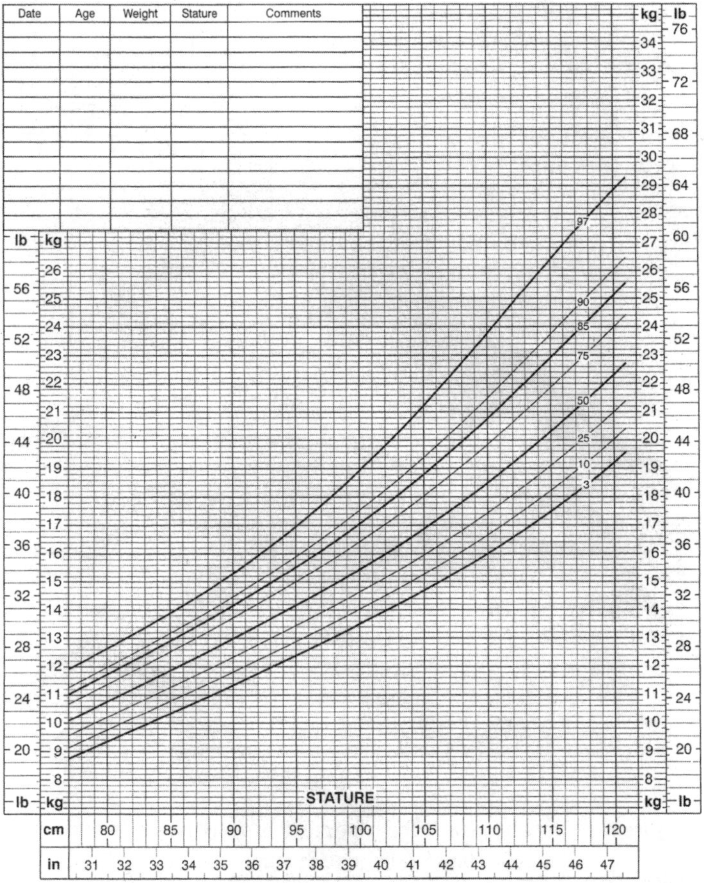

Published May 30, 2000 (modified 10/16/00).
SOURCE: Developed by the National Center for Health Statistics in collaboration with the National Center for Chronic Disease Prevention and Health Promotion (2000).
http://www.cdc.gov/growthcharts

CDC
SAFER • HEALTHIER • PEOPLE

SECTION 7

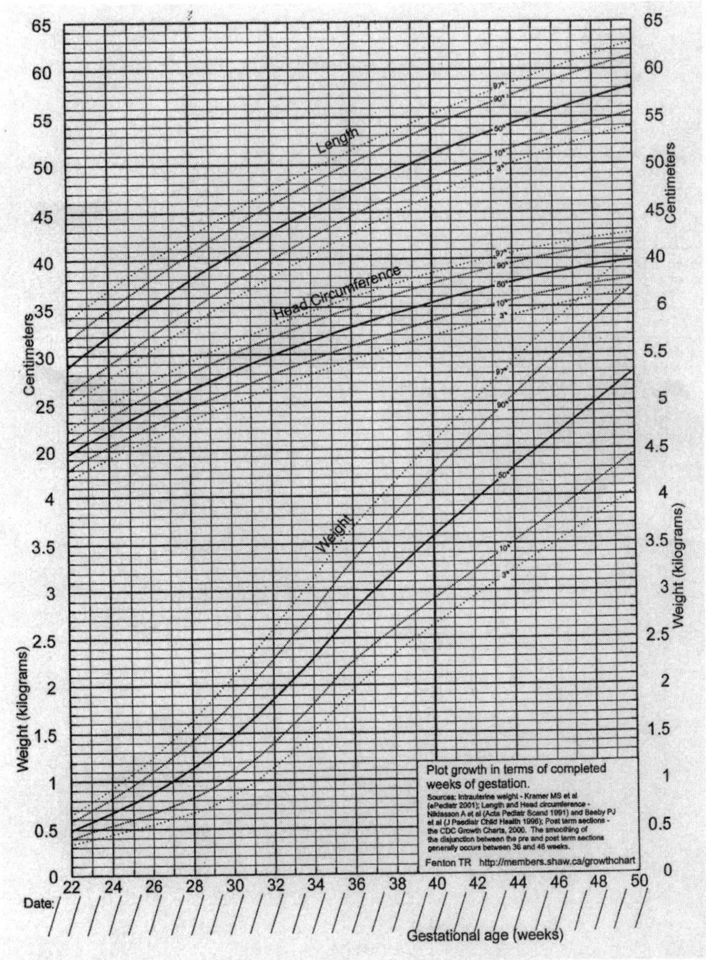

Figure S-1 A new growth chart for preterm babies: Babson and Benda's chart updated with recent data and a new format. *Pediatrics* (2003;3:13).

Appendix T: Heimlich Maneuver

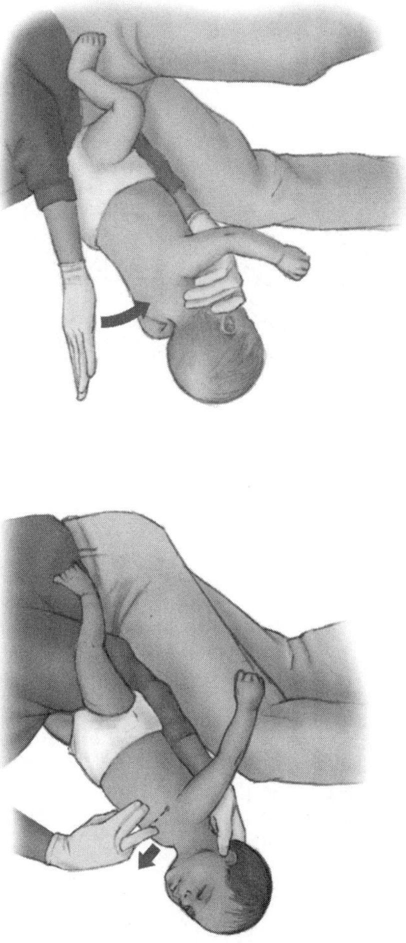

The key difference is to use less force with a child. With an infant, use gravity and back blows and chest thrusts (with fingers only), not abdominal thrusts.

1.

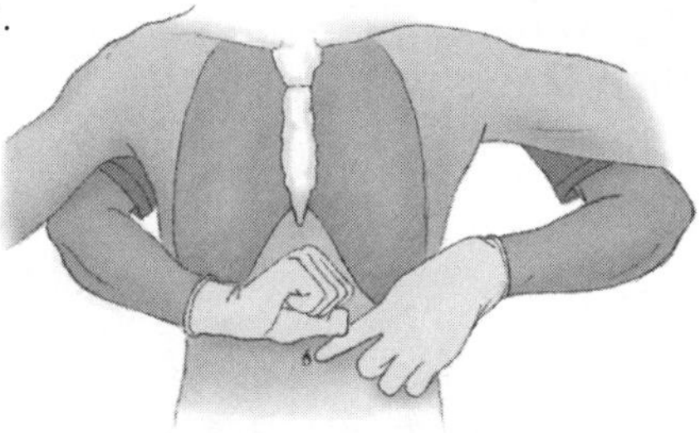

1. Tuck thumb into fist.

2.

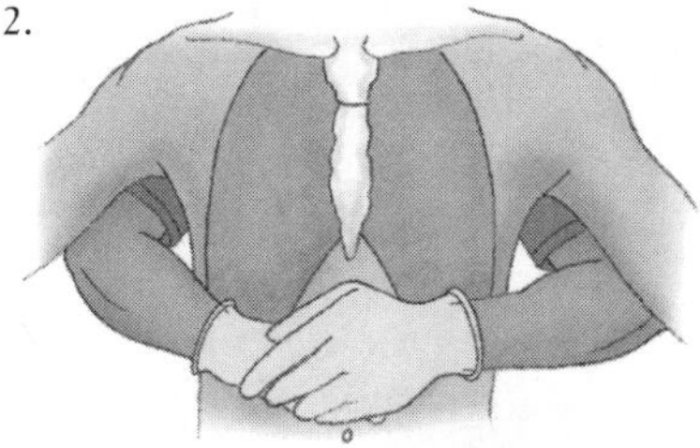

2. Place thumb side of fist against abdomen (midline below diaphragm). Cover fist with other hand.

3.

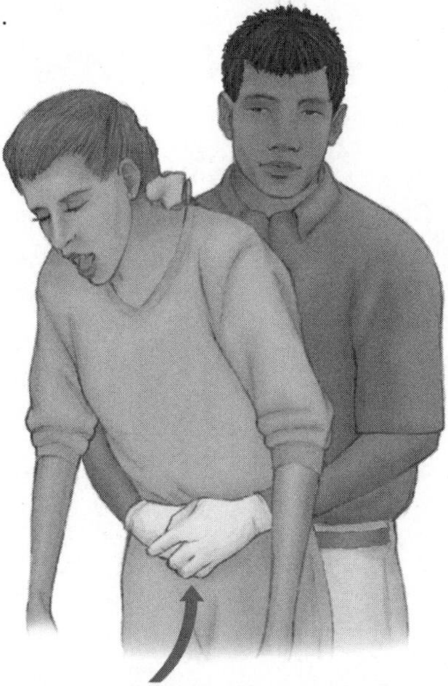

3. Thrust up and in toward diaphragm.

Appendix U: Herb Guide

Table U-1 Common Herbal Remedies

HERB Common and Latin Names	TRADITIONAL USAGE Internal and External Uses	Contraindications/ Precautions
Aloe (*Aloe vera*)	External use: wound healing, minor skin irritation, burns	Not recommended internally for pediatrics
Anise (*Pimpinella anisum*)	Internal use: common colds, coughs, bronchitis, indigestion	Rare allergic reactions to anise and its constituent anethole
Bilberry (*Vaccinium myrtillus*)	Internal use: diarrhea	None known
Calendula flowers (*Calendula officinalis*)	Internal use: inflammation of mouth and pharynx External use: wounds and burns	Rare allergic reactions through frequent skin contact
Catnip (*Nepeta cataria*)	Internal use: nervous disorders, sleep aid, common colds, colic	None known
Chamomile flowers (*Matricaria ehamomilla*)	Internal use: carminative, sleep aid External use: inflammation and irritations of the skin, wounds, burns	Rare allergic reactions
Cherry bark (*Prunus sp.*)	Internal use: coughs, common colds	None known
Comfrey leaf (*Symphytum officinale*)	External use: minor wounds, ulcers, inflammations, bruises, and sprains. Used as poultice for skin disorder	Not to be taken internally. Internal use promotes hepatotoxic effects.
Echinacea (*Echinacea angustifolia*) (*Echinacea purpurea*)	Internal use: common colds, flu, coughs, bronchitis, fever, immune stimulant External use: wounds, burns	Allergic reactions may occur with some individuals. Not recommended for individuals with autoimmune diseases

continues

SECTION 7

Table U-1 Common Herbal Remedies—*continued*

HERB Common and Latin Names	TRADITIONAL USAGE Internal and External Uses	Contraindications/ Precautions
Elder flowers (*Sambucus nigra*)	Internal use: common colds, antiviral, diaphoretic	None known
Eucalyptus (*Eucalyptus globulus*)	Internal use: expectorant, coughs, congestion of the respiratory tract	Nausea, vomiting, and diarrhea may occur after ingestion in rare cases. Eucalyptus preparations should not be applied to the face or nose of infants and very young children.
Fennel Seed (*Foeniculum vulgare*)	Internal use: carminative, indigestion, coughs, bronchitis, gastrointestinal afflictions	Allergic reactions may occur with some individuals.
Garlic (*Allium sativum*)	Internal use: common colds, bronchitis, fever External use: antibacterial, antifungal, ear infections	Intake of large quantities can lead to stomach complaints. Rare allergic reactions
Ginger (*Zingiber officinale*)	Internal use: carminative, antinausea, indigestion	None known
Goldenseal (*Hydrastis canadensis*)	Internal use: common colds, flu, inflammation of mucous membranes External use: antiseptic, antimicrobial, cuts, wounds, ear infections	Internal use can cause nausea, vomiting, diarrhea, and may disrupt intestinal flora. Internal use is not recommended for young children by many experts due to the herb's alkaloid (berberine and hydrastine) content.
Hops (*Humulus lupulus*)	Internal use: nervous disorders, sleep aid	Rare allergic reactions
Horehound (*Maffubium vulgare*)	Internal use: coughs	None known
Hyssop (*Hyssopus officinalis*)	Internal use: coughs, bronchitis	None known

Table U-1 Common Herbal Remedies—*continued*

HERB Common and Latin Names	TRADITIONAL USAGE Internal and External Uses	Contraindications/ Precautions
Lemon balm (*Melissa officinalis*)	Internal use: nervous disorders, sleep aid	None known
Licorice root (*Glycyrrhiza glabra*)	Internal use: coughs, bronchitis	Prolonged use with high doses may promote hypertension, edema, and hypokalemia
Marshmallow root (*Althaea officinalis*)	Internal use: coughs, bronchitis, sore throat	None known
Mullein leaf (*Verbascum thapsus*)	Internal use: coughs, bronchitis, common colds, flu	None known
Oat straw (*Avena sativa*)	External use: inflammation of the skin, itching	None known
Passion flower (*Passiflora incarnata*)	Internal use: nervous disorders, sleep aid	None known
Peppermint leaf (*Mentha piperita*)	Internal use: carminative, indigestion, nausea, gastrointestinal disorders, common colds, cough, bronchitis	Preparations containing peppermint oil should not be applied to the face or nose of infants or very young children.
Pleurisy root (*Asclepias tuberosa*)	Internal use: coughs, pleurisy	Excessive amounts can be toxic due to the herb's cardioactive steroid content that can lead to digitalis-like poisonings. High doses can promote vomiting.
St. John's wort (*Hypericum perforatum*)	Internal use: emotional upsets, including anxiety and depressive moods External use: cuts and abrasions	Safety of internal use with children has not been established. The safety and ethics of the use of herbal antidepressants with children without the consultation of a doctor is questionable.

continues

SECTION 7

Table U-1 Common Herbal Remedies—*continued*

HERB Common and Latin Names	**TRADITIONAL USAGE Internal and External Uses**	**Contraindications/ Precautions**
		Should not be taken by children already taking prescription medications for depression without first consulting a doctor. May cause sun sensitivity in some individuals.
Thyme (*Thymus vulgarus*)	Internal use: cough, bronchitis, common colds	None known
Valerian root (*Valeriana officinalis*)	Internal use: nervous disorders, sleep aid	The safety and ethics of the use of herbal sedatives with children without the consultation of a doctor is questionable.

Note: Clinical efficacy for each of these herbs has not necessarily been established.

Appendix V:
Infant Formulas

Table V-1 Standard Infant Formulas

	Enfamil with Iron per 100 kcals Mead Johnson	Similac with Iron per 100 kcals Ross	Carnation Good Start per 100 kcals Nestle	Parents Choice with Iron per 100 kcals Wyeth-Ayerst
Macronutrients				
Energy (kcals)	100	100	100	100
Protein (g)	2.1	2.07	2.2	2.2
Carbohydrate (g)	10.9	10.8	11.2	10.6
Fat (g)	5.3	5.4	5.1	5.3
Linoleic Acid (mg)	860	1,000	900	500
Vitamins				
Vit. A (IU)	300	300	300	300
Vit. D (IU)	60	60	60	60
Vit. E (IU)	2	1.5	2	1.4
Vit. K (IU)	8	8	8	8
Vit. C (mg)	12	9	9	8.5
Thiamine (μg)	80	100	60	100
Riboflavin (μg)	140	150	140	150
Vit. B6 (μg)	60	60	65	62.5
Vit. B12 (μg)	0.3	0.25	0.22	0.2
Niacin (μg)	1,000	1,050	750	750
Folic Acid (μg)	16	15	15	7.5
Pantothenic Acid (μg)	500	450	450	315
Biotin (μg)	3	4.4	2.2	2.2
Choline (mg)	12	16	12	15
Inositol (mg)	6	4.7	15	4.1
Minerals				
Calcium (mg)	78	78	75	63
Phosphorus (mg)	53	42	42	42
Magnesium (μg)	8	6	7	7
Iron (mg)	1.8	1.8	1.5	1.8
Zinc (mg)	1	0.75	0.8	0.8
Manganese (μg)	15	5	7	15

continues

Table V-1 Standard Infant Formulas—*continued*

	Enfamil with Iron per 100 kcals	Similac with Iron per 100 kcals	Carnation Good Start per 100 kcals	Parents Choice with Iron per 100 kcals
	Mead Johnson	**Ross**	**Nestle**	**Wyeth-Ayerst**
Copper (μg)	75	90	80	70
Iodine (μg)	10	6	10	9
Sodium (mg)	27	24	23	22
Potassium (mg)	108	105	98	83
Chloride (mg)	63	65	59	55.5
Other data				
Protein source	nonfat milk, whey	nonfat milk, whey	cow's milk, whey	nonfat milk, whey
% Calories protein	8.5	8	8.8	8.8
Carbohydrate source	Lactose	Lactose	Lactose	Lactose
% Calories carbohydrate	43.5	43	44.8	42.4

Table V-2 Soy Infant Formulas

	Isomil per 100 kcals	Prosobee per 100 kcals	Essentials Soy per 100 kcals	Parents Choice Soy per 100 kcals
	Ross	Mead Johnson	Nestle	Wyeth-Ayerst
Macronutrients				
Energy (kcals)	100	100	100	100
Protein (g)	2.45	2.5	2.8	2.7
Carbohydrate (g)	10.3	10.6	11.1	10.2
Fat (g)	5.46	5.3	5.1	5.3
Linoleic Acid (mg)	1,000	860	920	500
Vitamins				
Vit. A (IU)	300	300	300	300
Vit. D (IU)	60	60	60	60
Vit. E (IU)	1.5	2	3	1.4
Vit. K (IU)	11	8	8	8.3
Vit. C (mg)	9	12	16	8.3
Thiamine (μg)	60	80	60	100
Riboflavin (μg)	90	90	94	150
Vit. B6 (μg)	60	60	60	62.5
Vit. B12 (μg)	0.45	0.3	0.31	0.3
Niacin (μg)	1,350	1,000	1,300	750
Folic Acid (μg)	15	16	16	7.5
Pantothenic Acid (μg)	750	500	470	450
Biotin (μg)	4.5	3	7.8	5.5
Choline (mg)	12	12	12	13
Inositol (mg)	5	6	18	4.1
Minerals				
Calcium (mg)	105	105	105	90
Phosphorus (mg)	75	83	63	63
Magnesium (μg)	7.5	11	11	10
Iron (mg)	1.8	1.8	1.8	1.8
Zinc (mg)	0.75	1.2	0.9	0.8
Manganese (μg)	25	25	34	30
Copper (μg)	75	75	120	70
Iodine (μg)	15	15	15	9
Sodium (mg)	44	36	35	30

continues

SECTION 7

Table V-2 Soy Infant Formulas—*continued*

	Isomil per 100 kcals	Prosobee per 100 kcals	Essentials Soy per 100 kcals	Parents Choice Soy per 100 kcals
	Ross	Mead Johnson	Nestle	Wyeth-Ayerst
Potassium (mg)	108	120	116	105
Chloride (mg)	62	80	71	56
Other data				
Protein source	Soy protein isolate; L-Methionine	Soy protein isolate; L-Methionine	Soy protein isolate;	Soy protein isolate;
% Calories protein	10	10	11.2	10.8
Carbohydrate source	Corn syrup; sucrose	Corn syrup; solids	Corn maltodextrin; Sucrose	Corn syrup solids; Sucrose
% Calories carbohydrate	41	42	44.4	40.8

Sources: Data collected from manufacturers of specified formulas.

Table V-3 Protein Hydrolysate Formulas

	Nutramigen Lipil per 100 kcals Mead Johnson	Pregestimil per 100 kcals Mead Johnson	Alimentum Advance per 100 kcals Ross
Macronutrients			
Energy (kcals)	100	100	100
Protein (g)	2.8	2.8	2.75
Carbohydrate (g)	10.3	10.2	10.2
Fat (g)	5.3	5.6	5.54
Linoleic Acid (mg)	860	1,040	1,900
Vitamins			
Vit. A (IU)	300	380	300
Vit. D (IU)	50	50	45
Vit. E (IU)	2	4	3
Vit. K (IU)	8	12	15
Vit. C (mg)	12	12	9
Thiamine (μg)	80	80	60
Riboflavin (μg)	90	90	90
Vit. B6 (μg)	60	60	60
Vit. B12 (μg)	0.3	0.3	0.45
Niacin (μg)	1,000	1,000	1,350
Folic Acid (μg)	16	16	15
Pantothenic Acid (μg)	500	500	750
Biotin (μg)	3	3	4.5
Choline (mg)	12	12	12
Inositol (mg)	17	17	5
Minerals			
Calcium (mg)	94	115	105
Phosphorus (mg)	63	75	75
Magnesium (μg)	11	11	7.5
Iron (mg)	1.8	1.8	1.8
Zinc (mg)	1	1	0.75
Manganese (μg)	25	25	8
Copper (μg)	75	75	75
Iodine (μg)	15	15	15
Sodium (mg)	47	47	44
Potassium (mg)	110	110	118
Chloride (mg)	86	86	80

continues

Table V-3 Protein Hydrolysate Formulas—*continued*

	Nutramigen Lipil per 100 kcals Mead Johnson	Pregestimil per 100 kcals Mead Johnson	Alimentum Advance per 100 kcals Ross
Other data			
Protein source	Casein hydrolysate; Amino acids	Casein hydrolysate; Amino acids	Casein hydrolysate; Amino acids
% Calories protein	11	11	11
Carbohydrate source	Corn syrup solids; Modified corn starch	Corn syrup solids; Modified corn starch; Dextrose	Sucrose; Modified Tapioca Starch (70:30)
% Calories carbohydrate	41	41	41

Table V-4 Amino Acid-Based Formulas

	Elecare per 100 Kcals Ross	Neocate per 100 kcals Scientific Hosp. Supplies
Macronutrients		
Energy (kcals)	100	100
Protein (g)	4.76	3.7
Carbohydrate (g)	10.7	11.7
Fat (g)	3.01	4.5
Linoleic Acid (mg)	800	677
Vitamins		
Vit. A (IU)	273	409
Vit. D (IU)	42	87
Vit. E (IU)	2.1	1.14
Vit. K (IU)	6	9
Vit. C (mg)	9	9
Thiamine (μg)	210	93
Riboflavin (μg)	105	138
Vit. B6 (μg)	101	124
Vit. B12 (μg)	0.42	0.17
Niacin (μg)	1,680	1,544
Folic Acid (μg)	30	10
Pantothenic Acid (μg)	421	620
Biotin (μg)	4.2	3.1
Choline (mg)	8	13
Inositol (mg)	5.1	23
Minerals		
Calcium (mg)	108	124
Phosphorus (mg)	81	93
Magnesium (μg)	8	12
Iron (mg)	1.8	1.85
Zinc (mg)	1.1	1.7
Manganese (μg)	93	90
Copper (μg)	126	124
Iodine (μg)	7	15
Sodium (mg)	45	37
Potassium (mg)	150	155
Chloride (mg)	60	77
Other data		
Protein Source	Free L-amino acids	Free L-amino acids
% Calories protein	15	12
Carbohydrate source	Corn syrup solids	Corn syrup solids
% Calories carbohydrate	43	47

Table V-5 Standard Follow-up Formulas

	Similac 2 Advance per 100 kcals	Enfamil Next Step Lipil per 100 kcals	Good Start 2 Essentials per 100 kcals	Parents Choice 2 w/ Lipids per 100 kcals
	Ross	Mead Johnson	Nestle Nestle	Wyeth-Ayerst
Macronutrients				
Energy (kcals)	100	100	100	100
Protein (g)	2.07	2.6	2.6	2.6
Carbohydrate (g)	10.6	10.5	13.2	10
Fat (g)	5.49	5.3	4.1	5.4
Linoleic Acid (mg)	1,000	860	680	750
Vitamins				
Vit. A (IU)	300	300	250	370
Vit. D (IU)	60	60	60	65
Vit. E (IU)	3	2	2	2
Vit. K (IU)	8	8	8	9.9
Vit. C (mg)	9	12	9	13
Thiamine (μg)	100	80	80	150
Riboflavin (μg)	150	140	140	220
Vit. B6 (μg)	60	60	65	90
Vit. B12 (μg)	0.25	0.3	0.25	0.29
Niacin (μg)	1,050	1,000	900	1,020
Folic Acid (μg)	15	16	15	15
Pantothenic Acid (μg)	450	500	480	441
Biotin (μg)	4.4	3	2.2	2.9
Choline (mg)	16	12	12	15
Inositol (mg)	4.7	6	18	4
Minerals				
Calcium (mg)	118	195	120	120
Phosphorus (mg)	64	130	80	85
Magnesium (μg)	6	8	8	10
Iron (mg)	1.8	2	1.8	1.8
Zinc (mg)	0.75	1	0.8	0.88
Manganese (μg)	5	15	7	5.9
Copper (μg)	90	75	85	85
Iodine (μg)	6	10	10	10
Sodium (mg)	24	36	39	32
Potassium (mg)	105	130	135	125
Chloride (mg)	65	80	90	80

Table V-5 Standard Follow-up Formulas—*continued*

	Similac 2 Advance per 100 kcals	**Enfamil Next Step Lipil per 100 kcals**	**Good Start 2 Essentials per 100 kcals**	**Parents Choice 2 w/ Lipids per 100 kcals**
	Ross	**Mead Johnson**	**Nestle Nestle**	**Wyeth-Ayerst**
Other data				
Protein source	Nonfat milk; whey protein concentrate	Nonfat milk	Nonfat milk; whey protein concentrate	Nonfat milk; whey protein concentrate
% Calories protein	8	10.4	10.4	10.4
Carbohydrate source	Corn syrup solids; sucrose	Corn syrup solids lactose		Corn syrup solids; sucrose
% Calories carbohydrate	43	42	52.8	40

Appendix W: Activity of Insulin Preparations

Table W-1 Activity of Insulin Preparations

Type of Insulin	Examples	Onset of Action	Peak of Action	Duration of Action
Rapid-Acting	Humalog (lispro) Eli Lilly	15 minutes	30–90 minutes	3–5 hours
	NovoLog (aspart) Novo Nordisk	15 minutes	40–50 minutes	3–5 hours
Short-Acting (Regular)	Humulin R Eli Lilly Novolin R Novo Nordisk	30–60 minutes	50–120 minutes	5–8 hours
Intermediate-Acting (NPH)	Humulin N Eli Lilly Novolin N Novo Nordisk	1–3 hours	8 hours	20 hours
	Humulin L Eli Lilly Novolin L Novo Nordisk	1–2.5 hours	7–15 hours	18–24 hours

Intermediate- and Short-Acting Mixtures	Humulin 50/50 Humulin 70/30 Humalog Mix 75/25 Humalog Mix 50/50 Eli Lilly Novolin 70/30 NovoLog Mix 70/30 Novo Nordisk	The onset, peak, and duration of action for these mixtures would reflect a composite of the intermediate-, short-, or rapid-acting components with one peak of action.		
Long-Acting	Ultralente Eli Lilly	4–8 hours	8–12 hours	36 hours
	Lantus (glargine) Aventis	1 hour	none	24 hours

Source: Food and Drug Administration, http://www.fda.gov.

Appendix X: Micronutrients

Debra Wein, MS, RD, LDN, ACSM-HFI, NSCA-CPT

Table X-1 Function and Food Sources of Vitamins and Minerals

Nutrient	Functions Supporting Exercise	Food Source
Water-Soluble Vitamins		
Thiamine (B_1)	Coenzyme in cellular metabolism	Whole grains, legumes
Riboflavin (B_2)	Component of FAD+ and FMN of the electron transport chain	Most foods
Niacin	Component of NAD+ and NADP+	Lean meats, grains, legumes
Pyridoxine	Coenzyme in metabolism	Meat, vegetables, whole grains
Pantothenic acid	Component of coenzyme A (egacetyl-CoA, fatty acid acyl-CoA)	Most foods
Folacin	Coenzyme of cellular metabolism	Legumes, green vegetables, whole wheat
B_{12}	Coenzyme of metabolism in nucleolus	Muscle meat, eggs, dairy products
Biotin	Coenzyme of cellular metabolism	Meats, vegetables, legumes
Ascorbic acid	Maintains connective tissue, immune system	Citrus fruits, tomatoes, green peppers
Fat-Soluble Vitamins		
B-carotene (Pro vitamin A)		Dark green vegetables, yellow-orange vegetables, fruit
Retinol (A)	Sight, component of rhodopsin, maintains tissues	Milk, butter, cheese
Cholecalciferol (D)	Bone growth, and maintenance, calcium absorption	Eggs, dairy products
Tocopherol (E)	Antioxidant, protects cellular integrity	Seeds, green leafy vegetables, margarine
Phylloquinone (K)	Role in blood clotting	Green leafy vegetables, cereals, fruits, meats

Table X-1 Function and Food Sources of Vitamins and Minerals—*continued*

Nutrient	Functions Supporting Exercise	Food Source
Minerals		
Calcium (Ca^{2+})	Bone and tooth formation, muscle contraction, action potentials	Milk, cheese, dark green vegetables
Phosphorus (PO_3^-)	Bone and tooth formation, acid-base, chemical energy	Milk, cheese, yogurt, meat, poultry, grains, fish,
Potassium (K^+)	Action potential, acid-base, body water balance	Leafy vegetables, cantaloupe, lima beans, potatoes, milk, beans
Sulfur (S)	Acid-base, liver function	Proteins, dried food
Sodium (Na^+)	Action potential, acid-base, osmolality, body water balance	Fruits, vegetables, table salt
Chlorine (Cl^-)	Membrane potential, fluid balance	Fruits, vegetables, table salt
Magnesium (Mg^{2+})	Co-factor for enzyme function	Whole grains, green leafy vegetables
Iron (Fe)	Component of hemoglobin, myoglobin, and cytochromes	Eggs, lean meat, legumes, whole grains, green leafy vegetables
Fluoride (F)	Bone structure	Water, seafood
Zinc (Zn)	Components of enzymes of digestion	Most foods
Copper (Cu)	Component of enzymes of iron metabolism	Meat, water
Selenium (Se)	Functions with vitamin E	Seafood, meat, grains
Iodine (I)	Components of thyroid hormones	Marine fish and shellfish, dairy products, vegetables, iodized salt
Chromium (Cr)	Required for glycolysis	Legumes, cereals, whole grains
Molybdenum (Mo)	Co-factor for several enzymes	Fats, vegetables, oils, meats, whole grains

Appendix Y: MyPyramid

Anatomy of MyPyramid

One size doesn't fit all

USDA's new MyPyramid symbolizes a personalized approach to healthy eating and physical activity. The symbol has been designed to be simple. It has been developed to remind consumers to make healthy food choices and to be active every day. The different parts of the symbol are described below.

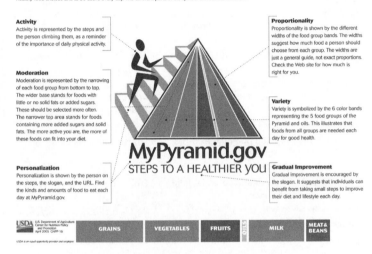

Activity
Activity is represented by the steps and the person climbing them, as a reminder of the importance of daily physical activity.

Moderation
Moderation is represented by the narrowing of each food group from bottom to top. The wider base stands for foods with little or no solid fats or added sugars. These should be selected more often. The narrower top area stands for foods containing more added sugars and solid fats. The more active you are, the more of these foods can fit into your diet.

Personalization
Personalization is shown by the person on the steps, the slogan, and the URL. Find the kinds and amounts of food to eat each day at MyPyramid.gov.

Proportionality
Proportionality is shown by the different widths of the food group bands. The widths suggest how much food a person should choose from each group. The widths are just a general guide, not exact proportions. Check the Web site for how much is right for you.

Variety
Variety is symbolized by the 6 color bands representing the 5 food groups of the Pyramid and oils. This illustrates that foods from all groups are needed each day for good health.

Gradual Improvement
Gradual improvement is encouraged by the slogan. It suggests that individuals can benefit from taking small steps to improve their diet and lifestyle each day.

Following the DASH Eating Plan

The DASH eating plan shown in the following pages is based on 2,000 calories a day. The number of daily servings in a food group may vary from those listed, depending on your caloric needs. Use this chart to help you plan your menus, or take it with you when you go to the store.

Table Y-1 Following the DASH Eating Plan

Food	Daily Servings (except as noted)	Serving Sizes	Examples and Notes	Significance of Food Group to the DASH Eating Plan
Grains and grain products	7–8	1 slice bread 1 oz. dry cereal* ½ cup cooked rice, pasta, or cereal	Whole-wheat bread, English muffin, pita bread, bagel, cereals, grits, oatmeal, crackers, unsalted pretzels, and popcorn	Major sources of energy and fiber
Vegetables	4–5	1 cup raw leafy vegetables ½ cup cooked vegetables 6 oz. vegetable juice	Tomatoes, potatoes, carrots, green peas, squash, broccoli, turnip greens, collards, kale, spinach, artichokes, green beans, lima beans, sweet potatoes	Rich sources of potassium, magnesium, and fiber
Fruits	4–5	6 oz. fruit juice 1 medium fruit ¼ cup dried fruit ½ cup fresh, frozen, or canned fruit	Apricots, bananas, dates, grapes, oranges, orange juice, grapefruit, grapefruit juice, mangoes, melons, peaches, pineapples, prunes, raisins, strawberries, tangerines	Important sources of potassium, magnesium, and fiber
Low-fat or fat-free dairy foods	2–3	8 oz. milk 1 cup yogurt 1½ oz. cheese	Fat-free (skim) or low-fat (1%) milk, fat-free or low-fat buttermilk, fat-free or low-fat regular or frozen yogurt, low-fat and fat-free cheese	Major sources of calcium and protein
Meats, poultry, and fish	2 or less	3 oz. cooked meats, poultry, or fish	Select only lean; trim away visible fats; broil, roast, or boil, instead of frying; remove skin from poultry	Rich sources of protein and magnesium

continues

Table Y-1 Following the DASH Eating Plan—*continued*

Food	Daily Servings (except as noted)	Serving Sizes	Examples and Notes	Significance of Food Group to the DASH Eating Plan
Nuts, seeds, and dry beans	4–5	1/3 cup or 1 1/2 oz. nuts 2 Tbsp or 1/2 oz. seeds 1/2 cup cooked dry beans, peas	Almonds, filberts, mixed nuts, peanuts, walnuts, sunflower seeds, kidney beans, lentils	Rich sources of energy, magnesium, potassium, protein, and fiber
Fats and oils‡	2–3	1 tsp soft margarine 1 Tbsp low-fat mayonnaise 2 Tbsp light salad dressing 1 tsp vegetable oil	Soft margarine, low-fat mayonnaise, light salad dressing, vegetable oil (such as olive, corn, canola, or safflower)	DASH has 27 percent of calories as fat, including fat in or added to foods
Sweets	5 per week	1 Tbsp sugar 1 Tbsp jelly or jam 1/2 oz. jelly beans 8 oz. lemonade	Maple syrup, sugar, jelly, jam, fruit-flavored gelatin, jelly beans, hard candy, fruit punch, sorbet, ices	Sweets should be low in fat

* Equals 1/2–1 1/4 cups, depending on cereal type. Check the product's Nutrition Fats label.

‡ Fat content changes serving counts for fats and oils: For example, 1 Tbsp of regular salad dressing equals 1 serving; 1 Tbsp of a low-fat dressing equals 1/2 serving; 1 Tbsp of a fat-free dressing equals 0 servings.

Appendix Z: Normal Nutritional Lab Values

Table Z-1 Selected Blood Tests Useful for Determining Nutritional Status

Nutrient	Laboratory Test	Acceptable Limits
1. Carbohydrate	Plasma glucose	70–120 mg[1]/100 ml[2]
2. Fat	a. Serum cholesterol	140–220 mg/100 ml
	b. Serum triglycerides	60–150 mg/100 ml
3. Protein	a. Visceral serum protein	above 6.5 gm[3]/100 ml
	b. Immune functions: (total lymphocyte count)	above 1,200
4. Fat-Soluble Vitamins		
Vitamin A	a. Serum vitamin A	20–45 μg[4]/100 ml
	b. Serum carotene	40–300 μg/100 ml
Vitamin D	a. Serum alkaline phosphatase	35–145 IU[5]/L[6]
	b. Plasma 25 hydroxy cholecalciferol	10–40 IU/L
Vitamin E	Plasma vitamin E	above 0.6 mg/100 ml
Vitamin K	Prothrombin time	12 seconds
5. Water-Soluble Vitamins		
a. Vitamin C	Serum ascorbic acid	above 0.3/100 ml
b. B complex:		
1. Thiamin	Red blood cell transketolase	0–15%
2. Riboflavin	Red blood cell glutathione	below 1.2
3. Niacin	Urinary nitrogen*	above 0.6 mg/gm creatinine
4. Vitamin B_6	Tryptophan load*	below 50 μg/24 hrs.
5. Vitamin B_{12}	Serum B_{12}	above 200 pg7/100 ml
6. Folacin	Serum folacin	above 6.0 ng8/100 ml

continues

Table Z-1 Selected Blood Tests Useful for Determining Nutritional Status—*continued*

Nutrient	Laboratory Test	Acceptable Limits
6. Minerals		
Iodine	Serum protein bound iodine (PHI)	4.8–8.0 μg/100 ml
Iron	a. Hemoglobin	male 14 mg/100 ml female 12 mg/100 ml
	b. Hematocrit	male 44% female 33%
Calcium	Serum calcium	9.0–11.0 mg/100 ml
Phosphorus	Serum phosphorus	2.5–4.5 mg/100 ml
Magnesium	Serum magnesium	1.3–2.0 mEq[7]/L[8]
Sodium	Serum sodium	130–150 mEq/L
Potassium	Serum potassium	3.5–5.0 mEq/L
Chloride	Serum chloride	99–110 mEq/L
Zinc	Plasma zinc	80–100 μg/100 ml

*Urine analysis rather than blood sampling

Measurement terminology:

1. mg (milligram) 1,000 mg = 1 gm (gram)
2. ml (milliliter) 1 ml = 1 cc (cubic centimeter)
3. gm (gram) 1,000 mg or 0.0001 kg (kilogram)
4. μg (microgram) 1,000 = 1 mg or 0.001 gm
5. IU (International Unit) not a metric measure
6. L (liter) 1,000 ml or 1,000 cc
7. pg (picogram) 10–12 gm
8. ng (nanogram) 10–9 gm

Table Z-2 Biochemical Evaluation of Nutritional Status

Test	Specimen	Reference Range	
Albumin	Serum		*g/dl*
		Premature:	3.0–4.2
		Newborn:	3.6–5.4
		Infant:	4.0–5.0
		Thereafter:	3.5–5.0
Calcium, ionized (iCa)	Serum, plasma, or whole blood (heparin)		*mg/dl*
		Cord:	5.0–5.0
		Newborn: 3–24 h:	4.3–5.1
		24–48 h:	4.0–4.7
		Thereafter:	4.48–4.92
		Or	2.24–2.46 mEq/l
Calcium, total	Serum		*mg/dl*
		Cord:	9.0–11.5
		Newborn: 3–24 h:	9.0–10.6
		24–48 h:	7.0–12.0
		4–7 days:	9.0–10.9
		Child:	8.8–10.8
		Thereafter:	8.4–10.2
	Urine, 24h	Ca in Diet	*mg/day*
		Ca Free:	5–40
		Low to average:	50–150
		Average (20m/mold):	100–300
B-Carotene	Serum		*μg/dl*
		Infant:	20–70
		Child:	40–130
		Thereafter:	60–200
Ceruloplasmin	Serum		*mg/dl*
		Newborn:	1–30
		6 mo–1 yr:	15–50
		1–12 yr:	30–65
		Thereafter:	14–40
Chloride	Serum or plasma (heparin)		*mmol/L*
		Cord:	96–104
		Newborn:	97–110
		Thereafter:	98–106

continues

SECTION 7

Table Z-2 Biochemical Evaluation of Nutritional Status—*continued*

Test	**Specimen**	**Reference Range**	
	CSF	118–132 mmol/L	
	Urine, 24h		*mmol/day*
		Infant:	2–10
		Child:	15–50
		Thereafter:	110–250
		(varies greatly with Cl intake)	
	Sweat		*mmol/L*
		Normal (homozygote):	0–35
		Marginal:	30–60
		Cystic fibrosis:	60–200
		Increases by 10 mmol/L during lifetime	
Cholesterol, total	Serum or plasma (EDTA or heparin)		*mg/dl*
		Cord:	45–100
		Newborn:	53–135
		Infant:	70–175
		Child:	120–200
		Adolescent:	120–210
		Recommended (desirable) range for	
		adults:	< 200
		adolescents:	< 170
Copper	Serum		*μg/dl*
		Birth–6 mo:	20–70
		6 yr:	90–190
		12 yr:	80–160
		Adult, M:	70–240
		Adult, F:	80–155
	Erythrocytes (heparin)	90–150 μg/dl	
	Urine (24h)	15–30 μg/day	
Creatinine Jaffe, kinetic, or enzymatic	Serum or plasma		*mg/dl*
		Cord:	0.6–1.2
		Newborn:	0.3–1.0
		Infant:	0.2–0.4
		Child:	0.3–0.7
		Adolescent:	0.5–1.0
		Adult, M:	0.6–1.2
		Adult, F:	0.5–1.1

Table Z-2 Biochemical Evaluation of Nutritional Status—*continued*

Test	Specimen	Reference Range	
	Urine 24h		*mg/kg/day*
		Infant:	8–20
		Child:	8–22
		Adolescent:	8–30
		Adult:	14–26
		or:	*mg/day*
		Adult, M:	800–2000
		Adult, F:	600–1800
Disaccharide absorption test	Serum		*mg/dl*
		Changes in glucose from fasting value:	
		Normal:	> 30
		Inconclusive:	20–30
		Abnormal:	< 20
Erythrocyte count	White blood (EDTA)	*millions of cells/mm*3 *(μl)*	
		Cord blood:	3.9–5.5
		1–3 d (cap):	4.0–6.6
		1 wk:	3.9–6.3
		2 wk:	3.6–6.2
		1 mo:	3.0–5.4
		2 mo:	2.7–4.9
		3–6 mo:	3.1–4.5
		0.5–2 yr:	3.7–5.3
		2–6 yr	3.9–5.3
		6–12 yr	4.0–5.2
		12–18 yr, M:	4.5–5.3
		F:	4.1–5.1
		18–49 yr, M:	4.5–5.9
		F:	4.0–5.2
Fat, fecal	Feces, 72 h	Coefficient of fat absorption (5)	
		Infant, breast-fed:	> 93
		Infant, formula-fed:	> 83
		> 1 yr:	≥ 95
Fatty acids Nonesterified (Free)	Serum or plasma (heparin)	Adults:	8–25 mg/dl
		Children and obese adults: < 31	

continues

SECTION 7

Table Z-2 Biochemical Evaluation of Nutritional Status—*continued*

Test	Specimen	Reference Range		
Ferritin	Serum		*μg/ml*	
		Newborn:	25–200	
		1 mo:	200–600	
		2–5 mo:	50–200	
		6 mo–15 yr:	7–140	
		Adult, M:	15–200	
		Adult, F:	12–150	
Folate	Serum		*μg/ml*	
		Newborn:	7.0–32	
		Thereafter:	1.8–9	
	Erythrocytes (EDTA)	150–450 μg/ml cells		
Glucose	Serum		*mg/dl*	
		Cord:	45–96	
		Premature:	20–60	
		Neonate:	30–60	
		Newborn, 1 d:	40–60	
		> 1 d:	50–90	
		Child:	60–100	
		Adult:	70–105	
Glucose Tolerance Test Serum (GTT)			*mg/dl*	
			Normal	*Diabetic*
Oral Dose:		Fasting:	70–105	> 115
Adult: 75 g		60 min:	120–170	> 200
Child: 1.75 g/kg of ideal weight up to maximum of 75 g		90 min:	100–140	> 200
		120 min:	70–120	> 140
Growth Hormone (hGH) (Somatotropin)	Serum or plasma (EDTA, heparin) fasting at rest		*μg/ml*	
		Cord:	10–50	
		Newborn:	10–40	
		Child:	< 5	
		Adult, M:	< 5	
		Adult, F:	< 8	

Table Z-2 Biochemical Evaluation of Nutritional Status—*continued*

Test	Specimen	Reference Range		
HDL-Cholesterol (HDLC)	Serum or plasma (EDTA)		*mg/dl*	
			Male	*Female*
		Mean	45	55
		Range		
		Cord blood:	5–50	5–50
		0–12 yr:	30–65	30–65
		15–19 yr:	30–65	30–70
		20–29 yr:	30–70	30–75
		30–39 yr:	30–70	30–80
		40+ yr:	30–70	30–85
		Values for blacks—20 mg/dl higher		
Hematocrit	Whole blood (EDTA)	*% of packed red cells (V red cells/V whole blood × 100)*		
Calculated from MCV and RBC (electronic displacement or laser)		1 d (cap):	48–69	
		2 d:	48–75	
		3 d:	44–72	
		2 mo:	28–42	
		6–12 yr:	35–45	
		12–18 yr, M:	37–49	
		F:	36–46	
		18–49 yr, M:	41–53	
		F:	36–46	
Hemoglobin (Hb)	Whole blood (EDTA)		*g/dl*	
		1–3 day (cap):	14.5–22.5	
		2 mo:	9.0–14.0	
		6–12 yr:	11.5–15.5	
		12–18 yr, M:	13.0–16.0	
		F:	12.0–16.0	
		18–49 yr, M:	13.5–17.5	
		F:	12.0–16.0	
	Serum or plasma (heparin, ACD)	< 10 mg/dl		
		< 3 mg/dl with butterfly setup and 18 g needle		
	Urine, fresh random	Negative		

continues

SECTION 7

Table Z-2 Biochemical Evaluation of Nutritional Status—*continued*

Test	Specimen	Reference Range		
Hemoglobin, glycosylated	Whole blood (heparin, EDTA, or oxalate)			
Electrophoresis		5.6–7.5% of total Hb		
Column		6.9% of total Hb		
HPLC		HbA_{1a} 1.6% total Hb		
		HbA_{1b} 0.8		
		HbA_{1c} 3–6		
Iron	Serum		*μg/dl*	
		Newborn:	100–250	
		Infant:	40–100	
		Child:	50–120	
		Thereafter, M:	50–160	
		F:	40–150	
		Intoxicated child:	280–2,250	
		Fatally poisoned child:	> 1800	
Iron-binding capacity total (TIBC)	Serum	Infant:	100–400 μg/dl	
		Thereafter:	250–400	
			mg/dl	
LDL-Cholesterol	Serum or plasma (EDTA)		*Male*	*Female*
		Cord blood:	10–50	10–50
		0–19 yr:	60–140	60–150
		20–29 yr:	60–175	60–160
		30–39 yr:	80–190	70–170
		40–49 yr:	90–205	80–190
		Recommended (desirable) range for adults: 65–175 mg/dl		
Lead	Whole blood (heparin)		*μg/dl*	
		Child:	< 30	
		Adult:	< 40	
		Acceptable for industrial exposure:	< 60	
		Toxic:	≥ 100	
	Urine 24 hr	< 80 μg/dl		

Table Z-2 Biochemical Evaluation of Nutritional Status—*continued*

Test	Specimen	Reference Range	
Mean corpuscular hemoglobin	Whole blood (EDTA)		*pg/cell*
		Birth:	31–37
		1–3 day (cap):	31–37
		1 wk–1 mo:	28–40
		2 mo:	26–34
		3–6 mo:	25–35
		0.5–2 yr:	23–31
		2–6 yr:	23–31
		6–12 yr:	25–33
		12–18 yr:	25–35
		18–49 yr:	26–34
Mean corpuscular hemoglobin concentration (EDTA)	Whole blood (EDTA)		*% Hb.cell or g Hb/dl RBC*
		Birth:	30–60
		1–3 (cap):	29–37
		1–2 wk:	28–38
		1–2 mo:	29–37
		3 mo–2 yr:	30–36
		2–18 yr:	31–37
		> 18 yr:	31–37
Mean corpuscular	Whole blood (EDTA)		*μm^3*
		1–3 day (cap):	95–121
		0.5–2 yr:	70–86
		6–12 yr:	77–95
		12–18 yr, M:	78–98
		F:	78–102
		18–49 yr, M:	80–100
		F:	80–100
Niacin (nicotine acid)	Urine 24 h	0.3–1.5 mg/day	
Phenylalanine	Serum		*mg/dl*
		Premature:	2.0–7.5
		Newborn:	1.2–3.4
		Thereafter:	0.8–1.8
			mg/day
	Urine 24 h	10 day–2 wk:	1–2
		3–12 yr:	4–18
		Thereafter:	trace–17

continues

Table Z-2 Biochemical Evaluation of Nutritional Status—*continued*

Test	Specimen	Reference Range	
Phosphatase, Alkaline (p-nitrophenyl phosphatase)	Serum		
SKI method 30°C			*U/L*
		Infant:	50–155
		Child:	20–150
		Adult:	20–70
Bowers and McComb, 30°C		25–90 U/L	
Phospholipid, total	Serum or plasma (EDTA)		*mg/dl*
		Newborn:	75–170
		Infant:	100–275
		Child:	180–295
		Adult:	125–275
Phosphorus, inorganic	Serum		*mg/dl*
		Cord:	3.7–8.1
		Premature (1 wk):	5.4–10.9
		Newborn:	4.3–9.3
		Child:	4.5–6.5
		Thereafter:	3.0–4.5
Potassium	Serum		*mmol/l*
		Newborn:	3.9–5.9
		Infant:	4.1–5.3
		Child:	3.4–4.7
		Thereafter:	3.5–5.2
	Plasma (heparin)	3.5–4.5 mmol/L	
	Urine, 24 h	2.5–125 mmol/day varies with diet	
Prealbumin (PA, tryptophan-rich, thyroxine-binding TBPA) R/D	Serum		*mg/dl*
		Cord:	13
		1 yr:	10
		Maternal:	23
		Adult:	10–40
Protein, total	Serum		*g/dl*
		Premature:	4.3–7.6
		Newborn:	4.6–7.4
		Child:	6.2–8.0
		Adult	
		Recumbent:	6.0–7.8
		0.5 g higher in ambulatory patients	

Table Z-2 Biochemical Evaluation of Nutritional Status—*continued*

Test	Specimen	Reference Range	
Electrophoresis			*g/dl*
		Albumin	
		Premature:	3.0–4.2
		Newborn:	3.6–5.4
		Infant:	4.0–5.0
		α_1-Globulin	
		Premature:	0.1–0.5
		Newborn:	0.1–0.3
		Infant:	0.2–0.4
		Thereafter:	0.2–0.3
		α_2-Globulin	
		Premature:	0.3–0.7
		Newborn:	0.5–0.5
		Infant:	0.5–0.8
		Thereafter:	0.4–1.0
		β-Globulin	
		Premature:	0.3–1.2
		Newborn:	0.2–0.6
		Infant:	0.5–0.8
		Thereafter:	0.5–1.1
		γ-Globin	
		Premature:	0.3–1.4
		Newborn:	0.2–1.0
		Infant:	0.3–1.2
		Thereafter:	0.7–1.2
		Higher in blacks	
Total	Urine, 24 h	1–14 mg/dl 50–80 mg/dl (at rest) < 250 mg/d after intense exercise	
Prothrombin time (PT) one-stage (quick)	Whole blood (Na citrate)	In general: 11–15a (varies with type of thromboplastin) Newborn: prolonged by 2–3 s	
Retinol-binding protein (RBP)	Serum plasma		*mg/dl*
		2–10 yr:	2.5–4.5
		16 yr and older, M:	4.5–9.0
		F:	2.5–9.0

continues

Table Z-2 Biochemical Evaluation of Nutritional Status—*continued*

Test	Specimen	Reference Range		
Riboflavin (vitamin B_2)	Urine, random, fasting		*μg/g* Creatinine	
		1–3 yr:	500–900	
		4–6 yr:	300–600	
		7–9 yr:	270–500	
		10–15 yr:	200–400	
		Adult:	80–269	
Sodium	Serum or plasma (heparin)		*mmol/L*	
		Newborn:	134–146	
		Infant:	139–146	
		Child:	138–145	
		Thereafter:	136–146	
	Sweat		10–40	
		Cystic fibrosis > 70		
Somatomedin C	Plasma	Vary with laboratory, for example, Nichols Institute		
			U/L	
			M	*F*
		0–2 yr:	0.10–0.72	0.10–1.7
		3–5 yr:	0.12–1.5	0.15–2.3
		6–10 yr:	0.19–2.2	0.44–3.6
		11–12 yr:	0.22–3.6	1.50–6.9
		13–14 yr:	0.79–5.5	0.81–7.4
		13–17 yr:	0.76–3.3	0.59–3.1
		15–17 yr:	0.76–3.3	0.59–3.1
		18–64 yr:	0.34–1.9	0.45–2.2
		Endocrine Sciences		
		Cord:	0.25–0.66	
		0–1 yr:	0.17–0.62	
		1–5 yr:	0.14–0.94	
		6–12 yr:	0.87–2.06	
		13–17 yr:	1.35–3.00	
		18–25 yr:	0.92–2.06	
		Thereafter:	0.70–2.04	

Table Z-2 Biochemical Evaluation of Nutritional Status—*continued*

Test	Specimen	Reference Range		
Thiamine (vitamin B_1)	Serum		0–2.0 μg/dl	
	Urine, acidified with HCl		μg/g creatinine	
		1–3 yr:	176–200	
		4–6 yr:	121–400	
		7–9 yr:	181–350	
		10–12 yr:	181–300	
		13–15 yr:	151–250	
		Thereafter:	66–129	
Transferrin	Serum	Newborn:	130–275 mg/dl	
		Adult:	200–400 mg/dl	
Triglycerides (TG)	Serum, after ≥ 12 h fast		*mg/dl*	
			Male	Female
		Cord blood:	10–98	10–98
		0–5 yr:	30–86	32–99
		6–11 yr:	31–108	35–114
		12–15 yr:	36–138	41–138
		16–19 yr:	40–163	40–128
		20–29 yr:	44–185	40–128
		Recommended (desirable) levels for adults:		
		Male:	40–160 mg/dl	
		Female:	35–135 mg/dl	
Tyrosine	Serum		*mg/dl*	
		Premature:	7.0–24.00	
		Newborn:	1.6–3.7	
		Adult:	0.8–1.3	
Urea nitrogen	Serum or plasma		*mg/dl*	
		Cord:	21–40	
		Premature (1 wk):	3–25	
		Newborn:	3–12	
		Infant/Child:	5–18	
		Thereafter:	7–18	
Vitamin A	Serum		*μg/dl*	
		Newborn:	35–75	
		Child:	30–80	
		Thereafter:	30–65	
Vitamin B_1, see Thiamine				

continues

Table Z-2 Biochemical Evaluation of Nutritional Status—*continued*

Test	Specimen	Reference Range	
Vitamin B_2, see Riboflavin			
Vitamin B_6	Plasma (EDTA)	3.6–18 ng/ml	
Vitamin B_{12}	Serum	Newborn: Thereafter:	175–800 pg/ml 140–700
Vitamin C	Plasma (oxalate, heparin, or EDTA)	0.6–2.0 mg/dl	
Vitamin D_2, 25 Hydroxy	Plasma (heparin)	Summer: Winter:	15–80 ng/ml 14–42
Vitamin D_3, 1,25-dihydroxy	Serum	25–45 pg/ml	
Vitamin E	Serum	5.0–20 μg/ml	
Zinc	Serum	70–150 μg/dl	

Source: Adapted with permission from *Nelson's Textbook of Pediatrics,* 13th ed., pp. 1535–1558, © 1989, W.B. Saunders Company.

Appendix AA: Nutrition Assessment Sheet

Nutritional Assessment and Diet History

Identification and Activity

1. Personal Data:
   Identifying number or name ______________________________
   Age _______ Sex _______ Marital status _______
   Race _______ Religious preference _______ Ethnic origin _______
   Education _______ (Highest completed grade/degree)
   Employment: type _______ hours _______ approximate income _______
   Unemployed _______ Public assistance _______ Other _______
   Family composition (all living at one residence, ages, and relationships)
   ____
   Person(s) most responsible for purchase, preparation of food ___________
   Housing: type _______ Facilities for storage, preparation of food _______

2. Health Data:
   A. Anthropometric: Height _______
   Present weight _______ (lbs.) _______ (kg)
   Usual weight _______ (lbs.) _______ (kg)
   Recent changes in weight _______
   Planned change? _______
   Triceps skin fold _______ (mm) Standard _______
   Midarm circumference _______ (cm) Standard _______
   B. Physical: Appearance of:
      1. Skin _______
      2. Hair _______
      3. Eyes _______
      4. Ears _______
      5. Nails _______
      6. Posture _______
      7. Mouth, tongue, lips
      ____
      8. Teeth: Dentures _______
      Edentulous _______
      Chews well _______
      Chews with difficulty _______
      9. Swallowing good _______ poor _______
      10. Any other pertinent physical data
      ____
   C. Laboratory: CBC _______ Hbg _______ Hct _______
   Serum levels of albumin/transferrin _______
   Urinary values _______
   Creatinine clearance _______
   Other _______
   D. Habits:
      1. Meals: number per day _______
      Snacks: number per day _______

SECTION 7

2. Alcohol: amount daily _______
   type _______
3. Smoking: amount daily _______
   type _______ (include cigars, pipes, and marijuana)
4. Drugs: amount daily _______
   specific kinds _______
5. Exercise: kind _______
   frequency _______ amount of time _______

E. Other
1. Gastrointestinal function:
   Appetite: good _______ fair _______ poor _______
   recent changes _______________________________
   Taste/smell: good _______ fair _______ poor _______
   recent changes _______________________________
   Indigestion: often _______ seldom _______ never _______
   If yes, list foods that cause _______________________
   List any foods that cause nausea/vomiting _______________
   List any foods that cause diarrhea _______________
   Bowel elimination: frequency _______ consistency _______
2. Emotional state:
   calm _______ agitated _______ anxious _______ depressed _______
   Other: (Explain) _______________

24-Hour Intake Record

1. Dietary History:
   A. Food Preferences Foods Acceptable Food Dislikes Food Allergies Other

   B. Meals: Usual Serving Size Time Where Special occasions weekends/ holidays

   Breakfast

   Lunch/dinner

   Dinner/supper

   Snacks

C. Vitamin, mineral supplements taken: kind _______ amount _______
Reason for taking ____

D. Usual preparation method (bake, boil, broil, fry, etc.)
1. Meats _______
2. Vegetables _______

Analysis

Nutritional Diagnosis/Planning

1. Review the assessment and diet history and list the potential needs for nutrition education.
2. Questions to guide the beginning practitioner:
   a. Was daily intake adequate in kcal, nutrients, kinds, and amounts of food? If *no*, indicate:
      1. Which food groups have been omitted or are in inadequate amounts?
      2. Which of the DRI/RDAs for major nutrients have not been met?
      3. Does the caloric intake provide for maintenance of normal weight?
         Too low? _______ Too high? _______
         For recovery from illness/injury? _______
   b. What foods need to be added/subtracted/substituted to meet the assessed needs of this person and maintain individuality?
   c. Identify areas of patient teaching that need to be included as you plan your nutrition care and interventions.

Explanatory Notes

The nutritional assessment should be a part of every health practitioner's relationship to the client. It is one of the tools that provide information to identify and meet client needs.

The purpose of nutritional assessment is to provide an essential part of the overall nursing assessment. Some people, because of their nutritional status at the time of disease or injury, may be at high risk for nutritional problems that affect the outcome of the disease process. This assessment may become critical in the overall recovery.

Some forms of food survey/intake should be obtained for every client at admission. If the client is unable to respond, information should be obtained from family or others who know the client's eating patterns, in order to individualize the diet. Some of the data may be collected from other recorded observations and tests.

The nutritional assessment and diet history can be used as a basis for planning a diet with a patient that will speed recovery, as well as for teaching sound nutrition principles and promoting health maintenance.

Appendix BB: Physical Indicators of Nutritional Status

Table BB-1 Physical Indicators of Nutritional Status

Body Area	Signs of Good Nutrition	Signs of Malnutrition
1. Head to neck		
a. Hair	a. Shiny	a. Dull, dry, thin, wirelike, sparse, brittle; scalp rough, flaky
b. Face	b. Skin smooth	b. Pale or mottled, dark under eyes, swollen, scaling or flakiness, lumpiness
c. Eyes	c. Bright	c. Dry membranes, redness, fissures at corners, red rimmed, fine blood vessels or scars at cornea
d. Lips	d. Smooth	d. Red, swollen, lesions or fissures
e. Tongue	e. Deep red	e. Scarlet or purplish color; raw, swollen, smooth
f. Teeth	f. Straight; none missing	f. Cavities, black or gray spots, erupting abnormally, missing
g. Gums	g. Firm, pink, smooth, no bleeding	g. Spongy, bleed easily, inflammation, receded, atrophied
2. Skin	2. Smooth, moist, uniform color	2. Dry, flaky, scaling, "gooseflesh," swollen, grayish, bruises due to capillary bleeding under skin, no fat layer under skin
3. Glands	3. No thyroid enlargement: no lumps at parotid juncture	3. Front of neck and cheeks become swollen, lumps visible at parotid; goiter visible if advanced hypothyroidism
4. Nails	4. Pink nail beds, smooth, firm, flexible, uniform shape	4. Brittle, ridged, pale nail beds, clubbed, spoon shaped

Table BB-1 Physical Indicators of Nutritional Status—*continued*

Body Area	Signs of Good Nutrition	Signs of Malnutrition
5. Muscle and skeletal system	5. Good posture, firm, well-developed muscles, good mobility; no malformations of skeleton	5. Flaccid, wasted muscles, weakness, tenderness, decreased reflexes, difficulty in walking Children: beading ribs, swelling at ends of bones, abnormal protrusion of frontal or parietal areas
6. Internal systems		
a. Gastrointestinal	a. Flat abdomen, liver not tender to palpate, normal size	a. Distended, enlarged abdomen, ascites, hepatomegaly (enlarged liver) Children: "potbelly"
b. Cardiovascular	b. Normal pulse rate; normal blood pressure	b. Pulse rate exceeds 100 beats/min., abnormal rhythm, blood pressure elevated, mental confusion, edema

While physical appearances give us clues to internal problems, they can be misleading. They may not be nutrition-related. Physical findings must be coupled with other indications (lab test, anthropometries, etc.) in order to validate them.

Table BB-2 Percentiles for Triceps Skinfold for Whites of the United States, Health and Nutrition Examination Survey I of 1971–1974

Age Group	Males n	5	10	25	50	75	90	95	Females n	5	10	25	50	75	90	95
1–1.9	228	6	7	8	10	12	14	16	204	6	7	8	10	12	14	16
2–2.9	223	6	7	8	10	12	14	15	208	6	8	9	10	12	15	16
3–3.9	220	6	7	8	10	11	14	15	208	7	8	9	11	12	14	15
4–4.9	230	6	6	8	9	11	12	14	208	7	8	8	10	12	14	16
5–5.9	214	6	6	8	9	11	14	15	219	6	7	8	10	12	15	18
6–6.9	117	5	6	7	8	10	13	16	118	6	6	8	10	12	14	16
7–7.9	122	5	6	7	9	12	15	17	126	6	7	9	11	13	16	18
8–8.9	117	5	6	7	8	10	13	16	118	6	8	9	12	15	18	24
9–9.9	121	6	6	7	10	13	17	18	125	8	8	10	13	16	20	22
10–10.9	146	6	6	8	10	14	18	21	152	7	8	10	12	17	23	27
11–11.9	122	6	6	8	11	16	20	24	117	7	8	10	13	18	24	28
12–12.9	153	6	6	8	11	14	22	28	129	8	9	11	14	18	23	27

13–13.9	134	5	5	7	10	14	22	26	151	8	8	12	15	21	26	30
14–14.9	131	4	5	7	9	14	21	24	141	9	10	13	16	21	26	28
15–15.9	128	4	5	6	8	11	18	24	117	8	10	12	17	21	25	32
16–16.9	131	4	5	6	8	12	16	22	142	10	12	15	18	22	26	31
17–17.9	133	5	5	6	8	12	16	19	114	10	12	13	19	24	30	37
18–18.9	91	4	5	6	9	13	20	24	109	10	12	15	18	22	26	30
19–24.9	531	4	5	7	10	15	20	22	1,060	10	11	14	18	24	30	34
25–34.9	971	5	6	8	12	16	20	24	1,987	10	12	16	21	27	34	37
35–44.9	806	5	6	8	12	16	20	23	1,614	12	14	18	23	29	35	38
45–54.9	898	6	6	8	12	15	20	25	1,047	12	16	20	25	30	36	40
55–64.9	734	5	6	8	11	14	19	22	809	12	16	20	25	31	36	38
65–74.9	1,503	4	6	8	11	15	19	22	1,670	12	14	18	24	29	34	36

Source: Reprinted with permission from Frisancho AR, "New norms of upper limb fat and muscle areas for assessment of nutritional status," in *American Journal of Clinical Nutrition* (1981; 34:2540–2545), Copyright © 1981, American Society for Clinical Nutrition.

SECTION 7

Table BB-3 Percentiles of Upper Arm Circumference (mm) and Estimated Upper Arm Muscle Circumference (mm) for Whites of the United States, Health and Nutrition Examination Survey I of 1971–1974

	Males													
	Arm Circumference (mm)							Arm Muscle Circumference (mm)						
Age Group	5	10	25	50	75	90	95	5	10	25	50	75	90	95
1–1.9	142	146	150	159	170	176	183	110	113	119	127	135	144	147
2–2.9	141	145	153	162	170	178	185	111	114	122	130	140	146	150
3–3.9	150	153	160	167	175	184	190	117	123	131	137	143	148	153
4–4.9	149	154	162	171	180	186	192	123	126	133	141	148	156	159
5–5.9	153	160	167	175	185	195	204	128	133	140	147	154	162	169
6–6.9	155	159	167	179	188	209	228	131	135	142	151	161	170	177
7–7.9	162	167	177	187	201	223	230	137	139	151	160	168	177	190
8–8.9	162	170	177	190	202	220	245	140	145	154	162	170	182	187
9–9.9	175	178	187	200	217	249	257	151	154	161	170	183	196	202
10–10.9	181	184	196	210	231	262	274	156	160	166	180	191	209	221
11–11.9	186	190	202	223	244	261	280	159	165	173	183	195	205	230
12–12.9	193	200	214	232	254	282	303	167	171	182	195	210	223	241

13–13.9	194	211	228	247	263	286	301	172	179	196	211	226	238	245
14–14.9	220	226	237	253	283	303	322	189	199	212	223	240	260	264
15–15.9	222	229	244	264	284	311	320	199	204	218	237	254	266	272
16–16.9	244	248	262	278	303	324	343	213	225	234	249	269	287	296
17–17.9	246	253	267	285	308	336	347	224	231	245	258	273	294	312
18–18.9	245	260	276	297	321	353	379	226	237	252	264	283	298	324
19–24.9	262	272	288	308	331	355	372	238	245	257	273	289	309	321
25–34.9	271	282	300	319	342	362	375	243	250	264	279	298	314	326
35–44.9	278	287	305	326	345	363	374	247	255	269	286	302	318	327
45–54.9	267	281	301	322	342	362	376	239	249	265	281	300	315	326
55–64.9	258	273	296	317	336	355	369	236	245	260	278	295	310	320
65–74.9	248	263	285	307	325	344	355	223	235	251	268	284	298	306

continues

Table BB-3 Percentiles of Upper Arm Circumference (mm) and Estimated Upper Arm Muscle Circumference (mm) for Whites of the United States, Health and Nutrition Examination Survey I of 1971–1974—*continued*

	Females													
	Arm Circumference (mm)							Arm Muscle Circumference (mm)						
Age Group	5	10	25	50	75	90	95	5	10	25	50	75	90	95
1–1.9	138	142	148	156	164	172	177	105	111	117	124	132	139	143
2–2.9	142	145	152	160	167	176	184	111	114	119	126	133	142	147
3–3.9	143	150	158	167	175	183	189	113	119	124	132	140	146	152
4–4.9	149	154	160	169	177	184	191	115	121	128	136	144	152	157
5–5.9	153	157	165	175	185	203	211	125	128	134	142	151	159	165
6–6.9	156	162	170	176	187	204	211	130	133	138	145	154	166	171
7–7.9	164	167	174	183	199	216	231	129	135	142	151	160	171	176
8–8.9	168	172	183	195	214	247	261	138	140	151	160	171	183	194
9–9.9	178	182	194	211	224	251	260	147	150	158	167	180	194	198
10–10.9	174	182	193	210	228	251	265	148	150	159	170	180	190	197
11–11.9	185	194	208	224	248	276	303	150	158	171	181	196	217	223
12–12.9	194	203	216	237	256	282	294	162	166	180	191	201	214	220

13–13.9	202	211	223	243	271	301	338	169	175	183	198	211	226	240
14–14.9	214	223	237	252	272	304	322	174	179	190	201	216	232	247
15–15.9	208	221	239	254	279	300	322	175	178	189	202	215	228	244
16–16.9	218	224	241	258	283	318	334	170	180	190	202	216	234	249
17–17.9	220	227	241	264	295	324	350	175	183	194	205	221	239	257
18–18.9	222	227	241	258	281	312	325	174	179	191	202	215	237	245
19–24.9	221	230	247	265	290	319	345	179	185	195	207	221	236	249
25–34.9	233	240	256	277	304	342	368	183	188	199	212	228	246	264
35–44.9	241	251	267	290	317	356	378	186	192	205	218	236	257	272
45–54.9	242	256	274	299	328	362	384	187	193	206	220	238	260	274
55–64.9	243	257	280	303	335	367	385	187	196	209	225	244	266	280
65–74.9	240	252	274	299	326	356	373	185	195	208	225	244	264	279

Source: Reprinted with permission from Frisancho AR, "New norms of upper limb fat and muscle areas for assessment of nutritional status," in *American Journal of Clinical Nutrition* (1981; 34:2540–2545), Copyright © 1981, American Society for Clinical Nutrition, Inc.

Table BB-4 Percentiles for Estimates of Upper Arm Fat Area (mm^2) and Upper Arm Muscle Area (mm^2) for Whites of the United States, Health and Nutrition Examination Survey I of 1971–1974

	Males													
	Arm Muscle Area Percentiles (mm^2)							Arm Fat Area Percentiles (mm^2)						
Age Group	5	10	25	50	75	90	95	5	10	25	50	75	90	95
1–1.9	956	1,014	1,133	1,278	1,447	1,644	1,720	452	486	590	741	895	1,036	1,176
2–2.9	973	1,040	1,190	1,345	1,557	1,690	1,787	434	504	578	737	871	1,044	1,148
3–3.9	1,095	1,201	1,357	1,484	1,618	1,750	1,853	464	519	590	736	868	1,071	1,151
4–4.9	1,207	1,264	1,408	1,579	1,747	1,926	2,008	428	494	598	722	859	989	1,085
5–5.9	1,298	1,411	1,550	1,720	1,884	2,089	2,285	446	488	582	713	914	1,176	1,299
6–6.9	1,360	1,447	1,605	1,815	2,056	2,297	2,493	371	446	539	678	896	1,115	1,519
7–7.9	1,497	1,548	1,808	2,027	2,246	2,494	2,886	423	473	574	758	1,011	1,393	1,511
8–8.9	1,550	1,664	1,895	2,089	2,296	2,628	2,788	410	460	588	725	1,003	1,248	1,558
9–9.9	1,811	1,884	2,067	2,288	2,657	3,053	3,257	485	527	635	859	1,252	1,864	2,081
10–10.9	1,930	2,027	2,182	2,575	2,903	3,486	3,882	523	543	738	982	1,376	1,906	2,609
11–11.9	2,016	2,156	2,382	2,670	3,022	3,359	4,226	536	595	754	1,148	1,710	2,348	2,574
12–12.9	2,216	2,339	2,649	3,022	3,496	3,968	4,640	554	650	874	1,172	1,558	2,536	3,580

13–13.9.	2,363	2,546	3,044	3,553	4,081	4,502	4,794	475	570	812	1,096	1,702	2,744	3,322
14–14.9	2,830	3,147	3,586	3,963	4,575	5,368	5,530	453	563	786	1,082	1,608	2,746	3,508
15–15.9	3,138	3,317	3,788	4,481	5,134	5,631	5,900	521	595	690	931	1,423	2,434	3,100
16–16.9	3,625	4,044	4,352	4,951	5,753	6,576	6,980	542	593	844	1,078	1,746	2,280	3,041
17–17.9	3,998	4,252	4,771	5,286	5,950	6,886	7,726	598	698	827	1,096	1,636	2,407	2,888
18–18.9	4,070	4,481	5,066	5,552	6,374	7,067	8,355	560	665	860	1,264	1,947	3,302	3,928
19–24.9	4,508	4,771	5,274	5,913	6,660	7,606	8,200	594	743	963	1,406	2,231	3,098	3,652
25–34.9	4,694	4,963	5,541	6,214	7,067	7,847	8,436	675	831	1,174	1,752	2,459	3,246	3,786
35–44.9	4,844	5,181	5,740	6,490	7,265	8,034	8,488	703	851	1,310	1,792	2,463	3,098	3,624
45–54.9	4,546	4,946	5,589	6,297	7,142	7,918	8,458	749	922	1,254	1,741	2,359	3,245	3,928
55–64.9	4,422	4,783	5,381	6,144	6,919	7,670	8,149	658	839	1,166	1,645	2,236	2,976	3,466
65–74.9	3,973	4,411	5,031	5,716	6,432	7,074	7,453	573	753	1,122	1,621	2,199	2,876	3,327

continues

Table BB-4 Percentiles for Estimates of Upper Arm Fat Area (mm^2) and Upper Arm Muscle Area (mm^2) for Whites of the United States, Health and Nutrition Examination Survey I of 1971–1974—*continued*

	Females													
	Arm Muscle Area Percentiles (mm^2)							Arm Fat Area Percentiles (mm^2)						
Age Group	5	10	25	50	75	90	95	5	10	25	50	75	90	95
1–1.9	885	973	1,084	1,221	1,378	1,535	1,621	401	466	578	706	847	1,022	1,140
2–2.9	973	1,029	1,119	1,269	1,405	1,595	1,727	469	526	642	747	894	1,061	1,173
3–3.9	1,014	1,133	1,227	1,396	1,563	1,690	1,846	473	529	656	822	967	1,106	1,158
4–4.9	1,058	1,171	1,313	1,475	1,644	1,832	1,958	490	541	654	766	907	1,109	1,236
5–5.9	1,238	1,301	1,432	1,598	1,825	2,012	2,159	470	529	647	812	991	1,330	1,536
6–6.9	1,354	1,414	1,513	1,683	1,877	2,182	2,323	464	508	838	827	1,009	1,263	1,436
7–7.9	1,330	1,441	1,602	1,815	2,045	2,332	2,469	491	560	706	920	1,135	1,407	1,644
8–8.9	1,513	1,566	1,808	2,034	2,327	2,657	2,996	527	634	769	1,042	1,383	1,872	2,482
9–9.9	1,723	1,788	1,976	2,227	2,571	2,987	3,112	642	690	933	1,219	1,584	2,171	2,524
10–10.9	1,740	1,784	2,019	2,296	2,583	2,873	3,093	616	702	842	1,141	1,608	2,500	3,005
11–11.9	1,784	1,987	2,316	2,612	3,071	3,739	3,953	707	802	1,015	1,301	1,942	2,730	3,690
12–12.9	2,092	2,182	2,579	2,904	3,225	3,655	3,847	782	854	1,090	1,511	2,056	2,666	3,369

13–13.9	2,269	2,426	2,657	3,130	3,529	4,081	4,568	726	838	1,219	1,625	2,374	3,272	4,150
14–14.9	2,418	2,562	2,814	3,220	3,704	4,294	4,850	981	1,043	1,423	1,818	2,403	3,250	3,765
15–15.9	2,426	2,518	2,847	3,248	3,689	4,123	4,756	839	1,126	1,396	1,886	2,544	3,093	4,195
16–16.9	2,308	2,567	2,865	3,248	3,718	4,353	4,946	1,126	1,351	1,663	2,006	2,598	3,374	4,236
17–17.9	2,442	2,674	2,996	3,336	3,883	4,552	5,251	1,042	1,267	1,463	2,104	2,977	3,864	5,159
18–18.9	2,398	2,538	2,917	3,243	3,694	4,461	4,767	1,003	1,230	1,616	2,104	2,617	3,508	3,733
19–24.9	2,538	2,728	3,026	3,406	3,877	4,439	4,940	1,046	1,198	1,596	2,166	2,959	4,050	4,896
25–34.9	2,661	2,826	3,148	3,573	4,138	4,806	5,541	1,173	1,399	1,841	2,548	3,512	4,690	5,560
35–44.9	2,750	2,948	3,359	3,783	4,428	5,240	5,877	1,336	1,619.	2,158	2,898	3,932	5,093	5,847
45–54.9	2,784	2,956	3,378	3,858	4,520	5,375	5,964	1,459	1,803	2,447	3,244	4,229	5,416	6,140
55–64.9	2,784	3,063	3,477	4,045	4,750	5,632	6,247	1,345	1,879	2,520	3,369	4,360	5,276	6,152
65–74.9	2,737	3,018	3,444	4,019	4,739	5,566	6,214	1,363	1,681	2,266	3,063	3,943	4,914	5,530

Source: Reprinted with permission from Frisancho AR,"New norms of upper limb fat and muscle areas for assessment of nutritional status," in *American Journal of Clinical Nutrition* (1981; 34:2540–2545), Copyright © 1981, American Society for Clinical Nutrition, Inc.

Appendix CC: Enteral Formula Selection

Table CC-1 Enteral Products Designed for Renal Disease

Product	Manufacturer	Kcals/mL	Protein (gm)	K (mEq)	P (mg)	Mg (mg)
Renal Formulas						
Magnacal Renal	Novartis	2.0	37.5	16	400	100
Nepro	Ross	2.0	35.0	14	343	108
NovaSource Renal	Novartis	2.0	37.0	14	325	100
Suplena	Ross	2.0	15.0	14	365	108
Nutri-Renal	Nestle	2.0	17.0	Negligible	Negligible	Negligible
Standard Concentrated Formulas						
Deliver 2.0	Novartis	2.0	37.5	21.5	555	200
NovaSource 2.0	Novartis	2.0	45.0	19	550	210
Nutren 2.0	Nestle	2.0	40.0	25	670	268
Two-Cal HN	Ross	2.0	42.0	31	538	213

*Per 1000 kcal.

Table CC-2 Enteral Formulas Designed for Hepatic Disease

Product	Manufacturer	Kcals/ mL	% CHO Kcals	% Fat Kcals	% Pro Kcals	Comments
Hepatic-Aid II	Hormel Healthlabs	1.2	57.3	27.7	15.0	• Increased levels of leucine and valine • Minimal phenylalanine, tryptophan, and tyrosine content • Contains negligible amounts of vitamins and minerals
NutriHep	Nestle	1.5	77.0	11.0	12.0	• Contains standard amounts of vitamins and minerals • 50% BCAA and 50% AAA • 66% of fat is MCT

Table CC-3 Enteral Formulas Designed for Diabetes Mellitus

Product	Manufacturer	Kcals/ mL	% CHO Kcals	% PRO Kcals	% FAT Kcals	Fiber (g/1000 mL)
Choice DM	Novartis	1.06	40.0	17.0	43.0	14.4
DiabetiSource AC	Novartis	1.0	36.0	20.0	44.0	4.3
Glucerna Select	Ross	1.0	22.8	20.0	49.0	21.1
Glytrol	Nestle	1.0	40.0	18.0	420	15.0
Resource Diabetic	Novartis	1.06	36.0	24.0	40.0	12.8

Table CC-4 Formulas Designed for Pulmonary Disease

Product	Manufacturer	Kcals/ mL	% CHO Kcals	% PRO Kcals	% FAT Kcals
COPD Formulas					
NovaSource Pulmonary	Novartis	1.5	40.0	20.0	40.0
NutriVent	Nestle	1.5	27.0	18.0	55.0
Pulmocare	Ross	1.5	28.2	16.7	55.1
Respalor	Novartis	1.5	40.0	20.0	40.0
ARDS Formula					
Oxepa	Ross	1.5	28.1	16.7	55.2

Appendix DD: Vitamin and Mineral Food Sources

Vitamins

Vitamin B-6
Bananas
Fish (most)
Liver
Meat
Nuts and seeds
Potatoes and sweet potatoes
Poultry
Whole-grain and fortified cereals

Vitamin B-12
Eggs
Fish and shellfish
Fortified cereals
Meat
Milk and milk products
Organ meats

Vitamin D
Egg yolk
Fortified cereals
Fortified milk
Liver
High-fat fish

Vitamin E
Margarine
Nuts and seeds
Peanuts and peanut butter
Vegetable oils
Wheat germ
Whole-grain and fortified cereals

Folate
Dark green vegetables
Dry beans, peas, and lentils
Enriched grain products
Fortified cereals
Liver
Orange juice
Wheat germ
Yeast

Vitamin K
Broccoli
Brussels sprouts
Cabbage
Leafy green vegetables
Mayonnaise
Soybean, canola, and olive oils

Minerals

Iodine
Iodized salt
Saltwater fish and shellfish

Magnesium
Cocoa and chocolate
Dark green vegetables (most)
Dry beans, peas, and lentils
Fish
Nuts and seeds
Peanuts and peanut butter
Whole grains

Phosphorus
Dry beans, peas, and lentils
Eggs
Fish
Meat
Milk and milk products
Nuts and seeds
Poultry
Whole grains

Zinc
Dry beans, peas, and lentils
Meat
Poultry
Seeds
Shellfish
Whole-grain and fortified cereals

Appendix EE: Information Resources

Academic

www.mayoclinic.com/findinformation/healthylivingcenter/index.cfm
Mayo Clinic health information

www.navigator.tufts.edu
Tufts University Nutrition Navigator

Aging

www.aoa.gov
Administration on Aging
One Massachusetts Avenue, Suites 4100 & 5100
Washington, DC 20201
(202) 619-0724

www.aarp.org
American Association of Retired Persons (AARP)
601 E Street NW
Washington, DC 20049
(800) 424-3410, (202) 434-2560

www.americangeriatrics.org
American Geriatrics Society
The Empire State Building
350 Fifth Avenue, Suite 801
New York, NY 10118
(212) 308-1414

www.aoa.gov/naic
Center for Communication and Consumer Services
Administration on Aging
330 Independence Avenue SW, Room 4656
Washington, DC 20201
(202) 619-7501

www.ncoa.org
National Council on the Aging
300 D Street SW
Suite 801
Washington, DC 20024
(202) 479-1200

www.nia.nih.gov
National Institute on Aging
Building 31, Room 5C27
31 Center Drive, MSC 2292
Bethesda, MD 20892
(301) 496-1752

www.nof.org
National Osteoporosis Foundation
1232 22nd Street NW
Washington, DC 20037-1292
(202) 223-2226

Alcohol and Drug Abuse

www.al-anon.alateen.org
Al-Anon/Alateen
1600 Corporate Landing Parkway
Virginia Beach, VA 23454-5617
(888) 425-2666

www.aa.org
Alcoholics Anonymous (AA)
Grand Central Station
P.O. Box 459
New York, NY 10163
(212) 870-3400

www.covesoft.eom/csap.html
Center for Substance Abuse Prevention
1010 Wayne Avenue, Suite 850
Silver Spring, MD 20910
(301) 459-1591 ext. 244; fax: (301) 495-2919

www.wsoinc.com
Narcotics Anonymous (NA)
P.O. Box 9999
Van Nuys, CA 91409
(818) 773-9999; fax: (818) 700-0700

www.health.org
National Clearinghouse for Alcohol and Drug Information (NCADI)
11426 Rockville Pike, Suite 200
Rockville, MD 20852
(800) 729-6686

www.ncadd.org
National Council on Alcoholism and Drug Dependence (NCADD)
20 Exchange Place, Suite 2902
New York, NY 10005
(800) 622-2255, (212) 269-7797; fax: (212) 269-7510

Canadian Government: Federal

www.agr.gc.ca
Agriculture and Agri-Food Canada
Public Information Request Services
Sir John Carling Building
930 Carling Avenue
Ottawa, Ontario K1A 0C5
(613) 759-1000; fax: (613) 759-6726

www.he-sc.gc.ca/food-aliment/ns-se/e_nutrition.html
Bureau of Nutritional Sciences
Nutrition Research Division
Sir Frederick G. Banting Research Centre
Tunney's Pasture (2203C)
Ottawa, Ontario K1A 0L2
(613) 957-0919; fax: (613) 941-6182

www.hc-se.gc.ca/food-aliment/ns-sc/e_nutrition.html
Bureau of Nutritional Sciences
Nutrition Evaluation Division
Sir Frederick G. Banting Research Centre
Tunney's Pasture (2203A)
Ottawa, Ontario K1A 0L2
(613) 957-0352; fax: (613) 941-6636

www.inspection.gc.ca
Canadian Food Inspection Agency
59 Camelot Drive
Ottawa, Ontario K1A 0Y9
(800) 442-2342, (613) 225-2342; fax: (613) 228-6601

www.cihi.ca
Canadian Institute for Health Information
377 Dalhousie Street, Suite 200
Ottawa, Ontario K1N 9N8
(613) 241-7860; fax: (613) 241-8120

www.cpha.ca
Canadian Public Health Association
400-1565 Carling Avenue
Ottawa, Ontario K1Z 8R1
(613) 725-3769 ext. 165; fax: (613) 725-9826

www.agr.ca/food/nff/enutrace.html
Functional Foods and Nutraceuticals Food Bureau
597-930 Carling Avenue
Ottawa, Ontario K1A 0C5

www.hc-sc.gc.ca
Health Canada
A.L. 0900C2
Ottawa, Ontario K1A 0K9
(613) 957-2991; fax: (613) 941-5366

www.nin.ca
National Institute of Nutrition
408 Queen Street, 3rd Floor
Ottawa, Ontario K1R 5A7
(613) 235-3355; fax: (613) 235-7032

Canadian Government: Provincial and Territorial

Consultant, Nutrition
Health and Wellness Promotion, Population Health, Department of Health and Social Services, Government of the Northwest Territories
Center Square Tower, 6th Floor
P.O. Box 1320
Yellowknife, NT X1A 219

Coordinator, Health Information
Resource Centre
Department of Health and Social Services
1 Rochford Street, Box 2000
Charlottetown, PEI C1A 7N8

Director, Health Promotion
Department of Health, Government of Newfoundland and Labrador
P.O. Box 8700
Confederation Building, West Block
St. John's, NF A1B 4J6

Director, Nutrition Services
Yukon Hospital Corporation
#5 Hospital Road
Whitehorse, YT Y1A 3H7

Executive Director
Health Programs
2nd Floor, 800 Portage Avenue
Winnipeg, MB R3G 0P4

Health Promotion Unit
Population Health Branch
Saskatchewan Health
3475 Albert Street
Regina, SK S4S 6X6

Nutritionist
Preventive Services Branch
Ministry of Health
1520 Blanshard Street
Victoria, BC V8W 3C8

Population Health Strategies Branch
Alberta Health
23rd Floor, TELUS Plaza, North Tower
10025 Jasper Avenue
Edmonton, AB T5J 2N3

Project Manager, Public Health Management Services
Health and Community Services
P.O. Box 5100
520 King Street
Fredericton, NB E3B 5G8

Public Health Nutritionist
Central Health Region
201 Brownlow Avenue, Unit 4
Dartmouth, NS B3B 1W2

Responsables de la sante cardiovasculaire et de la nutrition
Ministére de la Santé et des Services sociaux, Service de la Prevention en Santé
3e étage, 1075, chemin Sainte-Foy
Quebec G1S 2M1

Senior Consultant, Nutrition
Public Health Branch
Ministry of Health, 8th Floor
5700 Yonge St.
New York, Ontario M2M 4K5

Complementary and Alternative Nutrition

http://nccam.nih.gov/
National Center for Complementary and Alternative Medicine, NIH
NCCAM Clearinghouse
P.O. Box 7923
Gaithersburg, MD 20898-7923
(888) 644-6226

www.hc-sc.gc.ca/hpb/onhp/
Office of Natural Health Products
2936 Baseline Road, Tower A
Postal Locator: 3302A
Ottawa, Ontario K1A 0K9
(888) 774-5555; fax: (613) 946-1615

Consumer Organizations

www.diabetes.ca
Canadian Diabetes Association
15 Toronto Street, Suite 800
Toronto, Ontario M5C 2E3
(800) 226-8464; (416) 363-3373; fax: (416) 363-3393

www.cspinet.org
Center for Science in the Public Interest (CSPI)
1875 Connecticut Avenue NW, Suite 300
Washington, DC 20009
(202) 332-9110; fax: (202) 265-4954

www.consumersunion.org
Consumers Union
101 Truman Avenue
Yonkers, NY 10703-1057
(914) 378-2000

www.pueblo.gsa.gov
U.S. General Services Administration
Federal Citizen Information Center
Pueblo, CO 81009
(800) 688-9889; (888) 878-3256

www.ncahf.org
National Council Against Health Fraud, Inc. (NCAHF)
119 Foster Street
Peabody, MA 01960
(978) 532-9383

www.partnershipforcaring.org/HomePage
Partnership for Caring
1620 Eye Street NW, Suite 202
Washington, DC 20006
(800) 989-9455, (202) 296-8071; fax (202) 296-8352

www.quackwatch.com
Stephen Barrett, MD
P.O. Box 1747
Allentown, PA 18105
(610) 437-1795

Eating Disorders

www.anred.com
Anorexia Nervosa and Related Eating Disorders, Inc. (ANRED)
P.O. Box 5102
Eugene, OR 97405
(800) 931-2237

www.anad.org
National Association of Anorexia Nervosa and Associated Disorders (ANAD)
555 Vine Avenue
Highland Park, IL 60035
(847) 831-3438; fax: (847) 433-4632

www.nedic.ca
National Eating Disorder Information Centre
200 Elizabeth Street, CW 1-211
Toronto, Ontario M5G 2C4
(866) 633-4220, (416) 340-4156; fax: (416) 340-4736

www.nationaleatingdisorders.org
National Eating Disorders Association
603 Stewart Street, Suite 803
Seattle, WA 98101
(206) 382-3587

Food Safety

www.foodsafetyalliance.org
Alliance for Food & Farming
10866 Wilshire Boulevard, Suite 550
Los Angeles, CA 90024
(310) 446-1827; fax: (310) 446-1896

www.cfsan.fda.gov
FDA Center for Food Safety and Applied Nutrition
5100 Paint Branch Parkway (HFS-555)
College Park, MD 20740-3835
(888) 723-3366

www.epa.gov/opptintr/lead/nlic.htm
National Lead Information Center
422 South Clinton Avenue
Rochester, NY 14620
(800) 424-5323; fax: (585) 232-3111

www.npic.orst. edu/index.html
National Pesticide Information Center
Oregon State University
333 Weniger Hall
Corvallis, OR 97331-6502
(800) 858-7378; fax: (541) 737-0761

U.S. EPA Safe Drinking Water Hotline
(800) 426-4791

www.fsis.usda.gov
USDA Food Safety and Inspection Service (FSIS)
Food Safety Education Staff
Maildrop 5268
5601 Sunnyside Avenue
Beltsville, MD 20705
(301) 504-9605

USDA Meat and Poultry Hotline
(800) 535-4555

Infancy, Childhood, and Adolescence

www.aap.org
American Academy of Pediatrics
141 Northwest Point Boulevard
Elk Grove Village, IL 60007-1098
(847) 434-4000; fax: (847) 434-8000

www.birthdefects.org
Birth Defect Research for Children
930 Woodcock Road, Suite 225
Orlando, FL 32803
(407) 895-0802

www.cps.ca
Canadian Paediatric Society
100-2204 Walkley Road
Ottawa, Ontario K1G 4G8
(613) 526-9397; fax: (613) 526-3332

www.childrensfoundation.net
Children's Foundation
725 Fifteenth Street NW, Suite 505
Washington, DC 20005-2109
(202) 347-3300; fax: (202) 347-3382

www.KidsHealth.org
KidsHealth
The Nemours Foundation
1600 Rockland Road
Wilmington, DE 19803
(302) 651-4046

www.ncemch.org
National Center for Education in Maternal & Child Health
Georgetown University
Box 571272
Washington, DC 20057-1272
(202) 784-9770; fax: (202) 784-9777

International Agencies

www.fao.org
Food and Agriculture Organization of the United Nations (FAO)
Liaison Office for North America
Suite 300, 2175 K Street NW
Washington, DC 20437-0001
(202) 653-2400; fax: (202) 653-5760

www.ific.org
International Food Information Council Foundation
1100 Connecticut Avenue NW, Suite 430
Washington, DC 20036
(202) 296-6540; fax: (202) 296-6547

www.unicef.org
UNICEF
3 United Nations Plaza
New York, NY 10017
(212) 326-7000; fax: (212) 887-7465

www.who.int/home-page
World Health Organization (WHO) Regional Office
525 23rd Street NW
Washington, DC 20037
(202) 974-3000; fax: (202) 974-3663

Pregnancy and Lactation

www.acog.org
American College of Obstetricians and Gynecologists
Resource Center
409 12th Street SW
P.O. Box 96920
Washington, D.C. 20090-6920
(202) 638-5577

www.lalecheleague.org
La Leche League International
1400 N. Meacham Road
Schaumburg, IL 60173-4048
(847) 519-7730

www.modimes.org
March of Dimes Birth Defects Foundation
1275 Mamaroneck Avenue
White Plains, NY 10605
(888) 663-4637

Professional Nutrition Organizations

ADA, The Nutrition Line
(800) 366-1655

www.eatright.org
American Dietetic Association (ADA)
120 South Riverside Plaza, Suite 2000
Chicago, IL 60606-6995
(800) 877-1600

www.faseb.org/ascn
American Society for Clinical Nutrition
9650 Rockville Pike
Bethesda, MD 20814-3998
(301) 530-7110; fax: (301) 571-1863

www.asns.org
American Society for Nutritional Sciences
9650 Rockville Pike, Suite 4500
Bethesda, MD 20814
(301) 634-7050; fax: (301) 571-7892

www.nutritionalsciences.ca
Canadian Society for Nutritional Sciences
Centre de Recherche Institut Universitaire de Gériatrie de Montréal
4565, chemin Queen-Mary
Montreal, Québec H3W 1W5

www.dietitians.ca
Dietitians of Canada
480 University Avenue, Suite 604
Toronto, Ontario M5G 1V2
(416) 596-0857; fax: (416) 596-0603

http://hni.ilsi.org
ILSI Human Nutrition Institute (HNI)
One Thomas Circle, Ninth Floor
Washington, DC 20005
(202) 659-0524; fax: (202) 659-3617

www.ift.org
Institute of Food Technologists
525 West Van Buren, Suite 1000
Chicago, IL 60607
(312) 782-8424; fax: (312) 782-8348

www.nationalacademies.org/ nrc
National Academy of Sciences/ National Research Council (NAS/NRC)
2001 Wisconsin Avenue NW
Washington, DC 20001
(202) 334-2000

www.sne.org
Society for Nutrition Education
9202 North Meridian, Suite 200
Indianapolis, IN 46260
(800) 235-6690; fax (317) 571-5603

Sports Nutrition

www.acsm.org
American College of Sports Medicine (ACSM)
401 W. Michigan Street
Indianapolis, IN 46202-3233
(317) 637-9200; fax: (317) 634-7817

www.acefitness.org
American Council on Exercise (ACE)
4851 Paramount Drive
San Diego, CA 92123
(800) 825-3636, (858) 279-8227; fax: (858) 279-8064

www.cahperd.ca
Canadian Association for Health, Physical Education, Recreation, and Dance
403-2197 Riverside Drive
Ottawa, Ontario K1H 7X3
(613) 523-1348; fax: (613) 523-1206

www.csep.ca
Canadian Society for Exercise Physiology
185 Somerset Street West, Suite 202
Ottawa, Ontario K2P 0J2
(613) 234-3755; fax: (613) 234-3565

www.fitness.gov
President's Council on Physical Fitness and Sports
Department W
200 Independence Avenue SW, Room 738-H
Washington, DC 20201-0004
(202) 690-9000; fax: (202) 690-5211

www.runnersworld.com
Runners World
33 East Minor Street
Emmaus, PA 18098
(610) 967-5171

Sports Medicine and Science Council of Canada
1600 James Naismith Drive, Suite 306
Gloucester, Ontario K1B 5N4
(613) 748-5671; fax: (613) 748-5729

www.scandpg.org
Sports, Cardiovascular and Wellness Nutritionists (SCAN)
P.O. Box 60820
Colorado Springs, CO 80960-0820
(719) 635-6005; fax: (719) 635-3587

www.ideafit.com
The International Association for Fitness Professionals (IDEA)
6190 Cornerstone Court East, Suite 204
San Diego, CA 92121-3773
(800) 999-4332 ext. 7; fax: (858) 535-8234

www.veggie.org/
Veggie Sports Association

Supplements

http://dietary-supplements.info.nih.gov/databases/ibids.html
International Bibliographic Information on Dietary Supplements (IBIDS)

http://dietary-supplements.info.nih.gov
Office of Dietary Supplements
National Institutes of Health
6100 Executive Boulevard, Room 3B01, MSC 7517
Bethesda, MD 20892-7517
(301) 435-2920; fax: (301) 480-1845

Trade and Industry Organizations

www.aibonline.org
American Institute of Baking
1213 Bakers Way
P.O. Box 3999
Manhattan, KS 66505-3999
(800) 633-5137, (785) 537-4750; fax: (785) 537-1493

www.meatami.org
American Meat Institute
1700 North Moore Street, Suite 1600
Arlington, VA 22209
(703) 841-2400; fax: (703) 527-0938

www.beechnut.com
Beech-Nut Nutrition Corporation
100 S. 4th Street
St. Louis, MO 63102
(800) 233-2468

www.gssiweb.com
Gatorade Sports Science Institute
617 West Main Street
Barrington, IL 60010
(800) 616-4774

www.GeneralMills.com/corporate
General Mills
Number One General Mills Boulevard
Minneapolis, MN 55426
(800) 328-1144

www.gerber.com
Gerber Products Company
445 State Street
Fremont, MI 49413-0001
(800) 443-7237

www.heinz.com
H.J. Heinz Company
World Headquarters
600 Grant Street
Pittsburgh, PA 15219
(412) 456-5700

www.kelloggs.com
Kellogg Company
P.O. Box CAMB
Battle Creek, MI 49016
(800) 962-1413

www.kraftfoods.com
Kraft Foods
Consumer Response and Information Center
One Kraft Court
Glenview, IL 60025
(800) 323-0768

www.nationaldairycouncil.org
National Dairy Council
10255 West Higgins Road, Suite 900
Rosemont, IL 60018-5616
(847) 803-2000

www.pillsbury.com
Pillsbury Company
c/o General Mills
Number One General Mills Boulevard
Minneapolis, MN 55426
(800) 775-4777

www.pg.com
Procter & Gamble Company
One Procter and Gamble Plaza
Cincinnati, OH 45202
(513) 983-1100

www.sunkist.com
Sunkist Growers
Consumer Affairs, Fresh Fruit Division
14130 Riverside Drive
Sherman Oaks, CA 91423
(800) 248-7875

www.dannon.com
The Dannon Company
Dannon Consumer Response Center
P.O. Box 90296
Allentown, PA 18109-0296
(877) 326-6668

www.nutrasweet.com
The NutraSweet Company
P.O. Box 1280
South Bend, IN 46624-1280
(800) 323-5316

www.uffva.org
United Fresh Fruit and Vegetable Association
1901 Pennsylvania Avenue NW, Suite 1100
Washington, DC 20006
(202) 303-3400; fax: (202) 303-3433

www.usarice.com
USA Rice Federation
4301 North Fairfax Drive, Suite 305
Arlington, VA 22201
(703) 351-8161

Weight Management

http://nutrition.uvm.edu/bodycomp/
Body Composition Analysis Tutorials

www.overeatersanonymous.org
Overeaters Anonymous (OA)
World Service Office
P.O. Box 44020
Rio Rancho, NM 87174-4020
(505) 891-2664; fax: (505) 891-4320

www.shapeup.org
Shape Up America!
c/o WebFront Solutions Corporation
15757 Crabbs Branch Way
Rockville, MD 20855
(301) 258-0540; fax: (301) 258-0541

www.tops.org
TOPS (Take Off Pounds Sensibly)
4575 South Fifth Street
P.O. Box 070360
Milwaukee, WI 53207-0360
(800) 932-8677, (414) 482-4620

www.niddk.nih.gov/health/nutrit/win.htm
Weight-control Information Network
1 WIN Way
Bethesda, MD 20892-3665
(877) 946-4627, (202) 828-1025; fax: (202) 828-1028

www.weightwatchers.com
Weight Watchers International
Consumer Affairs Department/IN
175 Crossways Park West
Woodbury, NY 11797
(516) 390-1400

World Hunger

www.bread.org
Bread for the World
50 F Street NW, Suite 500
Washington, DC 20001
(800) 822-7323, (202) 639-9400; fax: (202) 639-9401

http://hunger.tufts.edu
Center on Hunger, Poverty, and Nutrition Policy
Tufts University School of Nutrition Science and Policy
136 Harrison Avenue
Boston, MA 02111
(617) 636-3736; fax: (617) 636-3871

www.freefromhunger.org
Freedom from Hunger
1644 DaVinci Court
Davis, CA 95616
(800) 708-2555; fax: (530) 758-6241

www.oxfamamerica.org
Oxfam America
26 West Street
Boston, MA 02111-1206
(800) 776-9326; fax: (617) 728-2594

www.worldwatch.org
Worldwatch Institute
1776 Massachusetts Avenue NW
Washington, DC 20036-1904
(202) 452-1999; fax: (202) 296-7365

U.S. Government

www.nutrition.gov
Online federal government information on nutrition

www.cdc.gov
Centers for Disease Control and Prevention
1600 Clifton Road
Atlanta, GA 30333
(800) 311-3435

FDA Consumer Information Line
(888) 463-6332

FDA Office of Nutritional Products, Labeling, and Dietary Supplements
HFS-800
RM4C096
College Park, MD 20740
(301) 436-23 73

www.ftc.gov
Federal Trade Commission (FTC)
CRC-240
Washington, DC 20580
(877) 382-4357

www.fda.gov
Food and Drug Administration (FDA)
5600 Fishers Lane
Rockville, MD 20857
(888) 463-6332, (301) 443-1544

www.fda.gov/medwatch/index.html
MedWatch
The FDA Safety Information and Adverse Event Reporting Program
US Food and Drug Administration
MedWatch Office
5600 Fishers Lane, HFD-410
Rockville, MD 20857
(301) 827-7240; fax: (301) 827-7241

www.nal.usda.gov/fnic
Food and Nutrition Information Center
National Agricultural Library, Room 105
10301 Baltimore Avenue
Beltsville, MD 20705-2351
(301) 504-5719; fax: (301) 504-6409

www.frac.org
Food Research and Action Center (FRAC)
1875 Connecticut Avenue NW, Suite 540
Washington, DC 20009
(202) 986-2200; fax: (202) 986-2525

www.healthfinder.gov
Gateway for health and nutrition information
Healthfinder
P.O. Box 1133
Washington, DC 20013-1133

www.nidr.nih.gov
National Institute of Dental and Craniofacial Research (NIDCR)
NIDCR Public Information & Liaison Branch
45 Center Drive, MSC 6400
Bethesda, MD 20892-6400
(301) 496-4261

www.niddk.nih.gov
National Institute of Diabetes & Digestive & Kidney Diseases
Office of Communications and Public Liaison
NIDDK, NIH
Building 31, Room 9A04
Center Drive, MSC 2560
Bethesda, MD 20892-2560

www.nih.gov/health
National Institutes of Health search engine and free access to Medline and PubMed databases

www.usda.gov
U.S. Department of Agriculture (USDA)
Washington, DC 20250
(202) 720-2791

www.dhhs.gov
U.S. Department of Health and Human Services
200 Independence Avenue SW
Washington, DC 20201
(877) 696-6775, (202) 619-0257

www.epa.gov
U.S. Environmental Protection Agency (EPA)
Ariel Rios Building
1200 Pennsylvania Avenue NW
Washington, DC 20460
(202) 272-0167

www.pueblo.gsa.gov
U.S. General Services Administration
Federal Communication Information Center
Pueblo, CO 81009
(800) 688-9889, (888) 878-3256

www.access.gpo.gov/su_docs
U.S. Government Printing Office
732 N Capitol Street NW #808
Washington, DC 20001
(866) 512-1800, (202) 512-2250; fax: (202) 512-2250

www.hhs.gov/
U.S. Department of Health and Human Services
200 Independence Avenue SW
Washington, DC 20201
(877) 696-6775, (202) 619-0257

www.usda.gov/cnpp
USDA Center for Nutrition Policy and Promotion
3101 Park Center Drive, Room 1034
Alexandria, VA 22302-1594
(703) 305-7600; fax: (703) 305-3400

Appendix FF: Food Sources of Selected Nutrients

Food sources of potassium ranked by milligrams of potassium per standard amount, also showing calories in the standard amount. (The adequate intake [AI] for adults is 4,700 mg/day potassium.)

Table FF-1 Food Sources of Potassium

Food, Standard Amount	Potassium (mg)	Calories
Sweet potato, baked, 1 potato (146 g)	694	131
Tomato paste, 1/4 cup	664	54
Beet greens, cooked, 1/2 cup	655	19
Potato, baked, flesh, 1 potato (156 g)	610	145
White beans, canned, 1/2 cup	595	153
Yogurt, plain, nonfat, 8 oz. container	579	127
Tomato puree, 1/2 cup	549	48
Clams, canned, 3 oz.	534	126
Yogurt, plain, low-fat, 8 oz. container	531	143
Prune juice, 3/4 cup	530	136
Carrot juice, 3/4 cup	517	71
Blackstrap molasses, 1 Tbsp	498	47
Halibut, cooked, 3 oz.	490	119
Soybeans, green, cooked, 1/2 cup	485	127
Tuna, yellowfin, cooked, 3 oz.	484	118
Lima beans, cooked, 1/2 cup	484	104
Winter squash, cooked, 1/2 cup	448	40
Soybeans, mature, cooked, 1/2 cup	443	149
Rockfish, Pacific, cooked, 3 oz.	442	103
Cod, Pacific, cooked, 3 oz.	439	89
Bananas, 1 medium	422	105
Spinach, cooked, 1/2 cup	419	21
Tomato juice, 3/4 cup	417	31
Tomato sauce, 1/2 cup	405	39
Peaches, dried, uncooked, 1/4 cup	398	96
Prunes, stewed, 1/2 cup	398	133
Milk, nonfat, 1 cup	382	83
Pork chop, center loin, cooked, 3 oz.	382	197
Apricots, dried, uncooked, 1/4 cup	378	78
Rainbow trout, farmed, cooked, 3 oz.	375	144
Pork loin, center rib (roasts), lean, roasted, 3 oz.	371	190
Buttermilk, cultured, low-fat, 1 cup	370	98

Table FF-1 Food Sources of Potassium—*continued*

Food, Standard Amount	Potassium (mg)	Calories
Cantaloupe, 1/4 medium	368	47
1%–2% milk, 1 cup	366	102–122
Honeydew melon, 1/8 medium	365	58
Lentils, cooked, 1/2 cup	365	115
Plantains, cooked, 1/2 cup slices	358	90
Kidney beans, cooked, 1/2 cup	358	112
Orange juice, 3/4 cup	355	85
Split peas, cooked, 1/2 cup	355	116
Yogurt, plain, whole milk, 8 oz. container	352	138

Source: Nutrient values from Agricultural Research Service (ARS) Nutrient Database for Standard Reference, Release 17. Foods are from ARS single nutrient reports, sorted in descending order by nutrient content in terms of common household measures. Food items and weights in the single nutrient reports are adapted from those in the 2002 revision of USDA Home and Garden Bulletin No. 72, Nutritive Value of Foods. Omitted from this table are mixed dishes and multiple preparations of the same food item.

Food sources of vitamin E ranked by milligrams of vitamin E per standard amount; also calories in the standard amount. (All provide greater than or equal to 10% of the RDA of vitamin E for adults, which is 15 mg a-tocopherol [AT] per day.)

Table FF-2 Food Sources of Vitamin E

Food, Standard Amount	AT (mg)	Calories
Fortified ready-to-eat cereals, ~ 1 oz.	1.6–12.8	90–107
Sunflower seeds, dry roasted, 1 oz.	7.4	165
Almonds, 1 oz.	7.3	164
Sunflower oil, high linoleic acid, 1 Tbsp	5.6	120
Cottonseed oil, 1 Tbsp	4.8	120
Safflower oil, high oleic, 1 Tbsp	4.6	120
Hazelnuts (filberts), 1 oz.	4.3	178
Mixed nuts, dry roasted, 1 oz.	3.1	168
Turnip greens, frozen, cooked, 1/2 cup	2.9	24
Tomato paste, 1/4 cup	2.8	54
Pine nuts, 1 oz.	2.6	191
Peanut butter, 2 Tbsp	2.5	192
Tomato puree, 1/2 cup	2.5	48
Tomato sauce, 1/2 cup	2.5	39
Canola oil, 1 Tbsp	2.4	124
Wheat germ, toasted, plain, 2 Tbsp	2.3	54
Peanuts, 1 oz.	2.2	166
Avocado, raw, 1/2 avocado	2.1	161
Carrot juice, canned, 3/4 cup	2.1	71
Peanut oil, 1 Tbsp	2.1	119
Corn oil, 1 Tbsp	1.9	120
Olive oil, 1 Tbsp	1.9	119
Spinach, cooked, 1/2 cup	1.9	21
Dandelion greens, cooked, 1/2 cup	1.8	18
Sardines, Atlantic, in oil, drained, 3 oz.	1.7	177
Blue crab, cooked–canned, 3 oz.	1.6	84
Brazil nuts, 1 oz.	1.6	186
Herring, Atlantic, pickled, 3 oz.	1.5	222

Source: Nutrient values from Agricultural Research Service (ARS) Nutrient Database for Standard Reference, Release 17. Foods are from ARS single nutrient reports, sorted in descending order by nutrient content in terms of common household measures. Food items and weights in the single nutrient reports are adapted from those in the 2002 revision of USDA Home and Garden Bulletin No. 72, Nutritive Value of Foods. Omitted from this table are mixed dishes and multiple preparations of the same food item.

Food sources of iron ranked by milligrams of iron per standard amount; also calories in the standard amount. (All are greater than or equal to 10% of the RDA for teen and adult females, which is 18 mg per day.)

Table FF-3 Food Sources of Iron

Food, Standard Amount	Iron (mg)	Calories
Clams, canned, drained, 3 oz.	23.8	126
Fortified ready-to-eat cereals (various), ~ 1 oz.	1.8–21.1	54–127
Oysters, eastern, wild, cooked, moist heat, 3 oz.	10.2	116
Organ meats (liver, giblets), various, cooked, 3 oz.[a]	5.2–9.9	134–235
Fortified instant cooked cereals (various), 1 packet	4.9–8.1	Varies
Soybeans, mature, cooked, 1/2 cup	4.4	149
Pumpkin and squash seed kernels, roasted, 1 oz.	4.2	148
White beans, canned, 1/2 cup	3.9	153
Blackstrap molasses, 1 Tbsp	3.5	47
Lentils, cooked, 1/2 cup	3.3	115
Spinach, cooked from fresh, 1/2 cup	3.2	21
Beef, chuck, blade roast, lean, cooked, 3 oz.	3.1	215
Beef, bottom round, lean, 0" fat, all grades, cooked, 3 oz.	2.8	182
Kidney beans, cooked, 1/2 cup	2.6	112
Sardines, canned in oil, drained, 3 oz.	2.5	177
Beef, rib, lean, 1/4" fat, all grades, 3 oz.	2.4	195
Chickpeas, cooked, 1/2 cup	2.4	134
Duck, meat only, roasted, 3 oz.	2.3	171
Lamb, shoulder, arm, lean, 1/4 " fat, choice, cooked, 3 oz.	2.3	237
Prune juice, 3/4 cup	2.3	136
Shrimp, canned, 3 oz.	2.3	102
Cowpeas, cooked, 1/2 cup	2.2	100
Ground beef, 15% fat, cooked, 3 oz.	2.2	212
Tomato puree, 1/2 cup	2.2	48
Lima beans, cooked, 1/2 cup	2.2	108
Soybeans, green, cooked, 1/2 cup	2.2	127
Navy beans, cooked, 1/2 cup	2.1	127
Refried beans, 1/2 cup	2.1	118
Beef, top sirloin, lean, 0" fat, all grades, cooked, 3 oz.	2.0	156
Tomato paste, 1/4 cup	2.0	54

[a] High in cholesterol.

Source: Nutrient values from Agricultural Research Service (ARS) Nutrient Database for Standard Reference, Release 17. Foods are from ARS single nutrient reports, sorted in descending order by nutrient content in terms of common household measures. Food items and weights in the single nutrient reports are adapted from those in the 2002 revision of USDA Home and Garden Bulletin No. 72, Nutritive Value of Foods. Omitted from this table are mixed dishes and multiple preparations of the same food item.

Non-dairy food sources of calcium ranked by milligrams of calcium per standard amount; also calories in the standard amount. The bioavailability may vary. (The AI for adults is 1,000 mg/day.)[a]

Table FF-4 Non-Dairy Food Sources of Calcium

Food, Standard Amount	Calcium (mg)	Calories
Fortified ready-to-eat cereals (various), 1 oz.	236–1,043	88–106
Soy beverage, calcium fortified, 1 cup	368	98
Sardines, Atlantic, in oil, drained, 3 oz.	325	177
Tofu, firm, prepared with nigari[b], ½ cup	253	88
Pink salmon, canned, with bone, 3 oz.	181	118
Collards, cooked from frozen, ½ cup	178	31
Molasses, blackstrap, 1 Tbsp	172	47
Spinach, cooked from frozen, ½ cup	146	30
Soybeans, green, cooked, ½ cup	130	127
Turnip greens, cooked from frozen, ½ cup	124	24
Ocean perch, Atlantic, cooked, 3 oz.	116	103
Oatmeal, plain and flavored, instant, fortified, 1 packet prepared	99–110	97–157
Cowpeas, cooked, ½ cup	106	80
White beans, canned, ½ cup	96	153
Kale, cooked from frozen, ½ cup	90	20
Okra, cooked from frozen, ½ cup	88	26
Soybeans, mature, cooked, ½ cup	88	149
Blue crab, canned, 3 oz.	86	84
Beet greens, cooked from fresh, ½ cup	82	19
Pak choi, Chinese cabbage, cooked from fresh, ½ cup	79	10
Clams, canned, 3 oz.	78	126
Dandelion greens, cooked from fresh, ½ cup	74	17
Rainbow trout, farmed, cooked, 3 oz.	73	144

[a] Both calcium content and bioavailability should be considered when selecting dietary sources of calcium. Some plant foods have calcium that is well absorbed, but the large quantity of plant foods that would be needed to provide as much calcium as in a glass of milk may be unachievable for many. Many other calcium-fortified foods are available, but the percentage of calcium that can be absorbed is unavailable for many of them.

[b] Calcium sulfate and magnesium chloride.

Source: Nutrient values from Agricultural Research Service (ARS) Nutrient Database for Standard Reference, Release 17. Foods are from ARS single nutrient reports, sorted in descending order by nutrient content in terms of common household measures. Food items and weights in the single nutrient reports are adapted from those in the 2002 revision of USDA Home and Garden Bulletin No. 72, Nutritive Value of Foods. Omitted from this table are mixed dishes and multiple preparations of the same food item.

Food sources of calcium ranked by milligrams of calcium per standard amount; also calories in the standard amount. (All are greater than or equal to 20% of the AI for adults 19–50, which is 1,000 mg/day.)

Table FF-5 Food Sources of Calcium

Food, Standard Amount	Calcium (mg)	Calories
Plain yogurt, nonfat (13 g protein/8 oz.), 8 oz. container	452	127
Romano cheese, 1.5 oz.	452	165
Pasteurized process Swiss cheese, 2 oz.	438	190
Plain yogurt, low-fat (12 g protein/8 oz.), 8 oz. container	415	143
Fruit yogurt, low-fat (10 g protein/8 oz.), 8 oz. container	345	232
Swiss cheese, 1.5 oz.	336	162
Ricotta cheese, part skim, ½ cup	335	170
Pasteurized process American cheese food, 2 oz.	323	188
Provolone cheese, 1.5 oz.	321	150
Mozzarella cheese, part-skim, 1.5 oz.	311	129
Cheddar cheese, 1.5 oz.	307	171
Fat-free (skim) milk, 1 cup	306	83
Muenster cheese, 1.5 oz.	305	156
1% low-fat milk, 1 cup	290	102
Low-fat chocolate milk (1%), 1 cup	288	158
2% reduced fat milk, 1 cup	285	122
Reduced-fat chocolate milk (2%), 1 cup	285	180
Buttermilk, low-fat, 1 cup	284	98
Chocolate milk, 1 cup	280	208
Whole milk, 1 cup	276	146
Yogurt, plain, whole milk (8 g protein/8 oz.), 8 oz. container	275	138
Ricotta cheese, whole milk, ½ cup	255	214
Blue cheese, 1.5 oz.	225	150
Mozzarella cheese, whole milk, 1.5 oz.	215	128
Feta cheese, 1.5 oz.	210	113

Source: Nutrient values from Agricultural Research Service (ARS) Nutrient Database for Standard Reference, Release 17. Foods are from ARS single nutrient reports, sorted in descending order by nutrient content in terms of common household measures. Food items and weights in the single nutrient reports are adapted from those in the 2002 revision of USDA Home and Garden Bulletin No. 72, Nutritive Value of Foods. Omitted from this table are mixed dishes and multiple preparations of the same food item.

Food sources of vitamin A ranked by micrograms Retinol Activity Equivalents (RAE) of vitamin A per standard amount; also calories in the standard amount. (All are greater than or equal to 20% of the RDA for adult men, which is 900 mg per day RAE.)

Table FF-6 Food Sources of Vitamin A

Food, Standard Amount	Vitamin A (µg RAE)	Calories
Organ meats (liver, giblets), various, cooked, 3 oz.[a]	1,490–9,126	134–235
Carrot juice, 3/4 cup	1,692	71
Sweet potato with peel, baked, 1 medium	1,096	103
Pumpkin, canned, 1/2 cup	953	42
Carrots, cooked from fresh, 1/2 cup	671	27
Spinach, cooked from frozen, 1/2 cup	573	30
Collards, cooked from frozen, 1/2 cup	489	31
Kale, cooked from frozen, 1/2 cup	478	20
Mixed vegetables, canned, 1/2 cup	474	40
Turnip greens, cooked from frozen, 1/2 cup	441	24
Instant cooked cereals, fortified, prepared, 1 packet	285–376	75–97
Various ready-to-eat cereals, with added vitamin A, ~ 1 oz.	180–376	100–117
Carrot, raw, 1 small	301	20
Beet greens, cooked, 1/2 cup	276	19
Winter squash, cooked, 1/2 cup	268	38
Dandelion greens, cooked, 1/2 cup	260	18
Cantaloupe, raw, 1/4 medium melon	233	46
Mustard greens, cooked, 1/2 cup	221	11
Pickled herring, 3 oz.	219	222
Red sweet pepper, cooked, 1/2 cup	186	19
Chinese cabbage, cooked, 1/2 cup	180	10

[a] High in cholesterol.

Source: Nutrient values from Agricultural Research Service (ARS) Nutrient Database for Standard Reference, Release 17. Foods are from ARS single nutrient reports, sorted in descending order by nutrient content in terms of common household measures. Food items and weights in the single nutrient reports are adapted from those in the 2002 revision of USDA Home and Garden Bulletin No. 72, Nutritive Value of Foods. Omitted from this table are mixed dishes and multiple preparations of the same food item.

Food sources of magnesium ranked by milligrams of magnesium per standard amount; also calories in the standard amount. (All are greater than or equal to 10% of the RDA for adult men, which is 420 mg per day.)

Table FF-7 Food Sources of Magnesium

Food, Standard Amount	Magnesium (mg)	Calories
Pumpkin and squash seed kernels, roasted, 1 oz.	151	148
Brazil nuts, 1 oz.	107	186
Bran ready-to-eat cereal (100%), ~ 1 oz.	103	74
Halibut, cooked, 3 oz.	91	119
Quinoa, dry, 1/4 cup	89	159
Spinach, canned, 1/2 cup	81	25
Almonds, 1 oz.	78	164
Spinach, cooked from fresh, 1/2 cup	78	20
Buckwheat flour, 1/4 cup	75	101
Cashews, dry roasted, 1 oz.	74	163
Soybeans, mature, cooked, 1/2 cup	74	149
Pine nuts, dried, 1 oz.	71	191
Mixed nuts, oil roasted, with peanuts, 1 oz.	67	175
White beans, canned, 1/2 cup	67	154
Pollock, walleye, cooked, 3 oz.	62	96
Black beans, cooked, 1/2 cup	60	114
Bulgur, dry, 1/4 cup	57	120
Oat bran, raw, 1/4 cup	55	58
Soybeans, green, cooked, 1/2 cup	54	127
Tuna, yellowfin, cooked, 3 oz.	54	118
Artichokes (hearts), cooked, 1/2 cup	50	42
Peanuts, dry roasted, 1 oz.	50	166
Lima beans, baby, cooked from frozen, 1/2 cup	50	95
Beet greens, cooked, 1/2 cup	49	19
Navy beans, cooked, 1/2 cup	48	127
Tofu, firm, prepared with nigari[a], 1/2 cup	47	88
Okra, cooked from frozen, 1/2 cup	47	26
Soy beverage, 1 cup	47	127
Cowpeas, cooked, 1/2 cup	46	100
Hazelnuts, 1 oz.	46	178
Oat bran muffin, 1 oz.	45	77

continues

Table FF-7 Food Sources of Magnesium—*continued*

Food, Standard Amount	Magnesium (mg)	Calories
Great northern beans, cooked, 1/2 cup	44	104
Oat bran, cooked, 1/2 cup	44	44
Buckwheat groats, roasted, cooked, 1/2 cup	43	78
Brown rice, cooked, 1/2 cup	42	108
Haddock, cooked, 3 oz.	42	95

[a] Calcium sulfate and magnesium chloride.

Source: Nutrient values from Agricultural Research Service (ARS) Nutrient Database for Standard Reference, Release 17. Foods are from ARS single nutrient reports, sorted in descending order by nutrient content in terms of common household measures. Food items and weights in the single nutrient reports are adapted from those in the 2002 revision of USDA Home and Garden Bulletin No. 72, Nutritive Value of Foods. Omitted from this table are mixed dishes and multiple preparations of the same food item.

Food Sources of Dietary Fiber ranked by grams of dietary fiber per standard amount; also calories in the standard amount. (All are greater than or equal to 10% of the AI for adult women, which is 25 grams per day.)

Table FF-8 Food Sources of Dietary Fiber

Food, Standard Amount	Dietary Fiber (g)	Calories
Navy beans, cooked, 1/2 cup	9.5	128
Bran ready-to-eat cereal (100%), 1/2 cup	8.8	78
Kidney beans, canned, 1/2 cup	8.2	109
Split peas, cooked, 1/2 cup	8.1	116
Lentils, cooked, 1/2 cup	7.8	115
Black beans, cooked, 1/2 cup	7.5	114
Pinto beans, cooked, 1/2 cup	7.7	122
Lima beans, cooked, 1/2 cup	6.6	108
Artichoke, globe, cooked, 1 each	6.5	60
White beans, canned, 1/2 cup	6.3	154
Chickpeas, cooked, 1/2 cup	6.2	135
Great northern beans, cooked, 1/2 cup	6.2	105
Cowpeas, cooked, 1/2 cup	5.6	100
Soybeans, mature, cooked, 1/2 cup	5.2	149
Bran ready-to-eat cereals, various, ~ 1 oz.	2.6–5.0	90–108
Crackers, rye wafers, plain, 2 wafers	5.0	74
Sweet potato, baked, with peel, 1 medium (146 g)	4.8	131
Asian pear, raw, 1 small	4.4	51
Green peas, cooked, 1/2 cup	4.4	67
Whole-wheat English muffin, 1 each	4.4	134
Pear, raw, 1 small	4.3	81
Bulgur, cooked, 1/2 cup	4.1	76
Mixed vegetables, cooked, 1/2 cup	4.0	59
Raspberries, raw, 1/2 cup	4.0	32
Sweet potato, boiled, no peel, 1 medium (156 g)	3.9	119
Blackberries, raw, 1/2 cup	3.8	31
Potato, baked, with skin, 1 medium	3.8	161
Soybeans, green, cooked, 1/2 cup	3.8	127
Stewed prunes, 1/2 cup	3.8	133
Figs, dried, 1/4 cup	3.7	93
Dates, 1/4 cup	3.6	126
Oat bran, raw, 1/4 cup	3.6	58
Pumpkin, canned, 1/2 cup	3.6	42
Spinach, frozen, cooked, 1/2 cup	3.5	30

continues

SECTION 7

Table FF-8 Food Sources of Dietary Fiber—*continued*

Food, Standard Amount	Dietary Fiber (g)	Calories
Shredded wheat ready-to-eat cereals, various, ~ 1 oz.	2.8–3.4	96
Almonds, 1 oz.	3.3	164
Apple with skin, raw, 1 medium	3.3	72
Brussels sprouts, frozen, cooked, 1/2 cup	3.2	33
Whole-wheat spaghetti, cooked, 1/2 cup	3.1	87
Banana, 1 medium	3.1	105
Orange, raw, 1 medium	3.1	62
Oat bran muffin, 1 small	3.0	178
Guava, 1 medium	3.0	37
Pearled barley, cooked, 1/2 cup	3.0	97
Sauerkraut, canned, solids, and liquids, 1/2 cup	3.0	23
Tomato paste, 1/4 cup	2.9	54
Winter squash, cooked, 1/2 cup	2.9	38
Broccoli, cooked, 1/2 cup	2.8	26
Parsnips, cooked, chopped, 1/2 cup	2.8	55
Turnip greens, cooked, 1/2 cup	2.5	15
Collards, cooked, 1/2 cup	2.7	25
Okra, frozen, cooked, 1/2 cup	2.6	26
Peas, edible-podded, cooked, 1/2 cup	2.5	42

Source: ARS Nutrient Database for Standard Reference, Release 17. Foods are from single nutrient reports, which are sorted either by food description or in descending order by nutrient content in terms of common household measures. The food items and weights in these reports are adapted from those in the 2002 revision of USDA Home and Garden Bulletin No. 72, Nutritive Value of Foods. Omitted from this table are mixed dishes and multiple preparations of the same food item.

Food Sources of Vitamin C ranked by milligrams of vitamin C per standard amount; also calories in the standard amount. (All provide greater than or equal to 20% of the RDA for adult men, which is 90 mg per day.)

Table FF-9 Food Sources of Vitamin C

Food, Standard Amount	Vitamin C (mg)	Calories
Guava, raw, 1/2 cup	188	56
Red sweet pepper, raw, 1/2 cup	142	20
Red sweet pepper, cooked, 1/2 cup	116	19
Kiwi, 1 medium	70	46
Orange, raw, 1 medium	70	62
Orange juice, 3/4 cup	61–93	79–84
Green pepper, sweet, raw, 1/2 cup	60	15
Green pepper, sweet, cooked, 1/2 cup	51	19
Grapefruit juice, 3/4 cup	50–70	71–86
Vegetable juice cocktail, 3/4 cup	50	34
Strawberries, raw, 1/2 cup	49	27
Brussels sprouts, cooked, 1/2 cup	48	28
Cantaloupe, 1/4 medium	47	51
Papaya, raw, 1/4 medium	47	30
Kohlrabi, cooked, 1/2 cup	45	24
Broccoli, raw, 1/2 cup	39	15
Edible pod peas, cooked, 1/2 cup	38	34
Broccoli, cooked, 1/2 cup	37	26
Sweet potato, canned, 1/2 cup	34	116
Tomato juice, 3/4 cup	33	31
Cauliflower, cooked, 1/2 cup	28	17
Pineapple, raw, 1/2 cup	28	37
Kale, cooked, 1/2 cup	27	18
Mango, 1/2 cup	23	54

Source: Nutrient values from Agricultural Research Service (ARS) Nutrient Database for Standard Reference, Release 17. Foods are from ARS single nutrient reports, sorted in descending order by nutrient content in terms of common household measures. Food items and weights in the single nutrient reports are adapted from those in the 2002 revision of USDA Home and Garden Bulletin No. 72, Nutritive Value of Foods. Omitted from this table are mixed dishes and multiple preparations of the same food item.

Appendix GG: BMI Chart

Table GG-1 Body Mass Index Table

	Normal						Overweight					Obese										Extreme Obesity														
BMI	**19**	**20**	**21**	**22**	**23**	**24**	**25**	**26**	**27**	**28**	**29**	**30**	**31**	**32**	**33**	**34**	**35**	**36**	**37**	**38**	**39**	**40**	**41**	**42**	**43**	**44**	**45**	**46**	**47**	**48**	**49**	**50**	**51**	**52**	**53**	**54**
Height (inches)	**Body Weight (pounds)**																																			
58	91	96	100	105	110	115	119	124	129	134	138	143	148	153	158	162	167	172	177	181	186	191	196	201	205	210	215	220	224	229	234	239	244	248	253	258
59	94	99	104	109	114	119	124	128	133	138	143	148	153	158	163	168	173	178	183	188	193	198	203	208	212	217	222	227	232	237	242	247	252	257	262	267
60	97	102	107	112	116	123	128	133	138	143	148	153	158	163	168	174	179	184	189	194	199	204	209	215	220	225	230	235	240	245	250	255	261	266	271	276
61	100	106	111	116	122	127	132	137	143	148	153	158	164	169	174	180	185	190	195	201	206	211	217	222	227	232	238	243	248	254	259	264	269	275	280	285
62	104	109	115	120	126	131	136	142	147	153	158	164	169	175	180	186	191	196	202	207	213	218	224	229	235	240	246	251	256	262	267	273	278	284	289	295
63	107	113	118	124	130	135	141	146	152	158	163	169	175	180	186	191	197	203	208	214	220	225	231	237	242	248	254	259	265	270	278	282	287	293	299	304
64	110	116	122	128	134	140	145	151	157	163	169	174	180	186	192	197	204	209	219	221	227	232	238	244	250	256	262	267	273	279	285	291	296	302	308	314
65	114	120	126	132	138	144	150	156	162	168	174	180	186	192	196	204	210	216	222	228	234	240	246	252	258	264	270	276	282	288	294	300	305	312	318	324
66	118	124	130	136	142	148	155	161	167	173	179	186	192	198	204	210	216	223	229	235	241	247	253	260	266	272	278	284	291	297	303	309	315	322	328	334
67	121	127	134	140	146	153	159	166	172	178	185	191	198	204	211	217	223	230	236	242	246	255	261	266	274	280	287	293	299	305	312	319	326	331	338	344
68	125	131	138	144	151	158	164	171	177	184	190	197	203	210	216	223	230	236	243	249	256	262	269	276	282	289	295	302	308	315	322	328	335	341	348	354
69	128	135	142	149	155	162	169	176	182	189	196	203	209	216	223	230	236	243	250	257	263	270	277	284	291	297	304	311	318	324	331	338	345	351	358	365
70	132	139	146	153	160	167	174	181	188	195	202	209	216	222	229	236	243	250	257	264	271	278	285	292	299	306	313	320	327	334	341	348	355	362	389	376
71	136	143	150	157	165	172	179	186	193	200	208	215	222	229	236	243	250	257	265	272	279	286	293	301	308	315	322	329	338	343	351	358	365	372	379	386
72	140	147	154	162	169	177	184	191	199	206	213	221	228	235	242	250	258	265	272	279	287	294	302	309	316	324	331	338	346	353	361	368	375	383	390	397
73	144	151	159	166	174	182	189	197	204	212	219	227	235	242	250	257	265	272	280	288	295	302	310	318	325	333	340	348	355	363	371	378	386	393	401	408
74	148	155	163	171	179	186	194	202	210	218	225	233	241	249	256	264	272	280	287	295	303	311	319	326	334	342	350	358	365	373	381	389	396	404	412	420
75	152	163	168	176	184	192	200	208	216	224	232	240	248	256	264	272	279	287	295	303	311	319	327	335	343	351	359	367	375	383	391	399	407	415	423	431
76	156	164	172	180	189	197	205	213	221	230	238	245	254	263	271	279	287	295	304	312	320	328	336	344	353	361	369	377	385	394	402	410	418	426	435	443

Source: Adapted from *Clinical Guidelines on the Identification, Evaluation, and Treatment of Overweight and Obesity in Adults. The Evidence Report.*

Appendix HH: Super Recipes

Fortified Food Recipes

Super Cereal #1

3½ cups oatmeal
2 cups light cream
2½ cups water
1 tsp. salt
4 Tbsp. margarine
10 Tbsp. brown sugar

Yield: 10 – ½ cup servings

1. Measure light cream, water, salt, and margarine into a saucepan; heat to a near boil.
2. Add oatmeal and cook until thick.
3. Add brown sugar and mix.

Estimated Nutrition Information per serving
Calories 380
Protein 8 gms.

Super Cereal #2

3½ cups oatmeal
4 cups evaporated milk
5 cups whole milk
2 cups dry milk powder
1½ cups melted margarine
1½ cups honey

Yield: 18 – ½ cup servings

1. Measure milk and cream into a saucepan; slowly heat to a near boil; stir often. Do not allow to burn.
2. Add melted margarine and mix.
3. Combine dry milk powder and contents of saucepan, stirring frequently.
4. Add oatmeal and continue to stir often.
5. Turn off heat; add maple syrup and stir.

Estimated Nutrition Information per serving
Calories 415
Protein 8 gms.

Super "Spuds"

3½ cups instant potato flakes
½ cup water
3½ cups light cream
5 Tbsp. butter/margarine
salt to taste

Yield: 10 – ½ cup servings

1. Heat water, light cream, salt, and margarine to near boiling in a saucepan.
2. Reduce heat; add potato flakes and whisk until moistened and fluffy. Add hot liquid if too firm.

Estimated Nutrition Information per serving
Calories 290
Protein 4 gms.

Super Chicken Soup

$2\frac{1}{4}$ cups diced onion
2 cups diced celery
1 cup roux
8 Tbsp. butter
6 cups leftover vegetables
1 cup pureed chicken
3 quarts chicken stock
6 cups evaporated milk
2 cups whole milk

Yield: 32 – ½ cup servings

1. Add butter, onion, and celery to large pot; sauté until tender. Add roux and stir.
2. Add vegetables, pureed chicken, and chicken stock. Bring to a boil and cook for ~ 10 minutes.
3. Utilizing a food processor, puree in batches the contents of the pot; place in another pot.
4. Add the evaporated milk and whole milk and simmer for ~ 20 minutes.

Estimated Nutrition Information per serving
Calories 142
Protein 8 gms.

Super Pudding

$2\frac{1}{4}$ cup dry instant pudding mix
$1\frac{3}{4}$ cups dry milk powder
5 cups whole milk
4 cups light cream
Flavor hints: vanilla extract, coffee syrup, almond extract

Yield: 18 – ½ cup servings

1. Prepare according to the directions on the package.

Estimated Nutrition Information per serving
Calories 205
Protein 4 gms.

Super Muffins

6 cups muffin mix
2 cups light cream
$1\frac{1}{2}$ cup sour cream
12 Tbsp. melted butter
Flavoring ideas: cinnamon, orange peel, lemon peel

Yield: 16 – 3 oz. muffins

1. Mix together muffin mix and flavoring.
2. Add remaining ingredients and stir together.
3. Using a #12 scoop of ⅓ cup, fill greased muffin pans.
4. Bake according to muffin mix directions, checking frequently so not to overbake.

Nutrition Information per serving
Calories 480
Protein 4 gms.

Appendix II: Sodium Content of Foods

Table II-1 Average Calculation Values for Sodium Content of Food Groups

Food Group	Approximate Sodium Content (mg)	Lower Sodium Choices
Milk—8 ounces	120 mg	
Bread—1 slice	135 mg	White/whole-wheat bread, puffed rice, puffed wheat, shredded wheat, plain pasta, or rice without added salt
Fruit—fresh, frozen, or dried without added sodium—one whole fruit or 1 cup	5 mg	Fresh apples, bananas, nectarines, oranges, peaches, pears, strawberries
Vegetables—fresh or frozen without salt—1 cup	15 mg	Fresh or frozen without salt, asparagus, green and waxed beans, squash, tomatoes
Meat, poultry, fish—fresh, unsalted—1 ounce	25 mg	Fresh meat, poultry, fish (not shellfish)
Egg—1	65 mg	
Fats and oils—1 teaspoon of butter or margarine,	50 mg	
1 teaspoon unsalted butter or margarine, oil	5 mg	Unsalted butter and margarine, oil

Index

A

Abdomen
burning sensation in, 250
cramping, short-bowel syndrome and, 257–258
discomfort, COPD and, 84
distention, adult tube feeding and, 232–233
Abdominal pain
cholecystitis or cholecystectomy and, 250
diverticulitis and, 238
gluten sensitive enteropathy and, 248–249
inflammatory bowel disease and, 247
lamotrigine and, 139
short-bowel syndrome and, 257–258
Academic information resources, 435*t*
Acquired immunodeficiency syndrome (AIDS)
lactation and, 52
nutrition care for adults with, 122–126
Acute nutrition care in adults. *See also* Acute nutrition care in children; Chronic nutrition care in adults
aspiration pneumonia, 190–192
cancer chemotherapy and radiation, 208–214
celiac disease or celiac sprue, 248–249
cholecystitis or cholecystectomy, 250–252
colostomy, 253–256
diverticulitis, 238–240
gastric bypass surgery, 193–207
gastroesophageal reflux disease, 241–242
ileostomy, 253–256
inflammatory bowel disease, 245–247
lactose intolerance, 243–244
liver disease, 260–265
parenteral nutrition, 215–220
renal calculi, 266–268, 269*t*
short-bowel syndrome, 257–259
troubleshooting with parenteral nutrition, 221–223
troubleshooting with tube feeding, 232–237
tube feeding guide, 224–231
Acute nutrition care in children, 272–273
ADHD medications, adults on, 132–133
Administration pumps, for enteral nutrition, 227
Adolescents. *See also* Pregnancy
information resources, 439*t*
normal nutrition, 14–17
pregnant, dietary reference intakes for, 46*t*, 307–308*t*
recommended DRIs 2000, 301–304*t*
Type I diabetes self-management by, 177
vegetarian diet and, 60–61
Adults. *See also* Acute nutrition care in adults; Chronic nutrition care in adults; Lactation; Pregnancy; Tube feeding, for adults
CPR procedures, 297*t*
normal nutrition, 18–23
older, normal nutrition, 24–32
pregnant, dietary reference intakes for, 46*t*
African Americans, foods commonly eaten by, 320–321*t*
Aging
information resources on, 435*t*
normal nutrition, 24–32
Air embolism, parenteral nutrition and, 221
Albumin, biochemical evaluation of nutritional status, 403*t*

INDEX

Alcohol, dietary
    abuse, information resources on, 435–436t
    by adults, 20–21
    Alzheimer's disease and, 76
    cerebrovascular accident or stroke and, 82
    congestive heart failure and, 87
    COPD and, 83
    fatty liver and, 260–261
    guidelines for Americans 2005, 300
    during lactation, 3, 48
    MAOIs and, 134
    by older adults, 27–28
    pregnancy and, 16, 40
Allergies. *See* Hypersensitivity
Alternate nutrition. *See also* Tube feeding
    cerebrovascular accident or stroke and, 81
Alternative nutrition, information resources on, 437–438t
Altman and Dittmer equations, for predicting energy requirements, 326t
Alzheimer's disease, 72–76
Amenorrhea, eating disorders and, 114–115
Amino acids
    infant formulas based on, 391t
    maximum, for PN formulation, 217
Analgesics, diet interaction with, 309
Anemia
    in adults, 22
    iron-deficiency, during pregnancy, 37
    iron-deficiency, in infants, 5
    iron-deficiency, in toddlers through pre-school age, 10
    postpartum, lactation and, 51
Angiotensin converting enzyme (ACE) inhibitors, diet interaction with, 313
Anorexia, 255, 265
Anti-anxiety agents, 130–131, 318
Antibiotics, 314–317
Anticoagulants, 314
Antidepressant medications, 134–137, 318
Antifungals, 314, 316–317
Antihistamines, 309
Antipsychotic drugs, 141–143
Antipyretics, 309
Anxiety disorders, 317–318. *See also* Anti-anxiety agents
Appetite, poor or decreased
    ADHD medications and, 132
    Alzheimer's disease and, 74
    cardiovascular disease and, 77
    cerebrovascular accident or stroke and, 81
    duloxetine and, 136
    HIV/AIDS infection and, 123
    during pregnancy, 36
    vegetarianism and, 60
Arabic foods, 323–324t
Arby's fast food, nutrient content of, 346t
Arginine, 89
Arthritis, 309–311
Artificial sweeteners, 38
Aspiration, adult tube feeding and, 230, 234
Aspiration pneumonia, 119, 190–192
Asthma, 311
Attention Deficient Hyperactivity Disorder (ADHD) medications, 132–133

B

Bacillary dysentery, 370t
Basal Energy Expenditure, 88, 127, 129, 190. *See also* Energy
Beans, peas, and lentils. *See also* Meat and meat substitutes
    exchange list for meal planning, 329t
Behavioral modifications or considerations
    for overweight or obese children, 166–167
    Type 1 diabetes in childhood and, 177–179
    Type 2 diabetes in childhood and, 182–183, 186–187
Beta blockers, 312
Binge eating, 116
Bloatedness or bloating, 211, 243–244, 248–249, 251–252
Blood pressure. *See also* Hypertension
    cerebrovascular accident or stroke and, 82
    MAOIs and, 134
Blood sugar. *See also* Glucose; Glycemic index; Hyperglycemia; Hypoglycemia
    elevated postprandial, diabetic diet and, 100–102
    exercise, diabetes and, 108
    high pre-meal, Type 1 diabetic diet and, 97–98

high pre-meal, Type 2 diabetic diet and, 98–99
low, before bed, diabetic diet and, 102
low pre-meal, Type 1 diabetic diet and, 99–100
low pre-meal, Type 2 diabetic diet and, 100
self-management testing goals, 113*t*
testing, self-management of diabetes with, 92
Blood urea nitrogen (BUN)
biochemical evaluation of nutritional status, 413*t*
nausea with chronic renal insufficiency and, 144–145
Body mass index (BMI), 162, 181, 289, 458*t*
Body weight. *See also* Weight gain; Weight loss
daily fluid needs and, 90
dysphagia and, 120, 121
ideal, aspiration pneumonia and, 190
ideal, malnutrition and, 129
during lactation, 47
maintenance in healthy adults, 18
maintenance with COPD, 83–84
malnutrition assessment and, 127
management, 158–160
management, guidelines for Americans 2005, 298
management in children, 162–168
management in children, Type 2 diabetes and, 181–182
management in older adults, 25–26
management, information resources, 443*t*
monitoring parenteral nutrition and, 218
during pregnancy, 34–36
sudden change in, adult tube feeding and, 236
sudden change in, parenteral nutrition and, 223
Bolus feeding, in enteral nutrition, 227–228
Bone health
in adults, 21
eating disorders and, 116
Boston Market fast food, nutrient content of, 346*t*
Bottle dependency, 7
Bottle feeding, 3
Botulism, 371*t*
Bradycardia
eating disorders and, 116
Bread exchange list for meal planning, 327*t*
Breakfast, skipping of
by school-age children, 12
Breast-feeding, 2–3
Bronchitis, chronic, 83–85
Bronchodilators
diet interaction with, 311
Bupropion, 136
Burger King fast food, nutrient content of, 346–347*t*
Burns
ideal body weight and, 129

C

Caffeinated beverages
Alzheimer's disease and, 76
during lactation, 3, 48
during pregnancy, 16, 34, 40
Caffeine, in foods and beverages, 282–283*t*
Calcium
biochemical evaluation of nutritional status, 403*t*
blood tests for determining nutritional status of, 402*t*
bone health and, 21
food sources of, 451*t*
non-dairy food sources of, 450*t*
Nutrition Facts label on, 360*t*
vegetarian sources of, 59–60
Calcium-based calculi, 266
Calicivirus, 372*t*
Calculations
dietary folate equivalents, 285
energy expenditures for various activities, 327*t*
energy from food, 284
estimated energy expenditure, 287–289
niacin equivalents, 284
osmolarity for PPN solutions, 217
for predicting energy requirements, equations for, 326*t*
resting energy expenditure, 288
retinol activity equivalents, 286
thermic effect of food, 288–289

INDEX

Caloric requirements. *See also* Energy
for adolescents, 14
chronic renal insufficiency and, 146
dialysis for end stage renal disease and, 152
during lactation, 47
for school age children, 11
sports nutrition and, 62
Calorie-free, legal definition of, 362*t*
Calories
of commonly consumed foods, 295–296*t*
on Nutrition Facts label, 359*t*
Campylobacter jejuni (campylobacteriosis), 367*t*
Canadian government information resources
federal, 436*t*
provincial and territorial, 437*t*
Cancer, 208–214
Capacities. *See also* Volumes
metric to U.S. conversions, 291
standard measurements of, 290
U.S. to metric conversions, 291
Carbamazepine, 138
Carbohydrates. *See also* Fruits; Milk products, dietary
acute diarrhea in infants and young children and, 273
blood tests for determining nutritional status of, 401*t*
of commonly consumed foods, 295–296*t*
content in a beverage, formula for, 68*t*
in diabetic diet, 95–96, 169–170, 184
food servings with 15 grams of, 112*t*
guidelines for Americans 2005, 299
nutrient content of exchanges, 345*t*
other, exchange list for meal planning, 333–334*t*
recommended dietary intakes during pregnancy, 46*t*
sports nutrition and, 63
Cardiopulmonary resuscitation (CPR) procedures, 297*t*
Cardiovascular disease (CVD), 77–79
cerebrovascular accident or stroke and, 82
diabetes and, 109
diet interactions with drugs for, 312–314
Carl's Junior fast food, nutrient content of, 347*t*
beta-Carotene. *See also* Vitamin A
biochemical evaluation of nutritional status, 403*t*
Catheters
clogged, parenteral nutrition and, 221
infection at insertion site, 222
insertion site care, 219
tip displacement or migration, 223
Celiac disease or celiac sprue, 248–249
Celsius (Centigrade) scale, conversion to Fahrenheit scale, 293
Cephalosporins, 315
Cereals and grains exchange list for meal planning, 328–329*t*
Cerebrovascular accident (CVA), 80–82
Ceruloplasmin, 403*t*
Cheese. *See* Meat and meat substitutes
Chewing problems. *See also* Dentition
cerebrovascular accident or stroke and, 80
Children. *See also* Adolescents; Infants or infancy
acute diarrhea in, 272–273
CPR procedures, 297*t*
food hypersensitivity and allergies, 40
information resources, 439*t*
overweight or obese, 162–168
recommended DRIs 2000, 301–304*t*
school-age, normal nutrition for, 11–13
toddler through pre-school age, normal nutrition for, 7–10
Type 1 diabetes and, 169–180
Type 2 diabetes and, 181–187
Chinese, foods commonly eaten by, 321*t*
Chloride
biochemical evaluation of nutritional status, 403–404*t*
blood tests for determining nutritional status of, 402*t*
Choking, 4, 9, 119. *See also* Heimlich maneuver
Cholecystectomy, 250–252
Cholecystitis, 250–252
Cholesterol. *See also* Dyslipidemia
cautions on Nutrition Facts label, 360*t*
diabetes in adults and, 93, 94, 96
high, cardiovascular disease and, 77
high, diabetes and, 110

legal definition of terms on Nutrition Label about, 364*t*
total, biochemical evaluation of nutritional status, 404*t*
Chronic diseases, prevention of, 18
Chronic nutrition care in adults
ADHD medications, 132–133
Alzheimer's disease, 72–76
anti-anxiety agents, 130–131
antidepressant medications, 134–137
antipsychotic drugs and diet interaction, 141–143
cardiovascular disease, 77–79
cerebrovascular accident, 80–82
chronic obstructive pulmonary disease, 83–85
chronic renal insufficiency or failure, 144–148
congestive heart failure, 86–87
decubitus ulcers, 88–89
dehydration, 90–91
diabetes, 92–111, 112*t*, 113*t*
dysphagia, 119–121
eating disorders, 114–118
end stage renal disease with dialysis, 150–156, 156*t*, 157*t*
HIV/AIDS infection, 122–126
malnutrition, 127–129
mood stabilizing agents, 138–140
weight management, 158–160
Chronic nutrition care in children
overweight or obesity, 162–168
Type 1 diabetes, 169–180
Type 2 diabetes, 181–187
Chronic obstructive pulmonary disease (COPD), 83–85
Clear-liquid diet, sample menu for, 276*t*
Closed systems, for enteral nutrition, 227
Clostridium botulinum, 371*t*
Cola products. *See also* Caffeinated beverages; Soda or soft drinks
bone health in adults and, 21
Colic, bottle feeding and, 5–6
Colitis, ulcerative, 245–247
Colostomy, 253–256
Combination foods exchange list for meal planning, 343*t*
Complementary feedings, for infants, 3–4
Complementary nutrition information resources, 437–438*t*
Condiments, as free foods, 342*t*
Congestive heart failure (CHF), 86–87
Constipation
adult tube feeding and, 232
Alzheimer's disease and, 75
antipsychotic drugs and, 142–143
cancer chemotherapy and radiation and, 209–210
carbamazepine and, 138
chronic renal insufficiency and, 147
colostomy or ileostomy and, 254–255
diabetes and, 105, 110
dialysis for end stage renal disease and, 153–154
duloxetine and, 136
eating disorders and, 114
gastric bypass surgery and, 194
in infants, 6
during pregnancy, 38
in toddlers through pre-school age, 10
topiramate and, 139
valproic acid and, 139
Consumer organizations, 438*t*
Continuous drip, for enteral nutrition, 228
Conversion factors, 292
Copper
biochemical evaluation of nutritional status, 404*t*
Wilson's Disease and, 262
Coronary artery bypass grafting (CABG), 77–79
Coronary artery disease (CAD), 77–79. *See also* Cardiovascular disease
cerebrovascular accident or stroke and, 82
Corticosteroids
diet interaction with, 310
Coughing, 119
Counseling
overweight or obese children, 162–164
CPR (cardiopulmonary resuscitation) procedures, 297*t*
Crackers
exchange list for meal planning, 329*t*
Cramping
abdominal, short-bowel syndrome and, 257–258
lactose intolerance and, 243–244

Creatinine
biochemical evaluation of nutritional status, 404–405*t*
Crohn's disease
nutrition care for adults with, 245–247
Cryptosporidium (cryptosporidiosis), 373*t*
Cultural or ethnic food considerations, 320–324*t*
CVD (cardiovascular disease), 297*t*
Cyclospora cayetanensis, 373*t*
Cystine
renal calculi and, 267

D

Dairy Queen fast food, nutrient content of, 347*t*
DASH diet or eating plan, 398
cerebrovascular accident or stroke and, 82
congestive heart failure and, 87
food groups, serving sizes, and examples, 399–400*t*
Decubitis ulcers, 88–89
Defined–hydrolyzed formula, for enteral nutrition, 225
Dehydration. *See also* Hydration
acute diarrhea in infants and young children and, 272–273
adult tube feeding and, 235–236
Alzheimer's disease and, 75–76
cancer chemotherapy and radiation and, 211
colostomy or ileostomy and, 253–254
diabetic diet and, 102
gastric bypass surgery and, 199
HIV/AIDS infection and, 125
nutrition care, 90–91
parenteral nutrition and, 222
prevention, by adults, 18–19
prevention, by older adults, 22
short-bowel syndrome and, 257
vomiting during pregnancy and, 34
Dental health
in older adults, 30
tooth enamel erosion, eating disorders and, 116–117
Dentition. *See also* Chewing problems
dysphagia and, 119, 121
improper, diabetes and, 107
malnutrition and, 127
Depression
Alzheimer's disease and, 75
diet interactions with drugs for, 317–318
malnutrition and, 127
Dextrose
maximum, for PN formulation, 217
Diabetes
Alzheimer's disease and, 76
cardiovascular disease and, 77
cerebrovascular accident or stroke and, 82
fatty liver and, 260
food servings with 15 grams of carbohydrates, 112*t*
insulin commonly used in the United States, 112*t*
lactation and, 52
nutrition care for adults with, 92–111
in older adults, 29
Type 1, diet therapy goals for, 93–94
Type 1, in childhood, 169–180
Type 2, diet therapy goals for, 94–95
Type 2, in childhood, 181–187
Dialysis for end stage renal disease
medications for, 157*t*
nutrition care for adults on, 150–156
renal laboratory values, 156*t*
Diarrhea
acute, in infants and young children, 272–273
adult tube feeding and, 232
antipsychotic drugs and, 143
cancer chemotherapy and radiation and, 209
carbamazepine and, 138
cholecystitis or cholecystectomy and, 250–251
chronic renal insufficiency and, 145
dialysis for end stage renal disease and, 151–152
gastric bypass surgery and, 196–197
gluten sensitive enteropathy and, 248–249
HIV/AIDS infection and, 122–123
inflammatory bowel disease and, 245–246
lactose intolerance and, 243–244
lithium and, 135, 138
short-bowel syndrome and, 257–258
topiramate and, 139
valproic acid and, 139

Diet and drug interactions. *See* Food/drug interactions
Dietary assessment
Type 2 diabetes in childhood and, 182
Dietary folate equivalents (DFE), calculation of, 285
Dietary guidelines for Americans 2005, 298–300
Dietary Reference Intakes (DRIs). *See also* Nutrient needs
for adolescents, 14
for individuals 2000, 301–304*t*
for infants, 5
for pregnant adolescents, 16, 307–308*t*
for pregnant women, 45*t*, 46*t*, 307–308*t*
for school age children, 11
for toddlers through pre-school age children, 8
tolerable upper intake levels, 305–306*t*
Disaccharide absorption test
biochemical evaluation of nutritional status, 405*t*
Disease-specific formula, for enteral nutrition, 225
Distractions at mealtimes
Alzheimer's disease and, 72
Diuretics
diet interaction with, 312
Diverticulitis
nutrition care for adults with, 238–240
Dizziness
gabapentin and, 139
gastric bypass surgery and, 198
nefazodone and, 136
Drinks, as free foods, 342*t*
Drooling
dysphagia and, 119
Drowsiness
duloxetine and, 136
mirtazapine and, 136
Drug abuse
information resources on, 435–436*t*
Drug/food interactions
carbamazepine and, 138
cerebrovascular accident or stroke and, 81
SSRIs and, 135
Drug/nutrient interactions
adult tube feeding and, 236
in parenteral nutrition, 223
Drugs, illicit
during lactation, 52
Drug-to-drug interactions, 319
Dry mouth, 139
antipsychotic drugs and, 141
bupropion and, 136
cancer chemotherapy and radiation and, 212–213
dialysis for end stage renal disease and, 153
duloxetine and, 136
lithium and, 135, 138
topiramate and, 139
tricyclic antidepressants and, 135
Duloxetine, 136
Dumping syndrome
gastric bypass surgery and, 193, 194
pregnancy, gastric bypass surgery and, 206, 207
Dysentery, bacillary, 370*t*
Dysgeusia
chronic renal insufficiency and, 147–148
dialysis for end stage renal disease and, 154–155
Dyslipidemia
diabetes in childhood and, 173
diabetic diet and, 103–104
HIV/AIDS infection and, 124–125
Dysphagia
HIV/AIDS infection and, 123
nutrition care for adults with, 119–121
Dysphasia
dysphagia and, 119

E

E. coli O157:H7, 368*t*
Eating disorders
adolescents, 15
information resources, 438*t*
nutrition care for adults with, 114–118
vegetarian diet and, 60–61
Eating utensils, use of
Alzheimer's disease and difficulty with, 73
malnutrition and difficulty with, 128
Edema
chronic renal insufficiency and, 146
during pregnancy, 36–37

INDEX

Electrolytes
  blood levels, parenteral nutrition and, 218
  imbalance, colostomy or ileostomy and, 253–254
  imbalance, short-bowel syndrome and, 257
  for parenteral nutrition, 217
Emotional disorders
  diet interactions with drugs for, 317–318
Emotional issues
  for overweight or obese children, 167–168
Emphysema, 83–85
End stage renal disease with dialysis
  medications for, 156*t*
  nutrition care for adults with, 150–156
  renal laboratory values, 156*t*
Energy. *See also* Caloric requirements; Resting energy expenditure
  equations, 326*t*
  estimated expenditure (EER), calculation of, 287–289
  expenditures for various activities, 327*t*
  from food, calculation of, 284
Engorgement
  during lactation, 49–50
Enteral nutrition
  for adults, 224–231
  formula selection for diabetes mellitus, 432*t*
  formula selection for hepatic disease, 431*t*
  formula selection for pulmonary disease, 433*t*
  formula selection for renal disease, 430*t*
  transitioning from parenteral nutrition to, 219–220
Enterostomy tubes, care for, 230
Esophagitis
  eating disorders and, 117
Esophagus
  burning sensation in, 241–242
Estimated energy expenditure (EER), calculation of, 287–289
Ethnic or cultural food considerations, 320–324*t*
Exercise or physical activity (PA). *See also* Inactivity
  by adolescents, 14
  by adults, 19
  constipation during chemotherapy and radiation and, 210
  diabetes and, 107–108
  in estimated energy expenditure, 287
  excessive, eating disorders and, 117
  excessive weight loss with gastric bypass surgery and, 203
  gastric bypass surgery and, 200
  guidelines for Americans 2005, 298
  malnutrition and, 127, 129
  by older adults, 26
  for overweight or obese children, 166
  as percentage of resting energy expenditure, 288
  by school age children, 13
  Type 1 diabetes in childhood and, 176
  Type 2 diabetes in childhood and, 184–185
  very slow weight loss with gastric bypass surgery and, 201–202
  weight management and, 158
  weight-bearing, bone health in adults and, 21
Extra
  legal definition on Nutrition Label of, 365*t*
Extravasation
  parenteral nutrition and, 221
Eye health
  in older adults, 29–30

F

Fahrenheit scale, conversion to Celsius (Centigrade) scale, 293
Fast foods
  exchange list for meal planning, 344*t*
  generic, nutrient content of, 348*t*
  nutrient content of, 346–355*t*
  nutrient content of Arby's, 346*t*
  nutrient content of Boston Market, 346*t*
  nutrient content of Burger King, 346–347*t*
  nutrient content of Carl's Junior, 348*t*
  nutrient content of Dairy Queen, 348*t*
  nutrient content of Hardees, 348–350*t*
  nutrient content of Jack in the Box, 350*t*
  nutrient content of Kentucky Fried Chicken, 350*t*

nutrient content of Long John Silver's, 350t
nutrient content of McDonald's, 350–352t
nutrient content of Pizza Hut, 352t
nutrient content of Subway, 352t
nutrient content of Taco Bell, 352–354t
nutrient content of Taco Time, 354t
nutrient content of Wendy's, 354–355t
Fat(s). *See also* HDL-cholesterol; LDL-cholesterol
accumulation of, HIV/AIDS infection and, 125
calories from, on Nutrition Facts label, 359t
cardiovascular disease and, 77
in diabetic diet, 96–97, 170–171
diverticulitis and, 240
exchange list for meal planning, 339–340t
guidelines for Americans 2005, 299
heart health in adults and, 19–20
inadequate intake of, eating disorders and, 116
legal definition of terms on Nutrition Label about, 363–364t
nutrient content of exchanges, 345t
saturated, amount providing 10% of calories, 281t
sources of, 356–357t
sports nutrition and, 63–64
total, amount providing 30% of calories, 281t
total, cautions on Nutrition Facts label, 360t
total, recommended dietary intakes during pregnancy, 46t
vegetarian sources of, 60
weight management and, 159
Fats
blood tests for determining nutritional status of, 401t
fecal, biochemical evaluation of nutritional status, 405t
Fat-free foods, 341t
Fatigue
duloxetine and, 136
gastric bypass surgery and, 199
Fat-soluble vitamins
blood tests for determining nutritional status of, 401t
function and food sources of, 396t
Fatty acids
biochemical evaluation of nutritional status, 405t
Fatty liver
alcohol and, 260–261
diabetes and, 260
overweight and, 260
TPN and, 261
Female athlete triad, 65–66
Ferritin
biochemical evaluation of nutritional status, 406t
Fiber
in diabetic diet, 171
dietary, food sources of, 455–456t
diverticulitis and, 239
gastric bypass surgery and, 194
legal definition of terms on Nutrition Label about, 364t
Nutrition Facts label on, 360t
Fiber, total
recommended dietary intakes during pregnancy, 46t
Fiber-enriched formula, for enteral nutrition, 225
Fiber-restricted diet, 278t
First year of life
normal nutrition, 2–6
Fish. *See also* Meat and meat substitutes
as fat source, 357t
Flatulence
cholecystitis or cholecystectomy and, 251
Fluid balance
with congestive heart failure, 86
with COPD, 84
Fluid intake. *See also* Dehydration; Hydration
aspiration pneumonia and, 191
carbamazepine and, 138
decubitus ulcers and, 88
duloxetine and, 136
edema with chronic renal insufficiency and, 146
gastric bypass surgery and, 194, 198
during lactation, 50
lithium and, 135, 138
malnutrition and, 129
for parenteral nutrition, 217
tricyclic antidepressants and, 135
weight management and, 158
Fluid overload
parenteral nutrition and, 222

Fluid retention
during pregnancy, 36–37
Folate
biochemical evaluation of nutritional status, 406*t*
dietary equivalents, calculation of, 285
food sources for, 434*t*
Food groups
guidelines for Americans 2005, 299
Food guide
for lactating women, 55*t*
Food insecurity
in older adults, 29
Food labels. *See also* Nutrition Facts label
health claims on, 366*t*
Food measurements
metric to U.S. conversions, 291
standard equivalents in, 291
U.S. to metric conversions, 291
Food safety
guidelines for Americans 2005, 300
information resources, 438–439*t*
during lactation, 50–51
liver disease and, 261
for older adults, 28–29
during pregnancy, 38–40
Food selection
healthful, for older adults, 26–27
for overweight or obese children, 164–165
Type 1 diabetes in childhood and, 171–172
Food taboos
during lactation, 52
Food variety
Alzheimer's disease and, 75
Foodborne illness
bacterial causes and symptoms, 368–371*t*
microbial, in adults, 20
prevention methods, 367
protozoal causes and symptoms, 373–374*t*
viral causes and symptoms, 371–372*t*
Food/drug interactions
analgesics/antipyretics for arthritis and pain and, 309
antihistamines for allergies and, 309
bronchodilators for asthma and, 311
cerebrovascular accident or stroke and, 81
corticosteroids for arthritis and pain and, 310
narcotic analgesics for arthritis and pain and, 310–311
NSAIDs for arthritis and pain and, 310
Food-related behaviors
abnormal, eating disorders and, 117
Footnotes
on Nutrition Facts label, 362*t*
Formulas, for enteral nutrition
choices in, 224–225
determining rate/volume for, 225
Fortified food recipes, 459–460*t*
Fractures
ideal body weight and, 129
Free foods
in diabetic diet, 172
exchange list for meal planning, 341–342*t*
Fresh
legal definition on Nutrition Label of, 365*t*
Fruit refusal
by school-age children, 12
Fruitarian diet
about, 58
Fruits
diverticulitis and, 239
weight management and, 158

G

Gabapentin, 139
Gallbladder disease, 262
Gallstones
gastric bypass surgery and, 204
Gas
bottle feeding and, 5–6
colostomy or ileostomy and, 254
lactose intolerance and, 243–244
Gastric bypass surgery
nutrition care for adults after, 193–207
Gastric residual volume
high, adult tube feeding and, 233
measuring, adult tube feeding and, 229
Gastroesophageal reflux disease (GERD)
nutrition care for adults with, 241–242

Gastroparesis
diabetes and, 105
General purpose intact (polymeric) formula, for enteral nutrition, 225
Geophagia
pregnancy and, 40
Giardia lamblia (giardiasis), 373*t*
Gilbert's Syndrome, 263
Glucose. *See also* Blood sugar; Glycemic index; Hyperglycemia; Hypoglycemia
biochemical evaluation of nutritional status, 406*t*
blood levels, in pediatric diabetes, 188*t*
blood levels, in Type 1 diabetes in childhood, 173–174
blood levels, parenteral nutrition and, 218
diagnostic criteria for impaired fasting tolerance and diabetes, 188*t*
elevated blood levels, parenteral nutrition and, 221
glycated hemoglobin levels and levels of, 113*t*
impaired fasting or impaired fasting tolerance (IFG), 109–110
maximum, for PN formulation, 217
pre-diabetes fasting, 109
Gluten sensitive enteropathy, 248–249
Glycemic index (GI). *See also* Blood sugar
of commonly consumed foods, 295–296*t*
glycemic load of specific foods and, 375*t*
sports nutrition and, 63
Good source
legal definition on Nutrition Label of, 365*t*
Grade A health claims, 366*t*
Grazing
by toddlers through pre-school age, 8
Growth charts
boys, 376*t*
girls, 377*t*
preterm babies, 378*t*
Growth hormone
biochemical evaluation of nutritional status, 406*t*
Growth, poor
in infants, 5
in school-age children, 11
in toddlers through pre-school age, 8–9

H

Hair loss, excessive
gastric bypass surgery and, 200–201
Hamburger disease, 368*t*
Hardees fast food, nutrient content of, 348–350*t*
Harris-Benedict equations
for Basal Energy Expenditure with aspiration pneumonia, 190
for Basal Energy Expenditure with malnutrition, 127
for predicting energy requirements, 326*t*
for resting energy expenditure, 288
HDL-cholesterol. *See also* Cholesterol
biochemical evaluation of nutritional status, 407*t*
diabetes in adults and, 93, 94, 96
Headaches
gastric bypass surgery and, 198
Healthy
legal definition on Nutrition Label of, 365*t*
Heart health
in adults, 19–20
Heartburn
cancer chemotherapy and radiation and, 211
gastric bypass surgery and, 199–200
during pregnancy, 36
valproic acid and, 139
Heimlich maneuver. *See also* Choking
for adults, 380
for infants, 379
Hematocrit
biochemical evaluation of nutritional status, 407*t*
Hemochromatosis, 262
Hemoglobin
biochemical evaluation of nutritional status, 407–408*t*
mean corpuscular, biochemical evaluation of nutritional status, 409*t*

Hepatic encephalopathy (HE), 263–264
Hepatitis A virus, 371–372*t*
Herbal remedies or supplements
 for adolescents, 16
 liver disease and, 261
 older adults, 22
 uses, contraindications, and precautions, 381–384*t*
High maternal weight
 during pregnancy, 35–36
Hindu food, 324*t*
Histamine blockers
 diet interaction with, 318–319
HIV/AIDS infection
 lactation and, 52
 nutrition care for adults with, 122–126
HMG-CoA reductase inhibitors
 diet interaction with, 313–314
Hunger
 extreme, gastric bypass surgery and, 202–203
 in older adults, 29
Hydration. *See also* Dehydration
 sports nutrition and, 64–65
Hyperemesis gravidarum
 during pregnancy, 34
Hyperglycemia. *See also* Blood sugar
 adult tube feeding and, 233–234
 diabetes in childhood and, 175
 during pregnancy, 34
Hypersensitivity
 diet interaction with antihistamines for, 309
 parenteral nutrition and, 222
 pediatric foods, diet during lactation and, 52
 pediatric foods, diet during pregnancy and, 40
Hypertension. *See also* Blood pressure
 Alzheimer's disease and, 76
 cardiovascular disease and, 77
 orthostatic, eating disorders and, 116
 portal, 263
Hypoglycemia. *See also* Blood sugar
 chronic renal insufficiency and, 148
 diabetes and, 105–107
 diabetes in childhood and, 174–175
 dialysis for end stage renal disease and, 155
 liver disease and, 264
 parenteral nutrition administration and, 218
 during pregnancy, 34
 reactive, gastric bypass surgery and, 204
Hypokalemia
 eating disorders and, 115
Hyponatremia
 with congestive heart failure, 86
Hypophosphatemia
 refeeding syndrome and, 115

I

IBW. *See* Body weight, ideal
Ileostomy
 nutrition care for adults with, 253–256
Inactivity. *See also* Exercise or physical activity
 in adults, 19
 cardiovascular disease and, 77
 estimated energy expenditure and, 287
Indian food, 324*t*
Indigestion
 colostomy or ileostomy and, 254
Infant formulas
 amino acid-based, 391*t*
 protein hydrolysate, 389–390*t*
 soy, 387–388*t*
 standard, 385–386*t*
 standard follow-up, 392–393*t*
Infants or infancy
 acute diarrhea in, 272–273
 CPR procedures, 297*t*
 information resources, 439*t*
 normal nutrition, 2–6
 recommended DRIs 2000, 301–304*t*
Infections
 adult tube feeding and, 235
 at catheter insertion site, 222
 diet interactions with drugs for, 314
 renal calculi and, 268
Inflammatory bowel disease (IBD)
 nutrition care for adults with, 245–247
Information resources, 435–445*t*
Insomnia
 ADHD medications and, 133
 antipsychotic drugs and, 143
 MAOIs and, 134
Insulin
 commonly used in the United States, 112*t*
 manipulation, eating disorders and, 118

preparations, activity of, 394–395*t*
resistance, HIV/AIDS infection and, 125
sick day guidelines for patients on, 110–111
Intake, adequate. *See* Nutrient needs
Intermittent drip, for enteral nutrition, 228
International agencies, information resources of, 439–440*t*
International Units, conversion to micrograms, 286
Iodine
food sources for, 434*t*
Irish, foods commonly eaten by, 323*t*
Iron. *See also* Hemochromatosis
biochemical evaluation of nutritional status, 408*t*
blood tests for determining nutritional status of, 402*t*
deficiency, gastric bypass surgery and, 205–206
food sources of, 449*t*
Nutrition Facts label on, 360*t*
vegetarian sources of, 60
Iron-deficiency anemia
in infants, 5
during pregnancy, 37
in toddlers through pre-school age, 10
Italians, foods commonly eaten by, 322*t*

J

Jack in the Box fast food, nutrient content of, 350*t*
Japanese, foods commonly eaten by, 321*t*
Jewish food, 324*t*
Jitteriness
ADHD medications and, 133
anti-anxiety agents and, 130
Juice
for adults, 18
determining carbohydrate content in, 68*t*
fruit, exchange list for meal planning, 331*t*
for infants, 4
reactive hypoglycemia with gastric bypass surgery and, 204
for school age children, 13
for toddlers through pre-school age children, 7

K

Kentucky Fried Chicken fast food, nutrient content of, 350*t*
Kilograms, conversions of pounds to, 294*t*
Koreans, foods commonly eaten by, 321*t*

L

Lactation, 440*t*
Do's and Don'ts, 2–3
food guide, 55*t*
food sources for nutrients needed in increased amounts during, 54*t*
nutrition during, 47–53
recommended DRIs 2000, 301–304*t*
Lacto-ovo diet
about, 57
vitamin B12 in, 59
Lactose intolerance
gastric bypass surgery and, 197–198
lactation and, 48
nutrition care for adults with, 243–244
Lamotrigine, 139
Large-bore tube, for enteral nutrition, 226
LDL-cholesterol. *See also* Cholesterol
biochemical evaluation of nutritional status, 408*t*
diabetes in adults and, 93, 94, 96
Lead
biochemical evaluation of nutritional status, 408*t*
Leg cramps
gastric bypass surgery and, 200
Length, metric and U.S. equivalents of, 290
Lentils, beans, and peas
exchange list for meal planning, 329*t*
Lifestyle modification
Type 2 diabetes in childhood and, 182–183
Light
legal definition on Nutrition Label of, 365*t*
Lightheadedness, sudden
gastric bypass surgery and, 198
Lipids
maximum, for PN formulation, 217
Listeria monocytogenes (listeriosis), 369–370*t*

INDEX

Lithium, 135, 138
Liver disease
nutrition care for adults with, 260–265
Long John Silver's fast food, nutrient content of, 350*t*
Low maternal weight
during pregnancy, 34–35
Low weight gain
during pregnancy, 34–35
Low-calorie
legal definition of, 362*t*
Lunch, school
school age children and, 12–13

M

Macrobiotic diet
about, 57
Macrolides
diet interaction with, 315
Maffeis et al. equations
for predicting energy requirements, 326*t*
Magnesium
blood tests for determining nutritional status of, 402*t*
food sources for, 434*t*
food sources of, 453–454*t*
Malnutrition. *See also* World hunger
early satiety and, 114
eating disorders and, 117
nutrition care for adults with, 127–129
physical indicators of, 418–419
MAOIs (monamine oxidase inhibitors), 134
McDonald's fast food, nutrient content of, 350–352*t*
Meal planning
combination foods exchange list for, 343*t*
fast foods exchange list for, 344*t*
fat exchange list for, 339–340*t*
free foods exchange list for, 341–342*t*
fruit exchange list for, 330–331*t*
meat and meat substitutes exchange list for, 335–339*t*
milk and milk product exchange list for, 332*t*
other carbohydrates exchange list for, 333–334*t*
starch exchange list for, 327–330*t*
Type 1 diabetes in childhood and, 171–172, 177
Type 2 diabetes in childhood and, 182–184
vegetable exchange list for, 334–335*t*
Meat and meat substitutes
exchange list for meal planning, 335–339*t*
as fat sources, 356–357*t*
nutrient content of exchanges, 345*t*
Mechanical soft diet
food permitted in, 277*t*
Medications. *See also specific type*
acute diarrhea in infants and young children and, 273
for chronic renal insufficiency, 149*t*
decubitus ulcers and, 88
for dialysis patients, 156*t*
during lactation, 3, 52
malnutrition and, 127, 128
during pregnancy, 40
Type 2 diabetes in childhood and, 185–186
Mediterranean food, 323*t*
Mercury contamination
in adults, 22–23
Metric prefixes, 289
Mexicans, foods commonly eaten by, 320*t*
Microbial contamination
adult tube feeding and, 235
Micronutrients/trace elements
function and food sources of, 396–397*t*
Micronutrient/trace element deficiencies or malabsorption
HIV/AIDS infection and, 125
Middle Eastern foods, 323*t*
Milk overabundance
during lactation, 49–50
Milk products, dietary
exchange list for meal planning, 332*t*
low intake during lactation and, 48
Milk supply, adequate
during lactation, 49
Minerals
blood tests for determining nutritional status of, 402*t*
deficiency, colostomy or ileostomy and, 256
deficiency, short-bowel syndrome and, 259

food sources for, 434t
function and food sources of, 397t
gastric bypass surgery and, 200
recommended dietary intakes during pregnancy, 45t
trace, for parenteral nutrition, 217
Mitrazapine, 136
Mobility impairment
cerebrovascular accident or stroke and, 80–81
Modular formulas, for enteral nutrition, 225
Mollusks
as fat source, 357t
Monamine oxidase inhibitors (MAOIs), 134
diet interaction with, 317
Monomeric formula, for enteral nutrition, 225
Monounsaturated fats exchange list, 339t
Mood disorders
diet interactions with drugs for, 317–318
Mood stabilizing agents
nutrition care for adults on, 138–140
More
legal definition on Nutrition Label of, 365t
Mormon food practices, 324t
Mother's diet
during lactation, baby reacting to, 48
Mouth sores
cancer chemotherapy and radiation and, 211–212
Muscle wasting
chronic renal insufficiency and, 146
dialysis for end stage renal disease and, 152–153
Muslim food practices, 324t
Myocardial infarction (MI), 77–79
MyPyramid guide, 398
for pregnant women, 44t

N

Narcotic analgesics
diet interaction with, 310–311
Nasally-placed tubes, care for, 230
Nasoduodenal (ND) route, for enteral nutrition, 226
Nasogastric (NG) route, for enteral nutrition, 226
Nasojejunal (NJ) route, for enteral nutrition, 226
National Cholesterol Education Program (NCEP), 77
National Dysphagia Diet, 80
Native Americans, foods commonly eaten by, 322t
Nausea
adult tube feeding and, 233
antipsychotic drugs and, 143
cancer chemotherapy and radiation and, 208
chronic renal insufficiency and, 144–145
diabetes and, 105
dialysis for end stage renal disease and, 150–151
duloxetine and, 136
gabapentin and, 139
gastric bypass surgery and, 193–194
HIV/AIDS infection and, 122
inflammatory bowel disease and, 246–247
lamotrigine and, 139
lithium and, 135, 138
liver disease and, 265
nefazodone and, 136
during pregnancy, 33–34
during pregnancy, shopping list to help stop, 43t
topiramate and, 139
valproic acid and, 139
Nefazodone, 136
Niacin
biochemical evaluation of nutritional status, 409t
Niacin equivalents (NE), calculation of, 284
Nipples, sore/cracked
during lactation, 50
Nitrates
diet interaction with, 313
Nitrogen, blood urea
biochemical evaluation of nutritional status, 413t
nausea with chronic renal insufficiency and, 144–145
Nitroimidazole
diet interaction with, 316
Nonalcoholic steatohepatitis (NASH)
overweight and, 260

Non-steroidal anti-inflammatory drugs (NSAIDs)
- diet interaction with, 310

Normal nutrition
- adolescents, 14–17
- adults, 18–23
- first year of life, 2–6
- infancy, 2–6
- during lactation, 47–53, 54*t*, 55*t*
- older adults, 24–32
- during pregnancy, 33–41
- school age (6–12 years) children, 11–13
- sports nutrition, 62–67
- toddler through pre-school age (1–6 years old), 7–10
- vegetarian diet, 56–61

Norovirus, 372*t*

Nutrient needs. *See also* Dietary Reference Intakes
- acute diarrhea in infants and young children and, 273
- with congestive heart failure, 86
- with COPD, 83
- with diabetes, 92–93
- guidelines for Americans 2005, 298
- during lactation, 47–48, 54*t*
- for older adults, 24–25
- during pregnancy, 37–38

Nutrients
- selected, food sources for, 446–457*t*
- of selected sports drinks, 69*t*

Nutrition Assessment and Diet History, 415–417

Nutrition Facts label
- calories and calories from fat, 359*t*
- footnotes, 362*t*
- get enough of these nutrients information, 360*t*
- health claims on, 366*t*
- legal definitions of terms used on, 362–365*t*
- limit these nutrients information, 360*t*
- Percent Daily Value (%DV), 361*t*
- sample label, 358*t*
- serving size and servings per container, 359*t*

Nutrition industry organizations, 442–443*t*

Nutrition, professional organizations, 440–441*t*

Nutritional status
- biochemical evaluation of, 403–414*t*
- physical indicators of, 418–419

O

Obesity
- in adolescents, 14–15
- cardiovascular disease and, 77
- in children, 162–168
- nutrition care for adults, 158–160

Older adults
- normal nutrition, 24–32

Open systems, for enteral nutrition, 227

Opportunistic infections
- HIV/AIDS infection and, 125

Oral feedings
- transitioning from parenteral nutrition to, 219–220
- transitioning from tube feeding to, 230

Oral hygiene
- Alzheimer's disease and, 76
- lithium and, 135, 138

Oral Rehydration Solution (ORS)
- acute diarrhea in infants and young children and, 272

Osmolarity
- calculation for PPN solutions, 217

Osteoarthritis
- in older adults, 31

Osteopenia
- eating disorders and, 116

Osteoporosis
- in older adults, 30
- prevention, in adults, 21

Other carbohydrates exchange list for meal planning, 333–334*t*

Oversight
- for adult tube feedings, 230–231, 236
- for parenteral nutrition, 220, 223

Overweight
- children, 162–168
- fatty liver or NASH and, 260
- nutrition care for adults, 158–160
- Type 2 diabetes in childhood and, 181–182

Oxygen saturation
- COPD and, 84

P

Pain
abdominal, diverticulitis and, 238
abdominal, gluten sensitive enteropathy and, 248–249
abdominal, inflammatory bowel disease and, 247
abdominal, lamotrigine and, 139
diet interactions with drugs for, 309–311
substernal, 241–242
Parenteral nutrition (PN)
for adults, 215–220
troubleshooting with, 221–223
Parenteral nutrition solutions
admixture types, 216
calculating osmolarity for PPN, 217
storage of, 216
understanding characteristics of, 216
Peas, beans, and lentils
exchange list for meal planning, 329*t*
Pediatric food hypersensitivities and allergies
diet during lactation and, 52
diet during pregnancy and, 40
Penicillin
diet interaction with, 314
Percent Daily Value (%DV)
on Nutrition Facts label, 361*t*
Percutaneous endoscopic gastrostomy (PEG), 226
Percutaneous endoscopic jejunostomy (PEJ), 226
Percutaneous gastrojejunostomy (PGJ), 226
Peripheral parenteral nutrition (PPN)
administration schedule, 218
choosing route or site for, 215–216
Phenylalanine
biochemical evaluation of nutritional status, 409*t*
Phosphatase, alkaline
biochemical evaluation of nutritional status, 410*t*
Phospholipid, total
biochemical evaluation of nutritional status, 410*t*
Phosphorus
blood tests for determining nutritional status of, 402*t*
food sources for, 434*t*
inorganic, biochemical evaluation of nutritional status, 410*t*
Physical activity. *See* Exercise or physical activity
Pica
pregnancy and, 40
Picky eating
by school-age children, 11–12
by toddlers through pre-school age, 7–8
Piero et al. equations
for predicting energy requirements in surgical infants, 326*t*
Pizza Hut fast food, nutrient content of, 352*t*
"Pocketed" food
dysphagia and, 119
Polymeric formula, for enteral nutrition, 225
Polyunsaturated fats exchange list, 340*t*
Portal hypertension, 263
Portion size
gastric bypass surgery and, 201, 202
malnutrition and, 128
on Nutrition Facts label, 359*t*
weight management and, 159
Portuguese, foods commonly eaten by, 322*t*
Postpartum anemia
lactation and, 51
Potassium, dietary
biochemical evaluation of nutritional status, 410*t*
blood tests for determining nutritional status of, 402*t*
food sources of, 446–447*t*
guidelines for Americans 2005, 299
for older adults, 27
Poultry. *See also* Meat and meat substitutes
as fat source, 357*t*
Pound to kilogram conversions, 294*t*
Prealbumin
biochemical evaluation of nutritional status, 410*t*
Pregnancy
adolescents, 16
after gastric bypass surgery, 206–207
information resources, 440*t*
nutrition during, 33–41
recommended dietary intakes, 45*t*, 46*t*, 307–308*t*

Pregnancy (*Continued*)
- recommended DRIs 2000, 301–304*t*
- recommended foods and portions, 44*t*
- recommended weight gain chart, 42*t*
- sample shopping list to help stop nausea during, 43*t*
- vegan diet and, 56

Premature infants
- growth charts, 378*t*
- plotting age of, 5, 9

Professional nutrition organizations, 440–441*t*

Progressive diets
- clear-liquid diet, 276*t*
- fiber-restricted diet, 278*t*
- mechanical soft diet, 277*t*

Protein
- aspiration pneumonia and, 191
- blood tests for determining nutritional status of, 401*t*
- decubitus ulcers and, 88, 89
- in diabetic diet, 96
- in diabetic diet, Type 1 in childhood, 170
- gastric bypass surgery and, 200–201
- malnutrition and, 129
- Nutrition Facts label on, 361*t*
- recommended dietary intakes during pregnancy, 46*t*
- sports nutrition and, 62
- total, biochemical evaluation of nutritional status, 410*t*
- vegetarian sources of, 59

Protein hydrolysate infant formulas, 389–390*t*

Prothrombin time
- biochemical evaluation of nutritional status, 411*t*

Pruritis
- chronic renal insufficiency and, 146–147
- dialysis for end stage renal disease and, 153

Psychological health
- of older adults, 28

Psychosocial considerations
- Type 1 diabetes in childhood and, 177–179
- Type 2 diabetes in childhood and, 186–187

Puerto Ricans, foods commonly eaten by, 320*t*

Pump-controlled feeding, in enteral nutrition, 228

Purine
- foods rich in, 269*t*
- metabolism, renal calculi and, 267

Q

Quinolones
- diet interaction with, 315

R

Raw foods diet
- about, 58

Reduced-fat foods, 341*t*

Reduced/less calorie(s)
- legal definition of, 362*t*

Refeeding syndrome
- adult tube feeding and, 235
- eating disorders and, 115
- parenteral nutrition and, 222

Religion, food restrictions or practices and, 324–325*t*

Renal calculi
- nutrition care for adults with, 266–268, 269*t*

Renal insufficiency or failure, chronic
- diabetes and, 104–105
- medications for, 149*t*
- nutrition care for adults with, 144–148

Resting energy expenditure (REE)
- calculation of, 288
- various activities and, 327*t*

Retinol activity equivalents (RAE), calculation of, 286

Retinol-binding protein
- biochemical evaluation of nutritional status, 411*t*

Rheumatoid arthritis
- in older adults, 31–32

Riboflavin
- biochemical evaluation of nutritional status, 412*t*

Russians, foods commonly eaten by, 323*t*

S

Salmonella (salmonellosis), 368–369*t*
Satiety, early
 eating disorders and, 114
Saturated fat(s)
 amount providing 10% of calories, 281*t*
 cautions on Nutrition Facts label, 360*t*
Saturated fats exchange list, 340*t*
Schofield equations
 for predicting energy requirements, 326*t*
School age (6en12 years) children
 normal nutrition, 11–13
Seasonings, as free foods, 342*t*
Sedation
 nefazodone and, 136
Selective serotonin reuptake inhibitors (SSRIs), 135
Serving size. *See also* Portion size
 on Nutrition Facts label, 359*t*
Seventh Day Adventist food practices, 325*t*
Sexual dysfunction
 MAOIs and, 134
Shellfish
 as fat source, 357*t*
Shigella (shigellosis), 370*t*
Short-bowel syndrome
 nutrition care for adults with, 257–259
Sick day guidelines
 for patients on insulin, 110–111
 Type 1 diabetes in childhood and, 175–176
Sleeplessness. *See* Insomnia
Small-bore tube, for enteral nutrition, 226
Smoking
 bone health in adults and, 21
 cardiovascular disease and, 77
 COPD and, 83
 during lactation, 52
Snacking
 by adolescents, 14
 dehydration and, 90
 for fruitarian diet, 56
 during pregnancy, 33
 by school-age children, 13
 for vegans, 56
 with vegetarian diets, 56–58
Snacks
 exchange list for meal planning, 329*t*
Social environment
 for older adults, 28
Soda or soft drinks. *See also* Caffeinated beverages
 bone health in adults and, 21
 for school age children, 13
Sodium, dietary
 biochemical evaluation of nutritional status, 412*t*
 blood tests for determining nutritional status of, 402*t*
 cautions on Nutrition Facts label, 360*t*
 content of various food groups, 461*t*
 diabetes in adults and, 94–95
 guidelines for Americans 2005, 299
 legal definition of terms on Nutrition Label about, 364–365*t*
 lithium and, 135, 138
 for older adults, 27
Soft diet, sample menu for, 278*t*
Somatomedin C
 biochemical evaluation of nutritional status, 412*t*
Soy infant formulas, 387–388*t*
Spitting up, by infants, 6
Sports. *See also* Exercise or physical activity
 adolescents, 15
Sports drinks
 determining carbohydrate content in, 68*t*
 selected, nutrient breakdown of, 69*t*
Sports nutrition, 62–67
 information resources, 441*t*
SSRIs (selective serotonin reuptake inhibitors), 135
Standard follow-up infant formulas, 392–393*t*
Standard infant formulas, 385–386*t*
Staphylococcus aureus (staphylococcal food poisoning), 370–371*t*
Starch exchange list for meal planning, 327–330*t*
Starchy foods prepared with fat
 exchange list for meal planning, 330*t*

Statins
diet interaction with, 313–314
Steatorrhea
liver disease and, 264
Stoma odor or blockages
colostomy or ileostomy and, 255
Stomach bloating after eating
gastric bypass surgery and, 196
Stomach conditions
diet interactions with drugs for, 318–319
Stomachaches
ADHD medications and, 133
Stools
frequent loose, colostomy or ileostomy and, 253–254
Stools, abnormal
gluten sensitive enteropathy and, 248–249
Stroke, 80–82
Struvite
renal calculi and, 268
Substernal pain, 241–242
Subway fast food, nutrient content of, 352*t*
Sugar substitutes
diabetes in childhood and, 177
Sugar-free foods, 341*t*
Sugars
Nutrition Facts label on, 361*t*
Sulfonamides
diet interaction with, 316
Super recipes, 459–460*t*
Supplements. *See also* Herbal remedies or supplements; Vitamins
Alzheimer's disease and, 75
aspiration pneumonia and, 192
decubitus ulcers and, 89
information resources, 442*t*
during lactation, 52
during pregnancy, 40
Surgery
ideal body weight and, 129
Swallowing difficulty
Alzheimer's disease and, 73–74
aspiration pneumonia and, 190, 191
cerebrovascular accident or stroke and, 80
nutrition care for adults with, 119–121
Sweating
duloxetine and, 136

T

Taco Bell fast food, nutrient content of, 352–354*t*
Taco Time fast food, nutrient content of, 354*t*
Taste
changes in, chemotherapy and radiation and, 212
HIV/AIDS infection and changes in, 126
impaired, chronic renal insufficiency and, 147–148
impaired, dialysis for end stage renal disease and, 154–155
malnutrition and, 128
Teenagers. *See* Adolescents
Temperature scales, Fahrenheit or Celsius (Centigrade), 293
Testosterone
eating disorders and lowered levels of, 115
Tetracyclines
diet interaction with, 316
Thai, foods commonly eaten by, 322*t*
Therapeutic Lifestyle Changes (TLC)
food lists for cardiovascular disease, 77–79
Thermic effect of food (TEF), calculation of, 288–289
Thiamine
biochemical evaluation of nutritional status, 413*t*
Thrush, oral
HIV/AIDS infection and, 123
Tiredness
gastric bypass surgery and, 199
Toddler through pre-school age (1–6 years old)
normal nutrition, 7–10
Tooth enamel
erosion, eating disorders and, 116–117
Topiramate, 139
Total fat
amount providing 30% of calories, 281*t*
recommended dietary intakes during pregnancy, 46*t*
Total parenteral nutrition (TPN)
administration schedule, 218
choosing route or site for, 215
fatty liver and, 261

Trade organizations, 442–443t
Trans fat(s)
  cautions on Nutrition Facts label, 360t
  Nutrition Facts label on, 361t
Transferrin
  biochemical evaluation of nutritional status, 413t
Triceps skinfold, percentiles for whites in U.S., 1971–1974, 420–421t
Tricyclic antidepressants, 135
Triglycerides
  biochemical evaluation of nutritional status, 413t
  blood levels, parenteral nutrition and, 218
  diabetes in adults and, 93, 94, 97
  elevated blood levels, parenteral nutrition and, 221
Tube feeding, for adults
  aspiration prevention, 230
  choosing formula types, 224–225
  choosing tube size, 226
  clogged tube, 234
  delivery routes, 225–226
  delivery systems, 227
  determining formula rate/volume, 225
  feeding schedule, 227–228
  indications/contraindications, 224
  initiation and advancement of, 228
  insertion site care, 230
  maintain tube patency, 229
  measuring gastric residual volume, 229
  monitoring, 228–229
  transitioning to oral feedings, 230
  troubleshooting with, 232–237
  tube displacement of migration, 236
Type 1 diabetes. *See also* Diabetes
  in childhood, 169–180
  diet therapy goals for, 93–94
Type 2 diabetes. *See also* Diabetes
  in childhood, 181–187
  diet therapy goals for, 94–95
Tyrosine
  biochemical evaluation of nutritional status, 413t

U

Ulcerative colitis
  nutrition care for adults with, 245–247
Ulcers, decubitus, 88–89
United States government information resources, 444–445t
Upper arm circumference, percentiles for whites in U.S., 1971–1974
  females, 424–425t
  males, 422–423t
Upper arm fat area, percentiles for whites in U.S., 1971–1974
  females, 428–429t
  males, 426–427t
Upper arm muscle area, percentiles for whites in U.S., 1971–1974
  females, 428–429t
  males, 426–427t
Upper arm muscle circumference, estimated for whites in U.S., 1971–1974
  females, 424–425t
  males, 422–423t
Upper intake levels (UL), tolerable, 305–306t
Uric acid
  renal calculi and, 267

V

Valproic acid, 138–139
Vegan diet
  about, 56–57
  during lactation, 51
Vegetable refusal
  by school-age children, 12
Vegetables
  diverticulitis and, 239
  exchange list for meal planning, 334–335t
  starchy, exchange list for meal planning, 329t
  weight management and, 158
Vegetarianism or vegetarian diet
  about, 56
  adolescents, 15
  adults, 22
  benefits of, 59
  breast-feeding and, 2
  during lactation, 51
Venlafaxine, 136
Vietnamese, foods commonly eaten by, 321t
Vision impairment
  cerebrovascular accident or stroke and, 80–81

Vitamins
for adolescents, 16
blood tests for determining nutritional status of, 401*t*
deficiency, colostomy or ileostomy and, 256
deficiency, short-bowel syndrome and, 259
function and food sources of, 396*t*
gastric bypass surgery and, 200
older adults, 22
for parenteral nutrition, 217
picky eating and, 8
recommended dietary intakes during pregnancy, 45*t*

Vitamin A
biochemical evaluation of nutritional status, 413*t*
calculating retinol activity equivalents, 286
deficiency, fat malabsorption and, 265
food sources of, 452*t*
Nutrition Facts label on, 360*t*

Vitamin B6
biochemical evaluation of nutritional status, 414*t*
food sources for, 434*t*

Vitamin B12
biochemical evaluation of nutritional status, 414*t*
deficiency, gastric bypass surgery and, 205
food sources for, 434*t*
vegetarian sources of, 59

Vitamin C
biochemical evaluation of nutritional status, 414*t*
decubitus ulcers and, 89
food sources of, 457*t*
Nutrition Facts label on, 360*t*

Vitamin D
bone health and, 21
conversion from International Units to micrograms, 286
deficiency, fat malabsorption and, 264–265
vegetarian sources of, 59–60

Vitamin D2
biochemical evaluation of nutritional status, 414*t*

Vitamin D3
biochemical evaluation of nutritional status, 414*t*

Vitamin E
biochemical evaluation of nutritional status, 414*t*
conversion from International Units to micrograms, 286
food sources for, 434*t*
food sources of, 448*t*

Vitamin K
food sources for, 434*t*

Vitamin K deficiency
fat malabsorption and, 264

Vitamins
food sources for, 434*t*

Volumes
enteral nutrition formulas for determination of rate and, 225
gastric residual, high, adult tube feeding and, 233
gastric residual, measuring, adult tube feeding and, 229
metric to U.S. conversions, 291
standard measurements of, 290
U.S. to metric conversions, 291

Vomiting
adult tube feeding and, 233
cancer chemotherapy and radiation and, 208–209
chronic renal insufficiency and, 145
diabetes and, 105
dialysis for end stage renal disease and, 151
gabapentin and, 139
gastric bypass surgery and, 195–196
gluten sensitive enteropathy and, 248–249
HIV/AIDS infection and, 122
lamotrigine and, 139
lithium and, 135, 138
liver disease and, 265
during pregnancy, 33–34
tooth enamel erosion and, 116–117
valproic acid and, 139

W

Water-soluble vitamins
blood tests for determining nutritional status of, 401*t*
function and food sources of, 396*t*

Weakness
gastric bypass surgery and, 199